Taking Action, Saving Lives

TAKING ACTION, SAVING LIVES

Our Duties to Protect Environmental and Public Health

Kristin Shrader-Frechette

OXFORD
UNIVERSITY PRESS

2007

OXFORD
UNIVERSITY PRESS

Oxford University Press, Inc., publishes works that further
Oxford University's objective of excellence
in research, scholarship, and education.

Oxford   New York
Auckland   Cape Town   Dar es Salaam   Hong Kong   Karachi
Kuala Lumpur   Madrid   Melbourne   Mexico City   Nairobi
New Delhi   Shanghai   Taipei   Toronto

With offices in
Argentina   Austria   Brazil   Chile   Czech Republic   France   Greece
Guatemala   Hungary   Italy   Japan   Poland   Portugal   Singapore
South Korea   Switzerland   Thailand   Turkey   Ukraine   Vietnam

Published by Oxford University Press, Inc.
198 Madison Avenue, New York, New York 10016

www.oup.com

Oxford is a registered trademark of Oxford University Press

Library of Congress Cataloging-in-Publication Data
Shrader-Frechette, K. S. (Kristin Sharon)
Taking action, saving lives : our duties to protect environmental
and public health / Kristin Shrader-Frechette.
p. cm.
Includes index.
ISBN 978-0-19-532546-1
1. Environmental health—Moral and ethical aspects.   I. Title.
RA566.S37 2007
362.1—dc22   2006052497

1 2 3 4 5 6 7 8 9
Printed in the United States of America
on acid-free paper

To Michael Cichon, M.D.,
a brilliant, compassionate, humble, and relentless healer,
for bringing back the lives of thousands, including mine.
You show the way.

Preface

Much of ethics has come unstuck from living, separated from the commitments, passions, and experiences that form character and ground behavior. Instead of learning from the lives of remarkable people—such as Juana Gutierrez, Thomas Jefferson, Wei Jingsheng, Rosa Parks, and Dhirendra Sharma—scholars often content themselves with deceptive abstractions that keep them from seeing things as they are. Even moral philosophers are often more concerned with justifying particular principles than with living them. Frequently they are preoccupied more with defining 'love' and 'community' then with embodying them, motivating them, and learning from those who live them. Philosopher Mary Midgley complains that many scholars frequently talk only to each other and only in dialects that nonspecialists do not understand. She claims philosophers often see themselves as critics of special argumentative skills in other philosophers, not as heirs to the whole task of philosophers who have come before them.

How can we reconnect philosophy with life? How can we *show* ethics, as well as write or speak about it? One way is not only to analyze ethical principles but also to tell stories that reveal character and ethical commitments. Without personal narratives to embody the virtues, many people would not be inspired to seek what is good. Without stories to illuminate ideals, few people would accept the demands they ought to make on their own lives. Narratives make ethical principles real. They capture the joys and struggles within and among us. They give us models for living. Inspired by the stories of ordinary people, this book retells them. It offers arguments, but it also traces the courage, moral support, and enlightenment that each of us receives from others.

Acknowledgments

Dad has an Alpha Romeo convertible. My brother Chris bought it used, redid the interior, and rebuilt the engine. He painted it red, Dad's color, then gave it to him. Dad loves to use it to take residents of a local senior home to their doctor appointments and on shopping trips. He says the little old ladies love it when he puts the top down. But he had to stop calling them "little old ladies." An exuberant eighty-five, he discovered all his passengers were younger than he.

The original self-made man, Dad is what you might call "a character." "Outspoken" is too mild a word to describe him. A retired General Electric engineer who often supervised university-trained engineers, he has no college degree. A math whiz and self-described "tinkerer," he is a completely self-taught mechanical engineer. Beginning as a machinist, then a tool-and-die maker, he worked his way up. He read voraciously, haunted the library, asked questions, learned from others and never saw a problem he could not solve.

Abandoned by his father while he was still a baby, Dad went with his mother to live with his grandmother. Speaking of his childhood, he says that sometimes he had only an apple to eat for the entire day. Yet he repeatedly describes himself as "fortunate" and "lucky." Each day, in exchange for tuition, he cleaned all the classrooms at the best Catholic high school in town. A kindly Boy Scout leader inspired him, became a father to him, and encouraged him to become an Eagle Scout. Several years ago, Dad gave our son Eric his faded-ribboned Eagle badge when Eric too received the award. For forty years Dad ran the Boy Scout troop at the local orphanage. For even longer he has been grafting vines and making wine from his own grapes. He gives bottles to family, friends, and the folks at the senior home. A powerful swimmer, he learned to snorkel in his late seventies, after three of his children had become scuba divers. Although he grew up in an inner-city slum, he has always known the names of every bird or insect, just from seeing or hearing them. And he has always been able to fix or build anything. Each week he still volunteers, repairing Braille writers at the state School for the Blind.

With Mom, Dad designed and built a house large enough for their own seven children—plus children the sisters sent, from the orphanage, because they needed special attention. Dad and Mom formally adopted some of these extra children. Working evenings and weekends for fourteen years, with occasional help from friends on big jobs, like laying the concrete foundation, we finished the house in 1960. Yet the "we" is a small one. We children helped rod the joints, after the bricks were laid, and we helped refinish the tongue-and-groove cherry paneling in our own bedrooms. Mom and Dad did everything else, side by side, except for the wiring. A German immigrant taught Dad how to lay bricks. And all of us helped pull large, flat stones out of a friend's rural creek bed. We filled the old trailer full of them, and from them, Dad created the large arched stone fireplace in the family living room.

Now retired, both my parents still teach, part-time, four days a week. For decades Dad has taught mathematics to apprentice tool-and-die makers, without college degrees, who are eager to work their way up, as he did. For decades, our stepmom Betty has taught GED in the poorest area of town. For decades, both have been hospice volunteers. Betty also helped start the flourishing hospice program at the state prison.

If there is any good in this book, it comes from my family and their example. They taught me how to make the possible real. My mother Mildred, who died in 1970, was raised in a black family in a rural Kentucky black neighborhood. For us children, visiting her "grandma" Catherine Jackman— the first black graduate from Centre College and the woman who took in my toddler mother when her parents became invalids—meant traveling two hours to "Colored Town," as everyone then called it. It had neither paved streets nor electricity. Civil-rights activists, Mom and Dad built their new home in the only then-integrated neighborhood of Jefferson County, Kentucky. Pulling the youngest children behind them in our red, rusted Flyer wagon, they marched in many demonstrations. For decades in Jefferson County, Mom was the white Godmother at many black Christenings. She was the first white member of the Kentucky N.A.A.C.P.—the National Association for the Advancement of Colored People. Diagnosed with an advanced, environmentally induced cancer at age forty-three, Mom died several months later. But she had earned a college degree, after several of her children had done so. When she died, she was teaching high school English at the poorest public school, largely minority, in Jefferson County.

Obviously this book would not have appeared without the lessons lived and learned in my own family. My parents lived the habits, virtues, public-interest advocacy, and environmental activism that these pages describe and praise. I owe them everything.

Thanks especially to Mom, Dad, Betty, Claudia, Marianna, and Eric Albert for all you do for the sick, the poor, prisoners, women, and the environment—and for what you challenge everyone to become. Thanks to our children Eric and Danielle for all you are. You make everything worthwhile.

Thanks most of all to my still-bearded, mathematician husband Maurice, a long-time peace- and civil-rights activist. You heard Martin Luther King's "I Have a Dream" speech, you have shared that dream, and that has made all the difference.

Thanks to Jim Childress, Lorraine Code, Kevin Elliott, Dan Hausmann, Rich Hiskes, Dale Jamieson, Hugh Lacey, Deborah Mayo, Sandy Mitchell, Colleen Moore, and Betty Shrader for constructive comments on earlier versions of this manuscript. Special thanks to Katie McCoy, Sharon Ostermann, Enrique Schaerer, Deanna Swits, and Jillian Vitter, for research, and to Tamara Baker, Margaret Jasiewicz, and Cheryl Reed for word processing. Whatever errors remain are my responsibility.

Contents

Taking Action, Saving Lives

Lives at Risk

Emily Pearson lived just East of Chicago, in the small town of Hammond, Indiana. A curly-headed blonde, she delighted her family and neighbors by playing "mother" to her newborn brother, Robbie. When she was 3 years old, suddenly everything changed. Emily was diagnosed with a rare brain cancer. Despite several rounds of chemotherapy and surgeries, she died in 1998— when she was only 7. Within weeks of Emily's diagnosis and only blocks away, the young Burns children—Nicole and Patricia—also were diagnosed with rare cancers, including one of the brain or central nervous system. Local doctors said the chances of having these rare cancers together, in their town of 80,000, were 1 in 16 billion. During the same time, 12 members of Hammond's Clark High School football team were diagnosed with testicular cancer. Relatively rare, it accounts for only about 1 percent of total cancers. The young men all lived on the north side of town, near Keil Chemical, a facility owned by Ferro Chemical.[1]

After her daughter's 1998 death, Gwen Pearson discovered that more local children were dying of rare cancers. Joel Cohen was diagnosed at age 3 and died a year later. Courtney Cerjewski was diagnosed at age 2 and died 2 years later. Stephanie Uhrina was diagnosed when she was 6 and died 2 years later. When Gwen Pearson and Kate Burns began comparing notes on local childhood cancers, they found 16 in only four blocks of single-residence homes near the Ferro Chemical plant. Saying the deaths "had to be stopped," in 1999 they founded Illiana Residents Against Toxico-Carcinogenic Emissions (IRATE). As more parents heard of IRATE and came to their meetings, Gwen and Kate soon had a list of more than 100 local children, all diagnosed with cancer. Most of the children were under age 3, and most had brain cancers. Yet because IRATE never did any systematic or door-to-door survey, Gwen and Kate say the actual number of childhood cancers is likely higher. They also believe the Ferro releases of ethylene dichloride (EDC) and ethylene monochloride (or vinyl chloride, VC) contributed to the pediatric deaths. Officials say Ferro's local releases of EDC peaked at 1.8 million pounds the year Emily Pearson was born, and scientists have linked EDC and VC to neurological, testicular, liver, and reproductive cancers and disorders.[2] In 1993, the year before Emily was diagnosed, the U.S. Environmental Protection Agency (EPA) said Ferro was the nation's top emitter of EDC and predicted the Hammond facility would cause at least 22 new cancers in the area. As a result, the government forced the plant to agree to release annually only 50,000 pounds of volatile organic compound like EDC and VC. Yet no one enforced the agreement. After the childhood cancers appeared in the 1990s, Ferro admitted to annually "losing" nearly 2 million pounds of EDC.[3]

Analyzing data from the government's local air-monitoring facility, several miles south of the plant, a Ferro toxicologist denied any connection between illegal company emissions and the children's cancers. In 2001 the U.S. Agency for Toxic Substances and Disease Registry (ATSDR) studied the same data. It also concluded that the EDC and VC "were not at concentrations likely to result in adverse health effects." Yet the ATSDR admitted, in the same report, that chemical concentrations measured at the local air-monitoring facility "may not fully capture maximum exposure" of the children. For one thing, the air-sampling station was several miles south of the chemical facility, not downwind from Ferro. No monitoring was done in residential areas, and none took account of either wind patterns or the "episodic and short duration of releases of EDC and VC" from the Ferro plant.[4]

The Indiana Department of Public Health agreed with ATSDR that "childhood cancer rates were not elevated in Lake County." It said 200 childhood cancers would have been expected for the county, and it had 243—not a statistically significant increase.[5] Yet the state compared countywide cancer averages, not cases near the plant, and it ignored all Illinois cancers, even though the Ferro facility sits very near the Indiana-Illinois border. The state likewise averaged all cancers, not the rare forms of brain and testicular cancer that appeared in residents living near the plant. All three procedures likely diluted exposures. Averages, in particular, can cover up a single high release that is enough to cause damaging health effects, especially in children. By taking biological-tissue samples from the children, the government could have obtained better health data, but no samples were taken. Nor did anyone admit that, because EDC and VC are volatile and easily evaporate, the local monitoring-station measures of them were likely underestimates. When VC is released to the air, it degrades rapidly and has an estimated half-life of 1.5 days. Depending on weather and distance, even downwind monitors might not fully capture releases of volatile organic compounds—especially if sampling was several miles from the chemical facility. Yet the Hammond monitors were upwind.[6]

On the one hand, ATSDR and Ferro were correct to say the data showed no clear connection among EDC, VC, and the children's deaths, especially since many affected families lived several miles from the plant. Besides, even if Ferro caused these deaths, it would be difficult to distinguish them from fatalities caused by other local industrial facilities. All the stricken families live within the narrow chemical corridor, extending eastward from Chicago toward Cleveland—called the new "Cancer Alley" of America. Responsible for one-third of all U.S. toxic-chemical releases, this south shore of the Great Lakes is loaded with petrochemical facilities, metal-fabrication plants, and waste incinerators. Just the 90-mile stretch East, from Chicago, Illinois, to Elkhart, Indiana, is home to 10 of the 12 highest-volume Great Lakes toxic polluters. Annually the United States releases about 8 pounds of toxic chemicals per person, but the overall Indiana average is nearly three times higher. By far the highest state releases are in this northern-Indiana "Cancer Alley."[7]

On the other hand, ATSDR and Ferro err in insisting the Ferro chemicals did no harm. Given the poor monitoring data and the nature of volatile organic compounds, the air-monitoring data obviously are inadequate to support this conclusion. Even EPA estimates contradict it. Besides, the hundreds of local childhood cancers are likely an underestimate, as already mentioned. Because the state's cancer database is 2–3 years behind, it counts only about 60 percent of total cancers and only those in Indiana. Officials should have improved their data and methods before drawing any conclusions about local cancers. Alternatively, they should have admitted that no reliable conclusions were possible. Instead, the government and Ferro committed an error in logic known as the appeal to ignorance. This error occurs whenever people assume that because current evidence (like monitoring data) does not prove harm, there is no harm. Yet from flawed or incomplete evidence—ignorance—no conclusion follows. More generally, the error occurs whenever people assume that "absence of evidence" for some effect—like high levels of pollution—is "evidence of absence" of harm. Yet failure to have evidence does not prove anything, one way or the other.

Why did no local scientists or engineers, from the branch campuses of Indiana University and Purdue University, come to the assistance of IRATE? Why didn't they detect the flawed ATSDR-Ferro-Indiana Department of Public Health studies? When asked these questions, Gwen Pearson gave a chilling response. She said university professors had told her that most of the local scientists either received research or consulting monies from the area's polluting industries or relied on them to hire their students and provide jobs.[8]

Overview: Three Lessons about Public Health and Ethics

The tragic deaths of Emily Pearson and the other northern Indiana children are important not only because they probably were preventable, and government reassurances were scientifically flawed. They also illustrate three important ethical points—about science, whistleblowing, and democracy.

This first point, that *flawed science often leads to flawed ethics*, is one that scientists frequently forget. They forget that public-health science has life-or-death consequences and is not just a theoretical exercise. The ATSDR engaged in a narrow, purely theoretical exercise that, so far as it went, was technically correct. There was no obvious connection between the monitored Ferro releases and the Hammond cancers. Yet ATSDR officials—who probably intended no harm—ignored the poor data, committed an appeal to ignorance, and neglected the health and ethical consequences of its doing incomplete science. Chapter 3 explores this point in more detail, showing how private-interest science often threatens both public health and ethics. *Private-interest science* is supposed science done in obviously flawed ways, to serve someone's private agenda, rather than to produce reliable results. Because of its flaws, private-interest science usually is not published in refereed scientific journals. Nevertheless, it can skew policy. The private-interest science of ATSDR and Ferro relied on flawed monitoring data and put more lives at risk. It also encouraged policies that ignored citizens' rights to know, to equal protection, to consent, and to life.

A second, more specific, ethical lesson of these tragic childhood deaths is that *when scientists swallow the whistle about private-interest science, they promote "private-interest ethics"* and insensitivity to public harm. Private-interest ethics allows behavior that serves someone's purely private agenda, like making money, but ignores the public good and what is right. Gwen Pearson's claims suggest that local university, the Indiana Department of Public Health, Ferro, and ATSDR scientists all followed private-interest ethics by swallowing the whistle and accepting flawed scientific reports. Yet Sigma Xi (the Scientific Research Society) is clear on this point. Whistleblowing is "a necessary part of maintaining the integrity of scientific research."[9] The American Association for the Advancement of Science says something similar. It claims scientists have a duty "to speak out where significant information concerning possible significant risks is being withheld or presented in such a way as to deceive or mislead persons who may be affected, and to refuse to work on such projects."[10]

A third ethical lesson of these childhood cancers is practical and personal, a conclusion to be defended later in the book. *Ordinary citizens have ethical responsibilities to use traditional democratic tools to help prevent threats to life and health.* Because two ordinary citizens, Kate Burns and Gwen Pearson, used these tools, they probably helped prevent additional childhood cancers. Demanding their rights as citizens, they urged their Washington congressman, Peter Visclosky, to bring in ATSDR. Using their rights of speech, press, and assembly, they contacted physicians, founded IRATE, and spoke out about what they found. They reached out to protect other northern Indiana families whose children had cancer. They provided information, promoted discussion, and supported other parents. Although Gwen and her husband have five young children of their own, and although Kate is a single parent, struggling financially, they did not wait for someone else to do the work of democracy. When Indiana Department of Public Health officials told them its database lagged behind and counted only about 60 percent of childhood cancers, they developed the IRATE website and began collecting childhood-cancer data themselves. They knew that local children might not have several years to wait for the state's health statistics to reveal community cancers. These parents became the change they sought. They helped make a difference between life and death. Gwen Pearson put it simply: "My daughter is dead. Nothing can bring her back. All I have left of her is what I can do for other children."[11]

As the Hammond case suggests, public-health ethics requires, at a minimum, policing private-interest science, blowing the whistle when necessary, and using the tools of democracy to help prevent threats to life and to human rights. One goal of this book is to encourage all citizens—especially scientists and other professionals—to accept these three ethical responsibilities. Although the book shows how private-interest science can be used to harm people, its main theme is ethical, not scientific. The issue is not the precise number of pollution-induced deaths or injuries, in part because this number can be controversial. The main issue is that any environmental deaths or injuries are too many—if they are easily preventable, inequitably distributed, victimize children most, or result from ignoring citizens' rights to know and to consent.

This first chapter outlines some of the major environmental threats to public health. It offers statistics from government and top scientific journals showing that pollution is far more serious than many of us realize. The next two chapters diagnose some of the reasons for widespread citizen failure to recognize these risks. Chapter 2 surveys a variety of media techniques—like public relations (PR) and advertising—that polluters sometimes use to "orchestrate ignorance." Because flawed science often underlies citizen misinformation about pollutants, chapter 3 outlines several ways that science may be manipulated, suppressed, or "privatized" by polluters who make misleading claims. Just as tobacco companies have misled people about the health effects of cigarettes, polluters sometimes have misled people about the health effects of pollution. The result? Manipulation of science and the media can jeopardize *disclosure* of health risks and threaten citizens' *rights to know* about, and *to consent* to, pollution.

Building on the severity and inequity of public-health risks (chapter 1) and the way polluters sometimes undercut rights to know and to consent to these risks—by manipulating media (chapter 2) or science (chapter 3), chapter 4 sketches an ethical response, the responsibility argument. It shows that because most citizens receive undeserved financial or medical benefits when minorities and poor people bear higher levels of pollution, citizens have *prima facie* ethical duties to help stop these harmful inequities. The responsibility argument also shows that because all citizens participate in some government and corporate institutions that jeopardize life or human rights through pollution, they have *prima facie* duties to help prevent these harms. (*Prima facie* duties are those that bind, in the absence of compelling arguments to the contrary.) Because the responsibility argument demands so much of citizens, chapter 5 answers key objections to it.

Chapter 6 provides practical suggestions for ways that citizens might implement the responsibility argument yet promote a healthy economy and technological growth. Many of these suggestions are recommendations of the American Public Health Association (APHA)—the oldest and largest organization of health professionals in the world. Founded about 130 years ago, APHA has more than 50,000 members. Annually since 1948, APHA has made about 20–30 new medical/public-health recommendations. For example, in 2004 APHA endorsed strategies to avoid antibiotics in meats, to require nutrition labels for fast food, and to enforce lead standards. In both 1978 and again in 2004, APHA recommended reforms such as an immediate, "deliberate" transition to "safe and renewable" energy sources. It argued that "dependence on fossil fuels and nuclear power is one of the greatest contemporary threats to human health." In 2003, APHA's recommendations included calls for independent testing of new drugs (rather than reliance merely on pharmaceutical-company claims); for a moratorium on concentrated animal-feed operations; and for better control of health-related advertising. In 2002, APHA's recommendations included reducing sodium food additives and protecting community and worker rights-to-know about toxic-chemical threats. Among other reforms, APHA's 2001 recommendations called for labeling genetically modified foods and intervening to stop minority health disparities. If U.S. policymakers had followed all APHA recommendations, probably this book would be unnecessary, and many threats to life and to human rights would have been prevented.[12]

As later chapters explain, citizens' duties to prevent life-threatening and rights-threatening harms obviously differ, according to each person's circumstances and abilities. Yet, equally obviously, everyone who contributes to these harms has duties to help prevent them. The main issue here is not the precise level of each person's responsibility for such harm, because this can be determined only after an extensive, case-by-case analysis. Rather, the point is that most citizens probably do less, than they ought, to prevent threats to life and to rights. Nor is the main issue whether typical citizens, like Gwen and Kate, are correct in all their scientific claims. Gwen and Kate are ordinary people, not scientists. The point is that ordinary, but active, democratic citizenship is what is most needed to help prevent both manipulation of science and the media, as well as pollutant threats to life and to human rights. The book also argues that public-health ethics does not require citizens to know infallibly that they are right, before speaking out. Instead it requires only that scientists and other citizens pursue open, democratic argument and interaction—the best means of discovering who is right. Nor is the key issue whether public-health advocates are successful, as Gwen and Kate were. They stopped Ferro's illegal EDC and VC emissions. The larger issue of this book is ethical, educational, and democratic. The bumper sticker is right; democracy is not a spectator sport. Because it is not, this book argues that citizens' educating themselves about pollution, exercising deliberative democracy, and helping prevent life-threatening and rights-threatening pollution is not mainly a matter of charity. Both justice and prudence require it.

Public Health and Deliberative Democracy

In arguing for citizens' duties to help prevent threats to life and to human rights, the book presupposes a commitment to "deliberative democracy," to full citizen involvement in self-government, as explained by Iris Marion Young and others.[13] Using open public debate about social problems like pollution, deliberative democracy has two distinct goals. One is substantive, to seek *distributive justice* in allocating material goods, such as public-health protection. The other goal is procedural, to seek *participative justice*—practices and policies that allocate decisionmaking *power* equitably among all citizens. Deliberative democracy thus presupposes both rights not to be harmed by things like pollution, as well as rights to equal participation in decisionmaking about how to prevent or manage such harms. Both rights are important because, as Young recognizes, when citizens protest some injury from pollution, as Gwen and Kate did, their worries are not only about *what* their risks are. They also worry about *how* those risks are imposed on them—why Ferro, the Indiana Department of Public Health, and ATSDR did not protect them. They seek not only equitable *distributions* of risk, like pollution, but also equitable *procedures* for allocating those risks. Citizens often bear unfair pollution burdens precisely because government procedures give them little voice in health-related decisions, and they are unable to exercise their rights to know and to consent.[14]

To understand deliberative democracy, consider three things that it is not. (1) It is not government based mainly on aggregating preferences. Aggregative or "show-of-hands" democrats conceive of *voting* as the primary political act. They believe democracy is little more than counting ballots. Deliberative democrats, however, believe primary political acts include not only voting but also full citizen *participation in authentic debate and deliberation,* in open-minded, respectful accommodation to the positions of others, so that democracy can be a personally and societally *transformative process.* Deliberative democrats say this process can make citizens more virtuous, society more just, and democratic agreement more legitimate and more representative of diverse points of view. But to achieve these goals, citizens must do more than vote. They must reciprocally interact with others, as equals, and reshape their self-interested preferences in the light of others' preferences. (2) Deliberative democracy is not fully realized anywhere, even in western Europe, Canada, and the United States—as the Hammond, Indiana, case reveals. Rather, deliberative democracy is a *normative ideal,* a dynamic, open-ended process realized to different degrees in different situations.[15]

(3) Deliberative democracy is not mainly a speculative political theory about justice, but a practical set of *processes and practices* through which citizens can reach consensus about justice. Deliberative democrats know that justice is achieved not mainly by invoking armchair reflections or principles but also by promoting political *practices* that seek five main goals: full and equal inclusion, participation, voting, understanding, and control over political agendas. To work toward these five practical ideals, deliberative democrats use traditional democratic actions—such as information-gathering, teach-ins, leafleting, meetings, lobbying, and debates. Yet, as Martin Luther King warned in his "Letter from Birmingham Jail," powerful people usually do not willingly give up power. Because they do not, Young and others recognize that deliberative democracy may not be possible in "societies with [serious] structural

inequalities." Amid such inequalities, citizen virtue often first requires sustained *democratic action* to promote conditions necessary for enfranchising the disenfranchised, conditions necessary for exercising deliberative democracy. Democratic action—including boycotts, circulating petitions, civil disobedience, demonstrations, exercising initiative and referenda, and whistleblowing—can help express public outrage at injustice, draw attention to it, and motivate other citizens to act against it. In using democratic action to express outrage, however, citizens err if they fall into mere pressure-group politics or interest-group activism. Rather than dedication to some partisan goal, what does the civic virtue of deliberative democracy require? It demands commitment to universal justice, to listening to others, to deliberating as soon as possible, and to avoiding blind rage, violence, and nihilism.[16]

What circumstances might require traditional democratic *action*, rather than only democratic deliberation? One of Iris Marion Young's examples concerns the World Trade Organization (WTO). Because the WTO operates in closed rather than public proceedings and gives people no access to the trade documents on which it votes, she says good citizens have no choice except to protest WTO threats to rights to know and to consent. She and others argue that the WTO—a "tool of transnational corporate power"—has been shown both to subvert democratically agreed-on health laws and to harm the poorest nations of the world. Given the severity of WTO threats and no democratic vehicles for alleviating them, Young concludes that virtuous citizens must protest their lack of voice. Her arguments show that citizen involvement in democratic *action* sometimes may be required, either to prevent institutions like the WTO from blocking deliberative democracy, or to promote conditions like access to information. Young's examples of deliberative democracy include public participation in Oregon's restructuring of its low-income health-care program and South Africans' participation in discussing their new constitution, which became law in 1996. Following Young's account, this book presupposes that citizen action also may be necessary either to draw attention to injustice or to help create conditions that are necessary for deliberative democracy and fulfilling human rights. Once citizens are made aware of injustice, they can help force society to use democratic deliberation both to evaluate various responses to it and to address injustice.[17]

Why the Pollution Emphasis? Themes and Limits of the Book

Urging citizens to use deliberative democracy and to implement the responsibility argument, this book asks people for two things, democratic responsibility and ethical responsibility. *Democratic responsibility* requires citizens to recognize that *they contribute to pollution harm* because they are members of institutions, like government, that sometimes cause this harm. As a consequence, they have duties either to remove themselves from such harm-causing institutions or to remain within them and help reform them. Such reform requires citizens to reclaim their civic birthright, engage in the traditional duties of active democratic citizenship, practice the civic virtue that democratic society preaches, and become "moral exemplars," like Gwen and Kate. *Ethical responsibility* requires citizens to recognize that, at others' expense, *they benefit from pollution harm*, from society's imposing unequal pollution burdens on poor people and minorities. As a consequence, they have duties to help stop this inequity and to compensate for what they have gained from it. To do so, again they must fulfill their duties of active, democratic citizenship.

In arguing that citizens have democratic and ethical duties to help prevent threats to life and to human rights, this book has six main themes. The first is that because private interests, like polluters who break the law, sometimes misuse and manipulate science, they sometimes promote private-interest ethics and threaten public health. After the first three chapters reveal *how* science and ethics are sometimes privatized, *what* citizens must do, in response, will be clearer. A similar theme appears in Asian philosophies like Zen Buddhism. Once people recognize the ways in which they are morally blind, their needed ethical responses will be clearer. Unless people come to this prior recognition of their moral blindness, they are unlikely to accept ethical arguments for how their behavior ought to change. This theme of moral blindness also appears in perhaps the most famous passage of moral philosophy ever written, Plato's Allegory of the Cave. According to Plato, most people are like prisoners, chained in a dark cave where they see only two-dimensional shadows on the wall, shadows they mistake for reality. To see correctly and behave ethically first requires leaving the cave. Yet few "chained" people are able to do this. Applied to public-health ethics, leaving the cave means shining the light of publicity and disinterestedness on how private-interest science and private-interest ethics sometimes imprison citizens, encourage moral blindness, limit knowledge, and thus threaten health and human rights.

A second theme, as the Buddhist proverb says, is that people cannot always change reality, but they can change the eyes that see it. This book argues for both: societal progress toward health-protective and rights-protective policies— and personal transformation in virtue. People may not achieve full democratic deliberation and transformation of every situation, but they personally can try to become the change they seek, as Gwen Pearson and Kate Burns did.

A third and related theme is that people ought not blame only government, corporations, labor unions, or other institutions for threats to their lives and health. Any institution that enjoys unchecked power, especially unchecked economic power, can be a threat to democracy. Whenever some institution enjoys unchecked power, democratic peoples ultimately should also blame themselves, and not merely scapegoat that institution. The problem is both the unchecked institutional power and lack of citizen attention to it. As later chapters show, examples of corporate abuses are plentiful because corporations fund most science, exercise the dominant global economic power, and donate 80 percent of U.S. campaign funds. However, at least in a wealthy democracy like that of the United States, the buck stops with the people. Ultimately, there is no one to do the work of democracy except the people themselves. Thus, to the degree that this volume is critical, it does not criticize mainly institutions, like corporations, but citizens' failures to shape and reform those institutions.

A fourth theme is the power and service of ordinary people, doing often-ordinary things, to reduce threats to life in their local communities. Each chapter begins with the stories of moral exemplars, like Gwen and Kate. A fifth theme is that whatever harms the environment ultimately harms people, because all living beings depend on the same environmental life-support systems. Although this book traces mainly pollutant impacts on people, the same pollutants also affect air, water, soil, and other species. Otherwise they would not affect humans. A final theme is that citizens must reclaim the sense of civic responsibility that has shaped their own traditions, like those of the American Revolution. Just as surviving the harsh New England winters helped teach the Pilgrims to be their sisters' and brothers' keepers, contemporary environmental- and public-health threats can help educate people about their democratic and ethical responsibilities.

Because no book can do everything, this one is limited in at least eight important ways. (1) Although those in developing nations obviously bear the worst health threats, this book emphasizes U.S. public health, for purely practical reasons to be explained later. (2) Although recent years have produced many public-health improvements, such as reduced U.S. use of tobacco, this book emphasizes only public-health threats from pollution. As this chapter argues later, this emphasis denies neither other health hazards nor significant public-health progress. Rather, the point is that further progress could save thousands of additional lives each year. For instance, a 2004 U.S. National Academies of Science (NAS) report concludes that universal U.S. health insurance could save 18,000 lives each year, and preventing food contamination could annually save another 5,000 people.[18]

There are many ethical reasons that this volume focuses only on pollutant-related, public-health threats. These include their magnitude, lay ignorance about them, their theoretical preventability, their often discriminatory impacts, their potential for human-rights violations, their frequent deliberate or criminal character, and the fact that they often result from acts of *committing* harm, not merely *omitting* to do good.

Regarding *magnitude*, even conservative estimates from the U.S. National Cancer Institute (NCI; see next section) show that industrial pollution contributes to at least 60,000 premature U.S. cancer fatalities annually—far more U.S. deaths than are attributable to lack of universal health insurance. Yet this cancer figure includes no pollution-related fatalities from noncancer causes, such as heart attacks or asthma deaths induced by particulate air pollution. Another reason for the pollution emphasis, as chapters 2 and 3 explain, is that many laypeople are *unaware* of the scientific evidence for large numbers of pollution-induced fatalities, although the U.S. Centers for Disease Control (CDC) say 90 percent of voters believe "that the environment plays a significant role in their health." Also, unlike many other threats to life, pollutants often are direct effects of *preventable* human actions. As the U.S. Office of Technology Assessment (OTA) has put it, "up to 90 percent of cancers are environmentally induced and theoretically preventable." Because life-threatening pollution frequently can be remedied, sometimes in obvious ways, it tends to be something for which people are more ethically responsible. Besides, as this chapter shows, pollution's most harmful effects tend to fall disproportionately on the most vulnerable among us—children, minorities, and poor people. The discrimination and environmental injustice involved in much pollution-induced harm give it a priority in public-health ethics. (*Environmental injustice* occurs whenever some people face greater pollution threats, for largely morally irrelevant or undeserved reasons, like their age, where they live, their skin color, or their poverty.) Still another reason for this book's emphasis on pollution-related (rather than other) health threats is that life-threatening pollution often involves human-rights violations. For example, because there is no National Health Tracking Act (see later chapters), there is only limited knowledge about many local pollution threats. As a result, citizens often cannot fulfill their rights to know and to consent to pollutant risks. Such human-rights problems are absent from many nonpollutant health risks. Life-threatening pollution also deserves special ethical attention because often it is the result of deliberate or criminal acts. Chapters 2–3 show that polluters frequently falsify emissions data or conduct fraudulent "scientific" studies. As a result, pollution threats have an ethical priority that noncriminal harms do not have. Pollution-related health threats likewise have an ethical priority because they often arise from acts of *commission* of harm, rather than from acts of *omission*—such as failure to provide health care or health education. While it is extremely important to provide universal health care, or to educate people about healthy lifestyles, ethically it is even more important to protect them against those who deliberately commit harm.[19]

(3) Besides dealing only with pollution-induced health threats, the book is limited in focusing on how pollution should force citizens to rethink their ethics. Following its third theme, the book's primary goal is not political but ethical—not criticizing or reforming *institutions*, but motivating *individuals* to accept responsibility for institutional harms to which they contribute and from which they benefit. Once citizens accept their democratic and ethical responsibilities, they themselves will reform their institutions in the ways that are needed. In a wealthy democracy, the buck stops with citizens. To varying degrees (that depend on their abilities and opportunities), citizens in wealthy democracies often have the environments, the governments, the communities, the corporations, and other institutions that they deserve.

(4) The book is likewise limited by being directed primarily at intelligent laypeople, not mainly scholarly specialists. Everyone must do the work of serving democracy and protecting life. (5) Because its main audience is intelligent laypeople, the book provides only basic defenses of key concepts, like collective responsibility. The notes often refer readers to journal articles for more technical analyses. (6) Although the book emphasizes personal moral responsibility to prevent threats to life and to human rights, chapter 6 offers only a few basic proposals for reforming particular policies and institutions.

More detailed recommendations are available from groups like the APHA. (7) While the book argues for a new paradigm of public-health ethics—the paradigm of preventing threats to life—its main goal is not ethical *theory* but ethical *practice*. Those interested mainly in ethical or scientific theory should look either to the notes or to other sources. The goal here is more specific: to motivate a personal ethical transformation, an individual journey that, joined with others' journeys, can eventually help reform institutions and therefore save lives. (8) Another limitation of the book is that the public-health ethics defended here focuses on why pollutant threats to life and health are tied to human-rights violations. The book does not go into a detailed examination of how other ethical theories, besides those of human rights, provide grounds for protecting life. While the full range of public-health ethics requires a variety of theories, especially for the "hard cases," such ethical "heavy lifting" is not needed here. Why not? The pollution threats to life and to human rights, surveyed here, are so serious that only elementary ethical considerations are needed to show that people have *prima facie* duties to do something about them. Thus, as chapter 4 explains (see the section entitled "Justice not Charity"), the book agrees with the APHA—that human rights provide "the ethical framework for public-health practice."

What are the elementary ethical considerations to be used here? They rely on example as well as on human-rights arguments. As philosopher Ludwig Wittgenstein recognized, people can understand a phenomenon in at least two ways: through practical examples or through precise definition.[20] British philologist and theologian C. S. Lewis said something similar. We learn ethics mainly indirectly, from the example of those around us. This is why he reminded us that being virtuous requires living among at least some virtuous people. Irish statesman Edmund Burke agreed: "Example is the school of humanity, and it will learn at no other."[21] Because normative ethics is about *how* people ought to *behave*, not just about *what* they ought to *believe*, much of this book relies on examples and illustrations. Each chapter not only shows how moral blindness keeps many people from recognizing threats to life but also introduces moral exemplars, people who have made a difference. Each chapter shows how ordinary citizens like Gwen Pearson and Kate Burns have done extraordinary things. They remind us that most of us know saints or heroes—relatives, teachers, or friends whose behavior shows us how to prevent threats to life and to human rights.

This book argues that there are many Gwen Pearsons and Kate Burns—but not yet enough to do the work of democracy and public health. Not enough are like Emelda West, a great-grandmother in her 70s. She helped campaign against toxic releases in her low-income Louisiana neighborhood. Not enough are like 23-year-old U.S. Veterans' Administration counselor Maude De Victor. She saw patterns of illness among Vietnam veterans, exposed to Agent Orange. When her superiors did nothing, she brought the problem to the attention of CBS news correspondent Bill Kurtis. The resulting exposé helped win health benefits for servicemen and earned Kurtis three Emmys and a coveted Peabody Award. When low-income residents of Pensacola, Florida, began experiencing eye, skin, and breathing difficulties from dioxin exposures from a local toxic dump, Margaret Williams began Citizens Against Toxic Exposures. Although the organization was unable to close the dump, it forced the government to relocate 358 families to a safer area. In 1990, when Waste Technologies Industries planned to build the world's largest toxic-waste incinerator on a West Virginia floodplain near an elementary school, Terri Swearingen responded. Worried because the government said the incinerator could annually emit 5 tons of lead, as well as dioxins, acids, and heavy metals, Swearingen asked for help from local citizens and university scientists. She led more than 20 civil-disobedience protests against the incinerator. In 1997, she received the prestigious Goldman Environmental Prize for her public-health leadership. When she received the award, Swearingen said simply: "I am not a scientist or a Ph.D. ... I am a mother... We have been forced to educate ourselves, and the final exam represents our children's future."[22]

Risks from Pollution: Cancer

Why are more people not like Gwen Pearson or Terri Swearingen? Perhaps they are not motivated to act because they do not recognize the ways that pollution often harms people. To motivate the ethics this volume defends, the rest of this chapter surveys some pollution harms. Once people see the magnitude and severity of many pollutant exposures, they are more likely to take steps to help reduce them.

One indicator of severe pollution is the escalating rate of *cancer incidence*, like that of Emily Pearson. Because of improved *cancer treatment*, people may not realize that cancer incidence is increasing about five times faster than cancer mortality is decreasing.[23] In the last 50 years, the percentage of cancer victims, still alive 5 years after diagnosis, has increased only 5 percent, from 49 to 54 percent. Despite this slight improvement in 5-year cancer *mortality*, and despite reduced cancers from cigarettes, overall cancer-*incidence* rates are increasing, especially among children. In the last 25 years, childhood-cancer incidence has increased 35 percent, while overall cancer incidence has increased 25 percent. Cancer is the leading killer of Americans under age 85.[24] In part as a result, sickness has increased in the United States. The 2005 report of the APHA shows that, on average, citizens' days of "limited physical activity" (sickness) have increased by 25 percent in the last decade—nearly 3 percent annually. The APHA data show that the average American now loses 2 days per month because of limited physical activity.[25]

Especially among childhood victims, like Emily Pearson, medical and scientific journals suggest that environmental pollution is now a major cause of increased cancer incidence and associated sickness.

- A 2002 study of 90,000 twins, published in the *New England Journal of Medicine*, distinguished genetically based, from environmentally induced, cancers. It concluded: "the overwhelming contribution to the causation of cancer in the population of twins that we studied was the environment."[26]

- Studies done by the U.S. NAS and the World Health Organization (WHO)—and published in medical journals like *Lancet*—show that increased environmental pollution causes increased cancer, heart trouble, respiratory diseases, asthma, allergies, and other ailments.[27]
- Apart from the effects of other air, water, and food pollutants, *Lancet* authors say that particulate air pollution alone annually causes 6.4 percent of children's deaths, age 0–4, in developed nations. In Europe, this means that air particulates, alone, kill 14,000 toddlers each year.[28]

Despite such statistics, there are both scientific and ethical reasons that this book does not take a position on the precise number of cancers and other fatalities caused by industrial pollutants. On the *ethical* side, the precise number is not necessary to the arguments presented here. Regardless of their number, any pollution-caused deaths are ethically indefensible if they are easily preventable, partly caused by discrimination, unequally distributed, borne more heavily by innocent children, or imposed in ways that violate citizens' human rights to life, to know, and to consent to pollutant risks.

On the *scientific* side, this volume takes no position on the precise numbers of pollution-induced cancers and other fatalities because the exact numbers are controversial. Cancer, for instance, typically occurs as a result of interactions among many environmental, genetic, personal, and viral factors, not just pollution. Genetics contributes to some cancers, and a mutation of the tumor-suppressor gene p53 has been implicated in about half of all cancers. Yet even genetically induced cancer often is not a purely natural occurrence. Current U.S. levels of chemical and radiological pollution repeatedly have been shown to induce the p53 mutation in humans.[29]

In 2005, U.S. National Academy of Sciences studies reaffirmed that precise causes for about half of all cancers are uncertain. Assuming that the 50 percent of known cancer causes are indicative of total causes, several hypotheses follow. One is that 5–10 percent of all cancers may be partly attributable to genetic inheritance—and another 5 percent to infections and viruses.[30] Up to 90 percent of cancer, says the U.S. OTA, is "environmentally induced and theoretically preventable."[31] As understood by the OTA, these "environmental" factors include things like smoking, sunlight, background radiation, and industrial pollutants. There are about 600,000 total U.S. cancer fatalities each year. Assuming that total environmental causes were 90 percent of all fatal cancers, this would amount annually to 540,000 deaths. Scientists say background radiation causes about 3 percent,[32] or 18,000 annual cancer fatalities. The U.S. CDC say cigarettes cause roughly another 30 percent (180,000 deaths), while about 33 percent (198,000) may be from personal environmental choices, such as lack of exercise. But that still leaves about 144,000 annual U.S. cancer deaths. Physician-researchers Paul Schulte and Philip Landrigan show that about 8 percent, or 50,000 annual U.S. cancer deaths, may be caused just by *occupational* exposure to workplace toxins.[33] What percentage may be attributable to nonoccupational exposure to industrial and agricultural pollutants?

As already mentioned, a decade ago the U.S. NCI attributed about 10 percent of U.S. cancer deaths (about 60,000 annually) to industrial pollution in the workplace, public areas, and consumer products; this figure was confirmed in 2005 U.S. National Academy of Sciences (NAS) studies.[34] Claiming this NCI figure was too low, some environmental scientists say these same pollutants cause up to 33 percent of all U.S. cancers.[35] Some U.S. Health, Education, and Welfare reports even say 38 percent of all cancers are caused by only five high-volume industrial carcinogens.[36] What explains the differences in these pollution-caused-death estimates? One factor is different ways of categorizing health hazards. A decade ago, the U.S. National Cancer Institute (NCL) attributed 35 percent of cancers to dietary factors, such as eating fatty or smoked foods, but NCI apparently did not include pesticide hazards as part of this dietary estimate. Yet carcinogenic pesticides, like chlordane and dieldrin, concentrate in animal fats and cause cancer in animals.[37] Studies by the U.S. NAS show that legal levels of food-borne pesticides cause at least 13,500 annual, preventable U.S. cancer deaths—a million premature deaths every 75 years.[38] Consequently, many cancers (that NCI ascribes to diet) actually may be attributable to chemical pollutants stored in fatty foods. The NAS estimate for fatalities from dietary pesticides is 2.2 percent of annual cancers. Together with the Landrigan-Schulte figure of 8 percent, this is 10.2 percent of annual cancer deaths, just from *dietary pesticides* and *workplace exposure* to toxins. This 10.2 percent does not count cancers caused by nondietary (e.g., air, water) and nonworkplace exposures. This suggests that total cancers induced by exposure to all agricultural and industrial pollutants could be between 11 and 15 percent of all cancers—60,000 to 90,000 deaths annually. Assuming that the conservative NCI and NAS figures are right, and total industrial and agricultural pollution causes only 10 percent of cancer fatalities, this number is still three times larger than annual U.S. murders. Something seems wrong.[39]

The U.S. National Institutes of Health (NIH) say the rates of U.S. cancers, now striking about one in three people, will double in the next 50 years.[40] Yet this estimate takes no account of continuing increases in radiological and chemical pollution. How many people will have to contract cancer or some environmentally induced disease before citizens realize that many people are killing themselves? As John Bailer of Harvard University School of Public Health puts it, more people are dying prematurely of cancer, and the increase is not just a matter of better diagnosis. To claim otherwise is "to mislead the American public."[41] Even improvements in cancer treatment may be illusory. Studies done in 2005 suggest that many of the claimed increases in cancer survival (measured 5 years after diagnosis) may come mainly from discovering tumors earlier, when they are smaller, and not from genuine increases in longevity.[42]

As already mentioned, since 1999 cancer has been the leading cause of premature death in the United States for all those under age 85. Heart disease is the leading killer of those over age 85. According to the NCI, 40 percent of cancers occur in those under age 65, so the disease is not just striking the elderly. It is the leading cause of death of women in their thirties. On average, its victims die 15 years prematurely. Annually cancer costs the United States at least $25 billion in lost workdays, economic failures, and medical bills.[43]

People may quibble about the precise percentage of cancer deaths associated with industrial pollutants. Environmentalists may say the conservative, 10-percent hypothesis of 60,000 annual deaths is too low by at least 25 percent, and industrialists may say it is too high by 5 percent. The preceding data, however, are enough to show that, *prima facie*, numbers of pollution-induced cancers are significant. Their significance is one reason that, in the last 5 years, the APHA has issued at least 20 recommendations designed in part to reduce pollutant-related contributions to cancer.[44] As already mentioned, however, the key issue here is *ethical*, not scientific—not the precise number of environmental cancers. As later chapters argue, and as the previous section suggested, because pollution-induced deaths represent at least seven crucial ethical problems, citizens have special duties to help prevent them.

Air Pollution

Cancer is not the only health threat sometimes caused by pollution. Air pollution, in particular, can induce neurological and developmental disorders, heart attacks, atherosclerosis, respiratory failure, asthma, inflammation, and lung disease. This is why, in the last half-century, the APHA has made about 100 different recommendations for reducing air pollution. These include calling for health-based air-pollution standards, toxics reduction, greater control of hazardous air pollutants, stricter standards for particulate air pollution, better asthma prevention, and so on.[45]

- In 1999, the WHO estimated that about 3 million people die prematurely each year because of both indoor and outdoor air pollution— more than 8,000 deaths each day.[46]

- One European Union scientific study calculated that between 25 and 40 percent of all United Kingdom deaths were "thought to be directly attributable to the effects of air pollution."[47]

- The APHA notes that there is an "epidemic" of asthma among U.S. "children and young adults under the age of 35.... Environmental factors known to exacerbate asthma...include ambient air pollution...and indoor environmental factors such as pesticides."[48]

- Mainly because of heart attacks, asthma, and cancer, polluted air costs European Union nations $161 billion annually in lost work days, deaths, and economic damages. European Union scientists say the average European loses about one year of life because of air pollution.[49]

While losing one year at the end of a long life may seem trivial, this figure is misleading. It really means that members of sensitive groups—like children—lose many years of life, while the most robust members of the population lose none. As the preceding APHA statement illustrates, pollution harms the youngest and the most vulnerable people first.

Scientists have known about the hazards of air pollution for nearly 50 years. Yet government has done little about them, partly for reasons outlined in the next two chapters. Even in the early 1960s, U.S. studies showed that air pollution increases mortality, lung cancer, and respiratory problems.[50] Nearly 40 years ago, economists writing in *Science* showed that a 50 percent reduction in air pollution could annually cut total U.S. health costs by 5 percent—and costs of illness and death by at least $2 billion. Yet little was done. A 1980 study showed that about 50,000 people died that year in the United States from air pollution alone, and the figure is even higher now. The latest (2007) data from *The Economist* show that more than 26 nations have better air quality than the United States, which has the worst ozone pollution in the developed world.[51]

The health costs of ignoring a half-century of scientific data on air pollution have been great. Scientists say that particulate pollution alone causes 50,000 to 100,000 premature U.S. deaths each year, especially among children. Even U.S. consultants, hired by the Bush administration in 2000, admit the severity of the problem. Although that administration weakened air-pollution regulations and enforcement, its consultants admitted that airborne-particulate pollution alone causes at least 30,000 annual, preventable U.S. deaths. A 2003 NCI study drew even more disturbing conclusions. Studying more than half a million people over 16 years in 156 cities, it showed there is no safe level of air pollution—that exposure to fine-particulate pollution is as risky as being overweight or exposed to cigarette smoke. Apart from cancer, effects of water and food pollution, or effects of other air pollutants, like volatile organic compounds—the NCI study says each 10 micrograms of fine-particulate pollution alone causes an 18-percent increase in heart-related deaths, an 8-percent increase in lung-related deaths, and a 4-percent increase in overall deaths.[52] Statistics from the CDC show cancer and heart disease each contribute to about a third of all U.S. deaths. This means that a particulate-induced, 18-percent increase in heart-related deaths is sizeable, particularly from only one pollutant in only one environmental medium.[53]

Consider what particulate pollution means for Chicagoans. In the Windy City, about 30,000 people die annually, including about 11,500 from heart trouble and 12,000 from cancer. Chicago's average annual fine-particulate air pollution (2.5 micrometers or less in diameter) is about 17 micrograms per cubic meter. According to the previous CDC data, these particulates cause roughly 3,000 annual preventable, heart-related Chicago deaths—eight per day. These 3,000 deaths include neither those from other (nonparticulate) airborne hazards, nor those from pesticide-laden food and contaminated water. Even before counting fatalities from other environmental causes, particulate air pollution alone causes about 10 percent of all Chicago deaths, mostly from heart attacks.[54]

Water Pollution

Polluted water also takes a toll. The WHO says 1.1 billion people—one-sixth of global inhabitants—do not have access to clean water.[55] Even in the United States, the APHA says "low levels of some 300 toxic substances, including many known or suspected carcinogens...have been found in the nation's water supply....A very substantial portion of the public's drinking water supply is obtained from sources contaminated by...industrial, agricultural, and municipal operations."[56]

- Yet, because the Safe Drinking Water Act is not fully enforced, the U.S. EPA says 45 million Americans drink unsafe water.[57]

- According to the U.S. EPA, approximately 56 percent of estuarine bodies, 45 percent of lakes, and 35 percent of rivers and streams in the nation are impaired—"unfit" for drinking, swimming, or fish consumption. This impairment comes mostly from pollutants like mercury, PCBs, chlordane, and dioxins, from sources like coal-fired plants, incinerators, and industrial stacks.[58]

- Largely because coal plants contaminate water and fish with mercury, in 2004 the U.S. CDC and EPA said 1 in 12 U.S. women of childbearing age had blood levels of mercury able to cause neurological and developmental harms to her unborn children. More recent 2006 studies, from the University of North Carolina, show that one in five U.S. women has blood-mercury levels that violate EPA limits. As of 2006, however, the United States continues to weaken mercury-pollution regulations.[59]

- Only two states (Wyoming and Alaska) have no restrictions on eating local fish because of their contamination.[60]

- About 14 million Americans drink water contaminated with the pesticides atrazine, cyanizine, simazine, alachlor, and metolachlor—which are implicated in cancer, birth defects, and genetic mutations.[61]

- U.S. NAS studies have found pesticides and their by-products (including aldicarb, 1,2-D, DBCP, alachlor, atrazine, and 2.4-D) in the groundwater of 34 states.[62]

- In violation of U.S. EPA standards, carcinogenic herbicides alone contaminate the drinking water of 4 million Americans.[63]

- Apart from all other water contaminants, only five common herbicides in drinking water cause about a million Americans to face cancer risks that are more than 10 times the federal standard.[64]

- Despite such statistics, and despite the fact that half of pesticide use is unnecessary and can be replaced by integrated pest management, use of pesticides in the United States has increased by more than 50 percent in the last three decades. It now amounts annually to 8 pounds per person.[65]

Arsenic contamination of drinking water is especially serious, partly because current U.S. EPA drinking-water standards for arsenic were set in 1942, before it was known to be a carcinogen. As a result, 35 million Americans face significant risks of diabetes, arteriosclerosis, and bladder, lung, and skin cancers because they drink water from community systems whose arsenic levels exceed 1 part per billion.[66] State of California scientists showed that currently allowed drinking-water standards for arsenic cause more than 1 cancer in every 100 people exposed.[67] Other drinking-water contaminants include trihalomethanes (water-disinfection by-products formed when water is purified, as with chlorine). These cause about 11,000 annual U.S. bladder and rectal cancers,[68] and they put 80–100 million Americans at risk.[69] In addition, although no dose of ionizing radiation is safe,[70] 19 million Americans drink tap water that violates current radon-safety standards; EPA says 81 million Americans have radiation-contaminated tap water posing "significant" cancer threats.[71]

Water contaminated with farm, sewage, or slaughterhouse waste likewise threatens U.S. health. As a result, in 2003 the APHA called for a moratorium on concentrated animal feed operations—facilities having more than 1,000 cattle, 2,500 hogs, or 100,000 hens. The APHA says such operations, which now house 54 percent of all U.S. livestock, lead to health threats from antibiotics, heavy metals, bacterial endotoxins, and volatile gases.[72]

- According to the EPA, more than 29 million Americans drink bacterially contaminated water that violates its health standards.[73]

- Bacterially contaminated tap water causes one in three U.S. gastrointestinal illnesses—often erroneously attributed to stomach flu.[74]

- In 14 states, 97 percent of water-treatment plants are contaminated with cryptosporidium or giardia, neither of which is controlled merely by adding chlorine.[75]

To avoid water-borne health threats, Americans spend nearly $2 billion per year for bottled water and home-treatment units. Yet home-treatment units are unregulated and not independently tested. Because bottled water must meet only tap-water standards, up to one-third of U.S. bottled water comes from public utilities whose water may be less healthy than what bottled-water drinkers have from their local utilities.[76]

Pollution Threats to Children

Although many adults have defenses against premature disease and death caused by air, water, and other pollution, children often do not.[77] Their developing organ systems, incomplete metabolic processes, and only partially developed detoxification systems are less able to withstand most toxins. Yet children, per unit of body mass, take in more air, water, and food (and thus more pollutants) than do adults. In addition, because many pollution regulations focus on cancer and only on adults, they ignore pollution-induced developmental and neurological disorders in children. Because "children are often more susceptible to environmental contaminants than adults," and government "policies and decisions" often fail to reflect this unique susceptibility," APHA says children have "particular need for special protection from pollutants."[78]

Even while they are still in the womb, children face higher pollution risks than adults. As the *New England Journal of Medicine* study of 90,000 identical twins (already mentioned) concluded, and as the WHO says, only "a small fraction of all childhood cancers" are associated with heredity, genetics, infections, and viruses. Instead, environmental pollutants appear "to play a major role."[79] The WHO says air pollution alone is associated with up to half of all childhood cancers.[80] The National Childhood Cancer Foundation, the Children's Oncology Group, and the U.S. NAS, among other groups, say childhood-cancer incidence and childhood developmental-neurological disorders are increasing rapidly. According to the NAS, each year in the United States, approximately 12,500 children are diagnosed with cancer. About half die. Each day, the equivalent of two average-size classrooms are diagnosed. As in Hammond, Indiana, childhood leukemias and tumors of the brain, nervous system, lymphatic system, kidneys, bones, and muscles are the most common. The U.S. NAS says cancer causes more deaths of children, aged 1–15, "than any other disease, more deaths than asthma, diabetes, cystic fibrosis and AIDS combined." Yet this annual 12,500 figure does not include the significant numbers of noncancer, pollution-induced disorders, including neurological and developmental injuries, endocrine disruption, genetic defects, birth defects, and heart, lung, and respiratory disorders.[81]

While 6,000 U.S. children die annually from cancer, 3,000 are killed by automobiles. Another roughly 1,400 are murdered each year, and about 1,100 children die annually from child abuse. Given these statistics, why do news reports give relatively little attention to pollution-induced childhood diseases like cancers, although they kill more children than automobiles, murder, or child abuse combined? As chapter 2 reveals, repeated media analyses show that because polluters control so much TV, radio, and newsprint advertising, they also influence news coverage. For instance, because chemical companies control major portions of U.S. media-advertising dollars, they frequently receive special news-media treatment. One result? Although pesticides and herbicides are designed to kill living things, there is relatively little media coverage of how these chemicals kill humans, especially children. There is virtually no media coverage of the fact that the APHA has repeatedly recommended phasing out chlorinated pesticides/herbicides and eliminating all chlorine compounds, except those in pharmaceuticals. The APHA says that because of their persistence in human tissues, these pesticides contaminate human breast milk and compromise many of the extraordinary benefits of breast-feeding.[82]

- Among pesticides listed as reproductive toxins by the state of California, two-thirds are still in use, including in schools. Parental exposure has been linked to their children's cancers—and to birth defects such as cleft palate, limb malformations, heart defects, facial and eye deformities, and incomplete bone development in the skull.[83]

- Most major classes of pesticides, including the organochlorines, organophosphates, carbamates, chlorophenoxy herbicides, and pyrethroids, have been shown to adversely affect the developing nervous system, to compromise the immune system, and to exacerbate risk of infection and disease.[84]

- U.S. NAS studies show that "exposure to neurotoxic compounds at levels believed to be safe for adults can result in permanent loss of brain function if it occurs during the prenatal and early childhood period of brain development."[85]

- For some pesticides, like organophosphate compounds, a lethal dose in immature animals can be only 1 percent of the lethal dose for adults.[86]

- *American Journal of Public Health* researchers have found that within a day following indoor treatment for fleas, infants absorbed 10 to 50 times more insecticide than what the EPA considers an acceptable exposure for adults.[87]

- According to U.S. NCI studies, childhood leukemias can increase by 400 percent in houses where pesticides are used at least once a week. They can increase by 600 percent for children whose families use garden pesticides at least once a month.[88]

- Childhood brain and lymph-system cancers can increase by 200 percent for children exposed to household exterminations—and by 500 percent for children whose pets have flea collars.[89]

- If their fathers work in agriculture, children can be 900 percent more likely to develop rare bone cancers.[90]

- Because of children's greater exposures and heightened vulnerability, the U.S. NAS says that following even U.S. government pesticide standards does not adequately protect children.[91]

Besides pesticides, children are especially at risk from industrial neurotoxins in air pollution.[92] This is partly because of their increased rates of respiration, their smaller airways, and their developing organs. Even in the United States, children are the largest and most vulnerable subgroup of the population that is harmed by air pollution.[93] A 2005 WHO study showed that current levels of air pollution, from sources like coal plants, oil refineries, manufacturing facilities, waste incinerators, and automobiles, are implicated in many childhood health threats. These include increased childhood mortality, lower birth weight, premature birth, intrauterine growth retardation, sudden infant-death syndrome, cancer, and birth defects. Scientists also say current U.S. levels of air pollution cause statistically significant U.S. increases in childhood inflammation, decreased immune function, impaired lung function, allergic responses, cardiac disease, and respiratory disease.[94]

As early as the 1960s, physicians showed that a 10 percent increase in particulate pollution alone can cause a 1-percent increase in infant mortality. But little was done to reduce particulates, and the nation has not followed most of the air-pollution recommendations of the APHA. Indeed, for the first time in 35 years, on February 2, 2006, the politically appointed head of the U.S. EPA rejected the recommendations of the EPA's Clean Air Scientific Advisory Committee, which called for strengthening particulate-air-pollution standards. Instead the EPA head rejected the internal-EPA and scientific-committee consensus. The state EPA of California said that the rejection was based on the White House Office of Management and Budget's making "last minute" insertions of "edits and opinions" that "misrepresent the scientific consensus." One result? The new standards, proposed by the scientific committee, would have cut particulate-induced deaths by about 50 percent, but instead the EPA head proposed rules that would reduce deaths by only 22 percent. Breathing problems now account for one-third of all U.S. infant deaths, and they are likely to continue increasing. Asthma is now the leading cause of childhood school absenteeism and the most common chronic childhood disease; in the last decade, asthma has increased by 40 percent in the United States—costing the nation about $6.2 billion in annual damage.[95] Similar problems exist in Europe, where 30 million people currently have asthma.[96] As already mentioned, airborne particulates alone now cause about 6.4 percent of annual U.S. deaths for children aged 0–4. Living only two months in a highly polluted city can increase infant mortality by 10 percent. Only eight nations, all in the developing world, have worse ozone pollution that the United States. About 27 million U.S. children under age 13, and half the pediatric asthma population, live in areas that violate EPA's ozone standards. What happens to these children? In 2005, Harvard, Yale, and New York University scientists showed that for every average-daily-ozone increase of 10 parts per billion, deaths increase 10 percent over the subsequent three days. For carbon monoxide, each increase in average background rates of 1 part per million increases risk of low birth weight by 19 percent.[97]

Part of children's vulnerability to dirty air comes from heavy metals. Each day coal utilities, waste incinerators, metal-processing facilities—and industries like those that manufacture paints, circuit boards, conductive fillers in plastics, heat-transfer media, and lubricants—release heavy metals like lead. Annual U.S. releases of lead are over 1 million tons.[98]

- While adults typically absorb only about 10–15 percent of lead entering their gastrointestinal tracts, pregnant women and children may absorb 50 percent.[99]

- For adults, drinking water contributes about 20 percent of average lead exposure, but the U.S. EPA says more than 85 percent of infants' blood lead may derive from drinking baby formula made with lead-contaminated water.[100]

- While 83 percent of U.S. homes have low or no levels of lead (parts per billion), the high levels in 17 percent of U.S. homes are sufficient to cause neurological and developmental risks to children.[101]

While some of this lead exposure comes from paint, chapter 4 shows that controlling pollution also could help reduce these lead exposures, but companies say it is cheaper, short term, not to do so. One result? The U.S. CDC say 900,000 children under age 5—4.4 percent of all U.S. children—have blood-lead levels able to cause *irreversible* cognitive, behavioral, internal-organ, blood-forming, and growth damage. These blood-lead levels also have been implicated in developmental damage, reduced IQ, delinquency, and criminality. Because children's defenses against lead are still developing, and because lead doses are cumulative, with no threshold for risk, any childhood or pregnancy exposure risks such damage—some of which is irreversible. The NAS says average background concentrations of lead in modern North Americans are 300 times higher than they were in the native North American people before European settlement.[102]

As already mentioned, even if all pollution laws were enforced, children would not be adequately protected from pollutants like lead. The American Academy of Pediatrics has warned that federal air-pollution standards have "little or no margin of safety for children engaged in active outdoor activity."[103]

- Columbia University researchers showed that even before they are born, children risk birth defects, genetic injuries, decreased birth weight, decreased length, and decreased head circumference because of mothers' exposures to carcinogens in ambient air.[104]

- Researchers have documented doublings of respiratory-related hospital admissions for preschoolers when even one local pollution source (a steel mill) was operating rather than closed.[105]

- During peak particulate-pollution months, although hospital admissions for adult respiratory problems can increase 40 percent, those for children can increase 300 percent.[106]

- Mortality rates also increase markedly as a function of air pollution, especially from ozone, sulfur dioxide, and particulates.[107]

Most U.S. water standards likewise fail to protect children and other vulnerable groups because they are based on health effects for average adults. Yet, based on average body weight, infants and children drink two to three times as much water as adults. And even inadequate U.S. water standards are not always enforced.[108] The U.S. EPA says 600,000 U.S. children annually drink tap water that violates its standards.[109] Outside the developed world, dirty water is even more dangerous for children. Mostly in developing nations, 5,000 children die daily from diarrhea, mainly from bacterially contaminated water.[110]

Environmental Justice and Pollution Risks to Minorities and Poor People

After children, poor people, and minorities, blue-collar workers often are most at risk from pollution. They are victims of environmental injustice— disproportional pollution burdens borne by some people because of discrimination based on age, income, race, or occupation. As the APHA confirms, environmental pollution likely causes the deaths of 100,000 blue-collar workers annually; minorities and poor people also are much more likely, than other people, to receive higher exposures to pollutants like synthetic chemicals.[111] The 30,000 U.S. children living in families at or below the poverty level are doubly at risk. Their families are less likely to have health-protective air filters and air conditioning. They also may eat contaminated fish, as poor people sometimes obtain food from polluted local waterways. The poor likewise are less likely to have under-the-sink water filters. Yet *American Journal of Public Health* studies show that U.S. homes with such filters can prevent 35 percent of the gastrointestinal illnesses that occur in filter-less homes. This 35 percent is "water-related and preventable"—but only for those who can afford the filters.[112]

Minorities and poor people also generally bear greater health risks, all things being equal, partly because poverty and racism force them to live where homes are cheapest and pollution tends to be highest. Their lack of socioeconomic power frequently causes their neighborhoods to be targeted for location of hazardous facilities, some of whose emissions may violate the law. Proportionately more landfills, power plants, toxic-waste dumps, bus and rail yards, sewage plants, and industrial facilities are sited in the neighborhoods of poor people and minorities. As a result, they bear higher levels of infectious disease, contaminated air, and contaminated tap water.[113] In Hammond, Indiana, where Gwen Pearson, Kate Burns, and their families lived, the mostpublicized children who died from central-nervous-system cancers were white and middle class.[114] Yet industry-reported Toxics Release Inventory and census-tract data show that average people of color in that Indiana county bear nearly eight times the levels of hazardous-chemical releases as do whites. Poverty-level families there bear more than three times the levels of toxic-chemical releases as those above the family poverty level of $12,575.[115] Examining the 593 sites on the U.S. EPA national-cleanup priority list (the Superfund), a U.S. NCI study found that in counties with Superfund sites, cancer death rates are higher, blacks live closer to the sites, and blacks have higher cancer rates than whites.[116] Dr. Glenn Paulson summarized the NCI results this way: "If you know where the chemical industry is, you know where the cancer hotspots are"—and where poor people and minorities live.[117]

Of course, environmental injustice is not the only reason for poorer health among minorities and poor people. Fewer educational opportunities, less access to medical care, and less insurance are among the other factors that put minorities and poor people at greater health risk. Nevertheless, as the APHA and later chapters argue, environmental injustice is a major cause of poor health. As already mentioned, it is one of at least seven *ethical considerations* showing that pollution-induced health threats deserve special scrutiny. These ethically relevant characteristics include the *magnitude* of pollution risks, lay *ignorance* about them, their frequent *preventability*, their typically *discriminatory impacts*, their often occurring through *human-rights violations*, through *deliberate* or *criminal acts*, and through *commission of harms* rather than omissions. As later chapters argue, environmental-justice threats are especially ethically troubling because they jeopardize human rights. People cannot fulfill their rights to life or to equal protection if they cannot breathe clean air and drink clean water—if "exposure to environmental risks varies based on race and...income," as the APHA emphasizes.[118]

In the United States, the percentage of people of color, living in counties with commercial hazardous-waste facilities, is three times higher than that in counties without these facilities.[119] U.S. people of color also live, in greater concentrations, in areas that have above-average numbers of air-polluting facilities and that fail to meet federal air-quality-attainment standards. In the United States, 52 percent of whites (but 71 percent of Hispanics) live in counties with high ozone concentrations. Only 5 percent of whites (but 10 percent of African-Americans and 15 percent of Hispanics) live in air that violates all four air-quality standards (carbon monoxide, sulfur dioxide, nitrogen dioxide, particulate matter). Similar statistics hold for other areas of the world. In the United Kingdom, for instance, half of all waste incinerators are in neighborhoods comprising the poorest 10 percent of the country. Such statistics illustrate the "managed inequality" in global health and human-rights protection.[120]

The APHA warns that children of color are especially at risk from pollution not only because of where they live but also because they are less likely to have health care to offset pollution. As a result, U.S. black and Hispanic children have much higher incidences of asthma than do white children. Black children, aged 5–14, are four times more likely than white children to die from asthma. They are three times more likely to be hospitalized for it, despite their lesser access to health care.[121] Among poverty-level U.S. black children, nearly one-third have blood-lead levels above the recommended health standard. Studies by the U.S. CDC show that blood-lead levels are consistently higher for black than white children; for younger than older children; and for children in lower, than higher, income families. They reveal that 8 percent of poverty-level children are lead poisoned, as compared to only 1 percent of children above the poverty level. About 11 percent of black children are lead poisoned, as compared with about 2 percent of white children.[122]

Even when different racial and socioeconomic groups are exposed to the same levels of pollutants, APHA data show that minority and poor children are likely to be affected worse than white or non-poverty-level children. Besides lack of health care, poorer economic conditions encourage poorer nutrition, poorer housing, and thus greater susceptibility to environmental pollution.

Repeatedly researchers have shown that mortality is strongly related to *income inequality*, rather than to median income, per capita income, or actual poverty levels. In short: what kills people is income inequality, not mainly poverty. One reason may be that the greater the societal and economic inequality, the more the rich can pay to avoid threats like pollution. The poor cannot. In democratic societies with greater economic equality, pollution typically decreases because more people can speak for and protect themselves, and others are less able to exploit them or force them to bear higher levels of pollution.[123]

Public-health effects of income inequality seem especially evident in the United States. It has the shortest average life expectancy, but the highest levels of income inequality, poverty, and percentage of children in poverty of any Western industrialized nation.[124] Such statistics—and the fact that income inequality rather than poverty increases mortality—help explain why poor people and minorities in the United States face more serious health threats, even where everyone is exposed to the same levels of pollutants.

- The U.S. death rate for 1- to 4-year-old children is double that of nations like Finland.

- Even when one controls for the higher U.S. murder rate, the U.S. death rate for 15- to 25-year-olds is double that of countries like Netherlands, Japan, Sweden, and the United Kingdom.

- The U.S. infant-mortality rate is triple that of many places, like Singapore.

- United States infant mortality is more than double the rate of democratic nations like Sweden, Japan, and Iceland.

- If U.S. infant-mortality rates were as good as in Singapore, 2,212 U.S. babies would be saved each year.

- Even Beijing, China, has an infant-mortality rate that is 4.6 per 1,000 live births, as compared to New York City's 6.5, and the U.S. rate of 7 per 1,000.[125]

Health disparities like these suggest that in the United States, poor people and minorities are more vulnerable (than others) to the same levels of pollution. Yet the preceding statistics show that poor people and minorities typically bear higher levels of pollution. In addition, nearly three times the percentage of U.S. blacks, as whites, are at the poverty level. Partly as a result, blacks have higher incidences of death and disease, especially for children.[126] For all cancers combined, black U.S. males have about a 50 percent higher cancer-mortality rate than white males, and black U.S. females have about a 30 percent higher cancer-mortality rate than white females. Even after one controls for other variables—like crime, medical coverage, and income—this inequality in mortality is only reduced, not eliminated. Such data suggest that universal health insurance alone will not equally protect U.S. minorities and poor people from cancer. As chapter 6 suggests, the solution is not to eliminate all toxic dumps or hazardous facilities but to minimize and equalize their burdens, especially by ensuring that they are sited without obvious violations of rights to know, to consent, to compensation, and so on. As the APHA has repeatedly noted, racism and environmental injustice (disproportionate pollution) also need to be confronted as factors in why U.S. minorities continue to bear higher health risks.[127]

Public Health in Developed versus Developing Nations

In the developing world, public-health threats, environmental injustice, and economic inequalities are even more serious than in the United States. Globally, 2.8 billion people, 46 percent of humanity, live below the World Bank's $2-per-day poverty level. This means they have less purchasing power than $2.15 per day had in the United States in 1993. Over 1.2 billion people live on less than $1 per day. As a result, each year 18 million people die prematurely. This is one-third of all human deaths—50,000 each day. These fatalities include 34,000 daily deaths of children under age 5. Deaths of children are roughly 70 percent of all global fatalities.[128]

One of the most troubling aspects of these deaths, as the APHA warns, is that developed nations like the United States have partly contributed to them. United States pesticide exports, pharmaceutical trials, extractive industries, and trade agreements are typical contributors.[129] Nearly one-third of U.S.-produced pesticides are banned or nonregistered for domestic use because of their dangers, yet they are exported to developing nations. There, the WHO says, they annually kill 40,000 people. They also often return illegally to the United States on imported food. Some U.S. drug companies likewise run risky clinical trials in developing nations, when they would never be allowed in the United States. Operating in poor nations, many U.S. extractive industries like oil, mining, and timber also have contributed to well-documented public-health threats. Even U.S. development assistance abroad sometimes has prevented fewer public-health threats than it might.[130]

The U.S. Agency for International Development (USAID), for instance, has given American companies hundreds of millions of dollars of taxpayer money to move their U.S. operations to low-wage, regulation-free "export-processing" zones in places like the Caribbean and Central America. During the senior Bush administration, one USAID–financed ad touted the benefits of hiring "Rosa Martinez" to work at her sewing machine, making textiles for U.S. markets for 33 cents per hour. In Mexico, for example, 90 percent of the products assembled in sweatshop maquiladoras are made in U.S.–owned facilities, for export to the United States. During the last two decades, these export-processing zones have provided cheaper textiles for U.S. consumers. They also have given U.S. apparel manufacturers profits that are much higher than average for the U.S. manufacturing sector. Yet according to the U.S. National Labor Committee and the U.S. Government Accountability Office (GAO), the U.S. oversight agency, these export-processing zones also have caused U.S. job losses as well as poor working conditions and poor wages abroad. The National Labor Committee and GAO say that "the funds spent on building export-processing zones were spent inappropriately." Over the last 15 years in the Caribbean, the countries with the steepest wage declines have been those with U.S. export-processing zones—nations that are the highest-volume exporters of apparel to the United States. Illustrating workplace environmental injustice, nearly all U.S.-government–sanctioned, export-processing, or sweatshop-zone employees are female; are coerced into working in unsafe conditions; and enjoy wages significantly lower than those paid men for comparable work in the same country. They are typically single mothers, earning 28 percent of the officially calculated living wage, and their families enjoy "significantly lower" standards of living than those not living in export-processing zones. They are fired if they become pregnant. They work in zones surrounded by barbed wire, are searched by armed guards, and toil 11–13 hours per day for at least 6 days each week. For their sewing, they are paid less than 1 percent of the retail price of the apparel when it is sold in the United States. After 3 or 4 years of harsh and unsafe working conditions, these young women return to their native countryside—worn out, sick, often unable to work. The National Labor Committee showed that frequently these apparel workers live in small (10-feet-by-20-feet) concrete dormitory rooms housing 12 workers. Why does the National Labor Committee say that about half of the young women abroad, who make clothing, shoes, and handbags for U.S. companies like Wal-Mart, often owe their employers money? They are forced to live in employer-owned dormitories, to buy food from employers, and to pay "placement" fees—all deducted from their paychecks.[131] To assist U.S. firms using taxpayer-funding to locate abroad in such export-processing zones, the National Labor Committee and GAO say that USAID officials have maintained blacklists of Central American groups that promote labor unions and workplace safety. Although U.S. president Clinton promised to overhaul USAID and to address workplace environmental injustice, he never succeeded. Congressional and labor officials say U.S. manufacturers fought the reform because they have become accustomed to USAID's promoting sweatshops, subsistence wages, unsafe workplaces, and blacklists. As a result, U.S. labor officials say U.S. industries, not poor nations, often remain the greatest beneficiaries of assistance from groups like USAID, the U.S. Overseas Private Investment Corporation (OPIC), the World Bank, and the International Monetary Fund. They say the World Trade Organization and the North American Free Trade Agreement (NAFTA) often have exacerbated these problems.[132]

Despite far more serious health problems in the developing world, some worsened by official U.S. policies like those for sweatshops, this book has four main reasons for focusing on U.S. public health. First, people are more likely to be motivated to do something about pollution and other public-health problems when they know they and their children are hurt, not just those in developing nations. Once they learn this lesson at home, and apply it to their own governments and institutions, they are more likely to apply it abroad. Second, theoretically at least, the United States has more political resources for addressing unequal health threats than does any other nation in the world. Later chapters show that these resources include the Bill of Rights, the Toxics Release Inventory, the Freedom of Information Act, and many nongovernmental organizations. Third, the United States has more money to address health threats, yet (as earlier paragraphs revealed) its health-related inequalities are greater than those of many Western democracies. Fourth, in part because the United States has more severe economic inequalities than most other Western democracies, it has more serious health inequalities that must be addressed.

Given these four practical reasons for beginning with U.S. rather than global public-health problems, this book presupposes a practical, two-step approach. The first presupposition is that U.S. public health can improve if ordinary people recognize that they and their children are at risk from pollution and other threats. The second presupposition is that, if U.S. citizens learn first to protect their own health, they will be better able to work for similar protections in developing nations.

The Health-Successes Objection

Some people, however, might question whether the developed world faces serious public-health problems. Are this chapter's pollution statistics misleading? Do they ignore important U.S. public-health improvements? Could more positive health statistics be assembled? Such questions might be called "the health-successes objection."

While this chapter's data do not deny obvious public-health improvements, the point here is not the relative balance of overall public-health successes and failures. Instead, this chapter's claims are much more specific. For example, (1) apart from various health successes, U.S. pollution-related health threats are both serious and increasing—needlessly killing tens of thousands of people a year, even according to the most conservative statistics. (2) These pollution-related health effects are disproportionately harming poor people, people of color, and children.[133] Building on these two factual points, later chapters make a specific ethical argument: Apart from public-health successes, any pollution-related deaths and injuries are too many, especially in the richest nation in the world, if they are easily preventable, deliberate or criminal, occurring because of violations of human rights to know and to consent, or imposed inequitably on vulnerable groups like children. As a consequence, citizens must act to minimize these threats, to change their own lives and, ultimately, to help reform the governments and institutions of which they are a part.

The health-successes objection is correct, however, in noting that many improvements in public health have occurred. After all, during 1990–2005, the United States experienced a 40 percent drop in the rate of motor-vehicle deaths, a 40 percent drop in incidence of infectious disease, a 24 percent drop in the rate of violent crime, and an 18 percent drop in the rate of cardiovascular disease. While nothing in this chapter denies such progress, the point here is similar to one made recently by the editors of the *American Journal of Public Health*: "Despite some significant improvements in health status in the last decade," the U.S. Department of Health and Human Services has failed "to achieve more than 15 percent of the [department's public-health] goals" mandated for the year 2000. This failure can be traced partly to pollution and partly to "excess mortality and morbidity experienced by the poor and by people of color."[134] Also, 2006 data show that the United States ranks below 30 other nations in its environmental performance, below 16 other nations in its environmental-health scores overall; and not in the top 27 nations regarding air-quality scores. In fact, the United States has the worst ozone pollution of all developed nations, and only eight nations (all in the developing world) are worse.[135]

One example of the failure to achieve 85 percent of United States–mandated, public-health goals is the apparent increase in annual toxic-chemical releases, as given in the Toxics Release Inventory. Comprised of reported, annual, industry releases of about 650 toxic chemicals, the Toxics Release Inventory shows that U.S. hazardous emissions and effluents are increasing, sometimes by as much as 5 percent annually.[136] Despite this apparent increase, independent aircraft measurements and gas-chromatograph data show that many companies underreport these toxic releases. Analyses from the U.S. EPA's inspector general, the U.S. GAO, state environmental officials, and watchdog groups all claim that industry sometimes releases up to 14 times more toxic chemicals than it reports.[137] In its latest available Toxics Release Inventory (2005), EPA admitted that the data "may reflect uncorrected facility reporting errors."[138] In addition, Toxics Release Inventory data do not cover all toxic releases, but only those for about 650 of 80,000 chemicals in use; besides, many companies required to report Toxics Release Inventory data do not do so, and reporting often is not enforced.[139]

Despite major public-health improvements, both Toxics Release Inventory data and this chapter's statistics provide *prima facie* data showing that many pollution-related health problems are not improving. Their magnitude is increasing, and they are inequitably distributed. Moreover, this chapter's data on these health threats are not from questionable sources but from government agencies, prestigious medical journals, and major associations of health professionals. As the APHA recently repeated: "Research has linked incidence and severity of cancer, asthma, Alzheimer's, autism, birth defects, endometriosis, infertility, and multiple sclerosis to environmental contaminants."[140] As already noted, these pollution-related deaths and injuries are the special focus of this book because they raise at least seven ethical problems that many other health problems do not raise. They signal not only poor health but also basic societal injustices that must be corrected.

The Longevity Objection

But how can there be basic societal injustices, associated with health effects of pollution, when people seem to be living longer and getting healthier? Even if pollution-related health threats are getting worse, how can they be serious if lifespans are increasing? Such questions might be called "the longevity objection."[141]

While partially correct in noting the increased U.S. lifespan, the longevity objection appears to misunderstand both the magnitude of this increase and its ethical significance. As the following paragraphs will show, the longevity objection errs ethically in ignoring at least six facts. These include ignoring the *causes* of increased longevity; *distributive inequities* in longevity; evidence for *increased disease* and days of limited activity (documented earlier); ethically significant differences between *deliberate harm* to others, versus merely failing to benefit them; disproportionately higher U.S. *expenditures* on health care; and disproportionately lower U.S. expenditures on *pollution control*, relative to many other developed nations.

The *causes* of increased longevity in developed nations are important to the longevity objection because public-health officials say most increases in longevity have come from things like antibiotics, better health care, and sewage treatment, all of which help mask the damage caused by pollution. Proponents of the longevity objection forget that people would be even healthier if pollution were reduced, if there were more access to medical care, and so on. The longevity objection thus relies on a fallacious argument that pollution is not ethically questionable because overall longevity is increasing. Yet pollution-induced decreases in longevity are real. They merely have been counterbalanced by factors like antibiotics. Using the longevity objection is like saying one ought not worry about the health of one's child because she is taller than she was last year. Height, like longevity, is not an adequate indicator of health. Using the longevity objection is like a worker's saying her employer's wage cuts are not ethically questionable because she herself has inherited money from a relative. Regardless of her inheritance (or her longevity), people have duties to pay just wages (and not to impose life-threatening pollution).

The biggest problem with the longevity objection, however, is its ignoring *distributive equity*. The longevity objection presupposes that if average longevity is increasing, pollution is not seriously harming health. This faulty inference errs because it confuses increased average longevity with increased longevity for the *most vulnerable* members of the population. Yet average U.S. longevity is increasing, while the longevity of many victims of environmental injustice is not. As the APHA noted in 2005, U.S. racial and socioeconomic disparities in health "have persisted for years, despite major advances in public health, biotechnology, economic wealth and prosperity, and the overall improvement in the health status of the American population over the last century."[142] Consequently, the APHA conclusions suggest that the supposed average increases in longevity may reflect the "healthy-survivor" effect, not improved longevity among those most at risk. (The healthy-survivor effect is that wealthier or healthier people, survivors, have longer lives, while members of vulnerable groups have shorter lives.) And, as already mentioned, even the slightly increased 5-year-survival of cancer victims may be misleading and merely a function of earlier diagnosis.[143] Five-year-survival likewise means little, since cancer disproportionately strikes children and kills average victims 15 years prematurely.

The longevity objection also errs in ignoring the fact that pollution is often the result of deliberately harmful, unethical, or criminal acts. It thus ignores all *ethical aspects* of death and disease statistics and instead focuses merely on the *average magnitude* of death and disease. This is like saying that because the average U.S. murder rate is decreasing, people ought not worry about the tens of thousands of annual murders. In both the longevity and the murder cases, the ethical issue is not merely the average increase or decrease in death. Rather, as already emphasized, the ethical issue is how many murders or pollution-induced deaths are (1) easily preventable; (2) inequitably imposed on vulnerable or innocent subgroups, like children; (3) caused by faulty enforcement; or (4) a result of failure to recognize equal human rights, and so on. Even if murder rates are going down, and even if longevity is improving, all deaths from causes like these four obviously ought to be avoided. Why? These deaths are not merely accidental or natural, but the result of unethical and unjust behavior. Society obviously has a greater ethical obligation to minimize deaths caused by injustice than to minimize those caused by accidents, natural events, or flawed personal choices. To see this point, consider another example.

Suppose a child, with a very high IQ, is exposed to a known neurotoxic pollutant by a manufacturer who cuts costs by failing to control emissions, as in the Ferro case. As a result, suppose the child experiences a 20-point IQ drop, yet remains slightly above average in intelligence. Just as the longevity objection is wrong, it would be wrong for someone to dismiss the child's neurotoxin exposure and decreased IQ, on grounds that she is still above average (or still enjoys greater longevity than others). Why? She has been harmed by others who have benefited from her harm. Besides, being above average is only a necessary, not a sufficient, condition for saying this bright child has not been harmed by the neurotoxin. It is not sufficient because, all things being equal, the 20-point IQ drop gives the child fewer educational, employment, and economic opportunities than she otherwise would have had. Regardless of longevity, environmental pollution likewise gives the most vulnerable people—children, particularly poor minority children—poorer health than they otherwise would have had. From an ethical point of view, the child's IQ and pollution victims' longevity should be assessed against what they might have been, without preventable pollution exposure, not against some average IQ or longevity. At least three reasons suggest it also would be ethically wrong, in the face of a child's pollutant-induced, 20-point IQ drop, to say that this pollution is not significant because other factors—like inadequate health care—have harmed her IQ more than the neurotoxin. One reason is that some harm (the neurotoxin) does not become harmless, just because the victim faces even more serious threats (poor health care). Second, the neurotoxin harm might be considered even worse, if it affects those already disenfranchised by society, those without adequate health care. Third, failure to provide equal health care to the child is a failure to enhance welfare, a failure to benefit her. Subjecting the child to neurotoxin pollution, however, is to deliberately harm her. As already mentioned, it is far more important ethically for society to prevent harms like pollution than to provide some benefit like health care or longevity.

From a purely practical point of view, another problem with the longevity objection is its failure to recognize that higher U.S. health-care *expenditures* are not causing proportionate increases in U.S. health and longevity. Instead, the modest U.S. increase in average longevity is partly a result of massively disproportionate health-care spending, not cleaner air and water. According to the latest (2004) WHO statistics, the United States spends more per capita on health care than any other nation in the world: $4,887 per person annually. *The Economist* 2007 data indicate that the United States spends 15.2 percent of its gross domestic product (GDP) on health—far more than any other nation. Despite such U.S. outlays, citizens in scores of developed nations have longer average lifespans. These nations include Australia, Canada, Denmark, Finland, France, Germany, Greece, Ireland, Italy, Japan, Luxembourg, the Netherlands, New Zealand, Norway, Spain, Sweden, and the United Kingdom. *The Economist* 2007 data indicate that 54 other nations have longer average lifespans than the United States. The average Japanese person lives to be 75, but the average American, 69. Yet Japan spends only about half ($2,627 annually) what the United States spends on per-capita health-care. On average, Australians will live to be 73, 4 years longer than Americans. Yet Australia annually spends only one-third ($1,741) what the United States spends ($4,887) per capita on health care. The same WHO statistics indicate that health-care costs are rising faster in the United States than anywhere, yet they are producing little increased longevity. In the last 5 years, even increased U.S. health expenditures have not closed the gap between the longevity rates for the United States and other nations that spend far less on health care. During this time, per capita health-care expenditures increased 12 percent in Japan but 24 percent in the United States. In Australia, they have remained about the same.[144]

Obviously, lack of universal health insurance contributes to poorer U.S. longevity, but health insurance is not the only issue. As already noted, the U.S. NAS says lack of health coverage causes about 18,000 annual preventable U.S. fatalities. Earlier government and academy statistics indicate that industrial pollution appears to cause at least 60,000 annual preventable deaths, just from cancer. These pollution-induced U.S. deaths are significant, in part, because the United States spends proportionately less on pollution control than many nations with better longevity rates. World Bank data show that the United States spends about 0.6 percent of its gross domestic product (GDP) on pollution control, while Japan and many European Union countries spend about double that percentage, 1.17 percent. With the world's longest lifespan, 6 years longer than that in the United States, Japan has long been praised for its decisive efforts to clean up pollution.[145] World Bank data also show that Japan recycles 54 percent of its paper and cardboard, but the United States only 8 percent. Japan recycles 50 percent of its glass, but the United States only 20 percent. Japan creates 394 kilograms of municipal waste per person per year, but the United States, 864 kilograms. The average Japanese inhales only 2 pounds of pollutants annually, but the average U.S. citizen 81 pounds. Japan annually releases 2.2 tons of carbon dioxide per person, but the United States 5.8 tons. Similar statistics hold for many United States and European Union comparisons. Whereas 15–18 percent of all travel in nations like Japan, Finland, and Denmark is on pollution-reducing public transportation, only 1 percent of U.S. travel is on public transport. Although the U.S. railway network is the longest in the world, triple its closest competitor, more than 20 nations exceed the United States in kilometer-per-person rail-travel per year. This is part of the reason that all nations in the UN Organization for Economic Cooperation and Development together release only about one-fourth of the per-capita carbon-dioxide as does the United States.[146] Even exposure to pesticide-laden food is different in European Union, versus U.S., communities. In Austria, Finland, Italy, Sweden, and Switzerland, for instance, the percentage of organically grown crops is 25 to 65 times higher than in the United States. Organically grown crops represent 5–13 percent of the total agricultural acreage in these five European nations, as compared to 0.2 percent in the United States.[147] Citizens in each of these five nations have lifespans, respectively, 2, 2, 3, 4, and 4 years longer than the average U.S. lifespan.[148] As the previous paragraph warned, while such aggregate national statistics do not show causality between improved pollution control and improved longevity, they do raise many questions that deserve further investigation, questions that may undercut the longevity objection.

One obvious question is why U.S. pollution-control and health-care expenditures appear to be an exception among many Western developed nations. They appear not to follow a traditional economic rule, articulated by World Bank economists and supported by World Bank data. This rule is that developed nations with higher per-capita income have lower average pollution. Pollution-abatement is cost-effective for rich nations because it saves lives and therefore dollars. In addition, wealthier people are willing to pay for healthier lives. Despite its wealth, however, the United States tends not to follow this rule, and it avoids obvious pollution-control expenditures that could save lives. Data from the U.S. CDC, for instance, show that pollution abatement could help save $13 billion in annual U.S. costs from asthma, $351 billion in annual U.S. costs from cardiovascular disease, and $240 billion in annual occupational disease and injury.[149] If World Bank and CDC data are correct, and if the United States is an exception in its pollution-control policies, then these are additional reasons for questioning both U.S. longevity rates and the fact that U.S. children, minorities, and poor people bear disproportionate pollution burdens.[150]

In response to the preceding longevity and pollution-control statistics, objectors might say that higher U.S. per-capita pollution is justified by higher U.S. manufacturing. While the higher-production claim is correct, it is beside the point. If the United States has higher production and profits, it also should have better pollution control, not worse. Yet U.S. pollution control is not proportionate to its output, as it is in many developed nations. Higher U.S. production also does not explain the weaker U.S. regulatory climate—less recycling, more pollution breathed by citizens, and a smaller percentage of the GDP spent on pollution control than in many other democracies. Consequently, higher levels of U.S. manufacturing do not help the longevity objection.

What do the preceding observations about longevity, health-care expenditures, and pollution control suggest? These responses to the longevity objection neither glorify life outside the United States nor attack U.S. values. They do not presuppose that countries with lower production, lower profits, higher pollution control, and longer lifespans than the United States are ethically superior. Nor do they presuppose that U.S. citizens receive no counterbalancing benefits in exchange for their lower pollution-control costs and shorter lifespans. Finally, these observations and responses to the longevity objection do not attempt to draw precise causal conclusions about longevity, based on aggregate national health and pollution-control expenditures. Obviously many factors are responsible for different longevity rates in different nations. Both high-tech U.S. medicine and lack of universal health care, not just pollution inequities, help explain higher U.S. health costs but relatively lower U.S. longevity. Compared to many other Western democracies, the United States often has better and more high-tech health care for the very wealthy, but worse health care for the very poor. Yet, as already argued, even when one controls for factors like unequal access to health care and unequal income, U.S. minorities continue to exhibit poorer health. As already mentioned, the APHA says at least one reason for this disparity is minorities' greater exposure to both racism and pollutants.

The point of this chapter and the preceding responses to the longevity objection is not to draw precise scientific and causal conclusions about longevity, pollution, and health expenditures. Instead, the five main points are ethical, as follows. (1) Regardless of pollution effects on longevity, U.S. children, minorities, and poor people enjoy poorer health than other U.S. groups. (2) The APHA suggests that both environmental injustice as well as poorer U.S. pollution-control, relative to other Western democracies, may be two of many factors in this poorer health, especially since the United States spends relatively less on pollution control than many nations whose citizens enjoy longer lifespans. Consequently, the United States may be violating human rights if it allows its most vulnerable citizens to bear the disproportionate health costs of its economic successes. (3) U.S. citizens may not be gaining longevity proportionate to their health-care expenditures. (4) Because of distributive injustices, higher average U.S. wealth may not compensate for poorer U.S. public health, relative to other Western democracies. A 2005 study by Harvard Medical School and Harvard Law School showed that half of all U.S. bankruptcies are caused by medical expenses. Even medical insurance does not prevent families from being "wiped out by an illness."[151] Because it does not, neither universal health insurance nor high average U.S. wealth alone may offset many of the pollution, human-rights, and public-health problems this chapter has described and to which the longevity objection attempts to respond. (5) As later chapters argue, although industrial pollution is not the top contributor to U.S. public-health problems, it may be one of most *ethically significant contributors* because of the seven factors already noted. These include pollution-related discriminatory impacts, violations of human rights, criminal acts, deliberate commissions of harm, and so on.

Conclusion

Despite medical and economic advances in the United States, many citizens apparently cannot rely only on government to ensure their equal protection from harm—to protect their lives, their health, and their human rights from pollution. The solution? Citizens need to avoid scapegoating offending institutions, politicians, and groups. Instead, they need to help ensure that these institutions avoid obvious conflicts of interest and obvious harms to the public good. Citizens also need to help create the environments, communities, and democracies they deserve. In part, citizens need to recognize the rights-related pollution abuses surveyed in the next two chapters, to consider the responsibility argument outlined in chapter 4, and to investigate the practical solutions summarized in chapter 6. In short, citizens need to reclaim their governments and institutions, to encourage economic growth that does not give polluters a free ride. Citizens need to reclaim their ethical and democratic responsibility to help prevent harm, just as Gwen Pearson and Kate Burns did. As Kentucky writer Wendell Berry put it,

> we are going to have to gather up the fragments of knowledge and responsibility that we have parceled out to the bureaus and the corporations and the specialists.... We are going to have to put those fragments back together again in our own minds and in our families and households and neighborhoods.[152]

Orchestrating Ignorance, Ignoring Consent

When Karen Silkwood joined Kerr-McGee's nuclear-fuel plant outside Oklahoma City in 1972, she was 26 and a divorced mother of four. Hired to grind plutonium for fuel pellets for fast-breeder nuclear reactors, she had attended a year of college on a scholarship. Better educated than most of the other lab technicians with whom she worked, she loved chemistry. In May 1974, however, Silkwood's enthusiasm began to wane when she saw a coworker collapse. Safety officers fumbled as they tried to revive him. They failed, then brought an oxygen tank into the laboratory. It was broken. After her coworker nearly died, Silkwood complained to managers about lax safety standards, but they did nothing. Leaders of the local union, the Oil, Chemical, and Atomic Workers (OCAW), however, heard her complaints. They recognized her education and recruited her to collect details of safety problems at the plant. In September 1974, when she and other local union members met with OCAW officials in Washington, D.C., Silkwood had a list of 39 items detailing accidents, contamination, poor training, and falsification of quality-assurance records. Alarmed, national union officials told Silkwood to get additional evidence to prove Kerr-McGee's health and safety violations. They told her to turn over her materials in 7 weeks to union representative Steve Wodka and the *New York Times*.[1]

One week before she was to give the evidence to OCAW, Silkwood became contaminated, even though she was not working in the lab. When the source of the puzzling radioactive contamination remained elusive, a Kerr-McGee decontamination squad was sent to her home. After the squad found plutonium throughout her house, including the highest readings from uneaten food in the refrigerator, Kerr-McGee sent Silkwood for contamination testing at Los Alamos National Laboratories. Following a week of testing, she returned to Oklahoma late on November 12, 1974. On November 13, at 8 p.m., she was scheduled to meet with national OCAW official Steve Wodka and *New York Times* reporter David Burnham. There she would turn over the manila folder containing all her evidence of Kerr-McGee health violations. She went to a union meeting earlier that evening. Fellow employees saw her leave, carrying the manila folder, for her 8 p.m. appointment. On the way to the meeting, however, Silkwood had a mysterious, fatal, one-car accident. With the help of four public-interest lawyers, her four young children sued Kerr-McGee. The court established that another vehicle had forced her car off the road, at high speeds, and into a concrete retaining wall. Courtroom testimony also showed that, immediately after the accident, Kerr-McGee quality-control supervisors and document-control managers came to the remote accident site. Both claimed they were there, together, "by chance." Testifying in court, highway patrolmen at the crash scene said that although a large packet of manila-folder materials, some with Kerr-McGee insignia, were in Silkwood's car immediately after the accident, they were missing the next day. Police records also showed that after a dispatcher told emergency vehicles to hurry to the site of Silkwood's accident, because someone was pinned in the car, other police soon radioed them to turn around, delaying medical help. The trial likewise uncovered FBI and CIA files showing that Silkwood was murdered and that her phone was tapped by Kerr-McGee. According to courtroom testimony, the company knew that she was ready to "blow the whistle" on safety violations of one of the world's largest energy conglomerates. Two weeks before she died, in an October 1974 phone call, Silkwood tearfully told her sister, "Someone is trying to do something to me."[2]

After Silkwood's death, *Paris Match* called her the world's first antinuclear martyr,[3] and the U.S. Nuclear Regulatory Commission verified 20 of her 39 health-and-safety allegations against Kerr-McGee. The court concluded that she and her apartment "had been deliberately contaminated." In May 1979, an Oklahoma jury ordered Kerr-McGee to pay $10.5 million in punitive damages to Silkwood's children. Kerr-McGee appealed, but in 1986 finally paid them a settlement of $1.4 million.[4]

Chapter Overview

Karen Silkwood was an ordinary citizen. Although she was a financially strapped divorcee with four children and no college degree, she tried to protect fellow radiation workers. First she attempted to "go through channels" to correct safety violations, but when her supervisors repeatedly did nothing, she became a whistleblower. Retaliating, Kerr-McGee appears to have deliberately contaminated and harassed her. Yet at her own expense and on her own time, Silkwood worked to collect evidence about Kerr-McGee's health and safety violations. The corporate and government institutions she challenged, however, had both billion-dollar assets and protections against public scrutiny of their unethical behavior.

Why was Kerr-McGee able to avoid public scrutiny for so long? Using lessons from the Silkwood case, this chapter outlines some of the unethical

strategies that polluters sometimes employ to mislead citizens about pollution risks. The chapter helps answer a question raised by chapter 1: If life-
threatening pollutants are so serious, why don't more people know about
them? The short answer is that most citizens do not have Silkwood's firsthand experiences of safety violations and coverups. The long answer is that
citizen ignorance frequently is not an accident. Polluters can orchestrate it.
As a result, public-health risks often are not adequately disclosed, and citizens cannot fulfill their rights to know and to give or withhold consent to
them. Illustrating how orchestrated ignorance can undercut informed consent, this chapter surveys 10 polluter strategies for misleading citizens about
health risks. These include special interests' unduly influencing federal regulators, using advisors with conflicts of interest, committing white-collar
crimes, manipulating the media through PR and advertising, promoting polluter self-policing, and using campaign contributions and lobbying to thwart
regulations. Showing how polluters sometimes cover up their illegal behavior
and thus why citizens are misled about it, the chapter helps explain why many
readers might have been surprised by the pollution-caused health threats surveyed in the previous chapter. Such coverups frequently occur because of regulatory capture.

Karen Silkwood and Nuclear-Regulatory Capture

Regulatory capture is the phenomenon in which regulated industries frequently
control or at least unduly influence government regulators and their watchdog
agencies. It is accomplished by many means described in this and subsequent
chapters, including bribes, retaliation, information suppression, campaign donations, and lobbying. The U.S. nuclear industry, including the case of Silkwood, provide a powerful illustration of regulatory capture that began more
than half a century ago. Since the 1940s and 1950s, the radiation doses of many
of the 600,000 nuclear workers, like Karen Silkwood, have been falsified
or ignored by corporations like Westinghouse and Martin Marietta. Nearly
500,000 U.S. atomic veterans, exposed during more than 100 U.S. nuclear-
weapons tests in the 1950s and 1960s, also were victims of the regulatory
capture. So were thousands of unknowing civilian victims of deliberate U.S.
radiation experiments—including Native Americans, children, and residents of
facilities for the mentally retarded. Until the 1990s, the U.S. government ac-
knowledged neither its harms to all these nuclear-pollution victims, nor the fact
that their radiation exposures often violated international ethical agreements
regarding both disclosure and consent.[5]
    Although the United States has recently offered compensation to many vic-
tims of radioactive pollution and coverup, this chapter suggests that nuclear-
regulatory capture continues. It began about 30 years before the 1974 Karen Silkwood tragedy, when the U.S. Atomic Energy Commission (AEC) was
charged with both promoting and regulating military and commercial uses of
nuclear fission. Trying to convince citizens that atomic energy was safe, the

AEC commissioned the 1956 taxpayer-funded Brookhaven Report. It concluded the opposite and showed that a nuclear accident could cause 150,000 fatalities, catastrophic economic damages, and destruction of an area the size of Pennsylvania. As a result, the AEC suppressed the report. It was not released until 1974, after the Freedom of Information Act was passed. During the 20 years that the report was suppressed, the AEC claimed atomic energy was safe and licensed more than 100 U.S. nuclear plants. The industry, however, knew better. It refused to open the first U.S. reactor in 1955 unless government both assumed responsibility for permanent radioactive-waste storage and provided liability protection against accidents. Government did both. It passed the U.S. Price-Anderson Act, providing industry with liability protection against 98 percent of total possible damage claims from the public. It also agreed to cover the bulk of the costs of permanent radioactive-waste storage.[6]

Critics immediately challenged the Price-Anderson Act as evidence of regulatory capture. They said it violated citizens' due-process rights, prohibited their suing negligent nuclear industries for full damages, and had a liability limit covering less than 2 percent of possible nuclear-accident claims. Noting the $500-billion costs of Russia's 1986 Chernobyl nuclear catastrophe, critics argue that it was not a worst-case accident. They say that because Chernobyl-caused cancer fatalities (estimated to be about 475,000) have not yet peaked, the accident's costs will increase further. Yet because Price-Anderson currently limits U.S. nuclear liability to about $10 billion, the critics say innocent victims could bear 98 percent of nuclear-accident costs, even if a company were negligent. Critics also point to nuclear-exclusion clauses on all homeowners-insurance policies. Likewise, they say that Hurricane Katrina, which hit the Gulf Coast in 2005, involved no radiation hazards yet caused about 1,200 deaths and $200 billion in damages. Why should government admit that a U.S. nuclear accident could kill 150,000 people—100 times more people than Katrina—yet prohibit the public from recovering more than $10 billion total in nuclear damages? If a U.S. nuclear accident caused damages 100 times greater than Katrina, critics say, a negligent utility could bear only one-half of 1 percent of the accident's cost. Innocent citizens, however, could lose everything and bear 99.5 percent of the cost. How did the U.S. Supreme Court respond to Price-Anderson? After a constitutional challenge, the Court responded in part that the law does not violate citizens' due-process rights because a catastrophic nuclear accident is unlikely.[7]

If an accident were truly unlikely, however, industry would neither need nor demand the Price-Anderson Act. Private insurers claim that nuclear risks are far higher than the one-in-five probability of a core melt that the U.S. government claims for the lifetime of all U.S. civilian reactors. Because obtaining private insurance would make commercial nuclear power prohibitively expensive, critics say government has given industry a "free ride" at citizens' expense. They also claim that, for decades, the captured AEC withheld safety data, falsified records, suppressed scientific information, failed to do adequate tests, and violated the civil liberties of nuclear critics. Using federal rights to preempt state vetoes of atomic plants, the AEC dismissed critics' charges by arguing that nuclear plants were essential to commerce. By 1974, however, the AEC was so embroiled in health and safety lawsuits that government abolished it and created a new agency, the Department of Energy (DOE).[8]

The 30-year-old DOE, however, has many of the same problems as the AEC. The U.S. National Academy of Sciences (NAS), the inspector general, the Office of Technology Assessment (OTA), and the U.S.-government oversight agency, the Government Accountability Office (GAO), all criticize DOE for lax safety, regulatory capture, and information suppression. Despite more than $100 billion in continuing U.S. taxpayer subsidies, no new commercial reactors have been ordered since 1974. Industry contractors like Martin Marietta and Westinghouse run DOE's 3,500 nuclear facilities. All use a system of "self-regulation" that government oversight agencies have criticized repeatedly. Congress, the NAS, the GAO, and the OTA have condemned these DOE-controlled facilities for repeated contamination, fires, explosions involving radioactive materials, and "significant and potentially widespread problems with... not adhering to nuclear-safety procedures."[9] Congressional investigators have said worker dose-monitoring programs are "inaccurate, and in many cases nonexistent."[10] In 1986, the GAO discovered that 90 percent of DOE nuclear facilities had contaminated groundwater that exceeded regulatory standards by a factor of up to 1,000. In response, virtually nothing was done. Again, in 1998, the GAO said: "We have long criticized DOE for weaknesses in its self-regulation of the environmental safety, and health at its own facilities.... Widespread environmental conmental contamination at DOE facilities... provides clear evidence that [DOE] self-regulation has failed."[11] Yet today these facilities remain totally self-regulated. GAO Officials say "DOE's credibility... [is] almost zero."[12]

Criticism of DOE's regulatory capture has been especially harsh in the last 15 years. Congress, the GAO, the OTA, and the NAS point to nuclear-industry falsification of worker-exposure records and coverup of contamination and safety problems. They claim DOE facilities even illegally exposed the public—including 13,000 children—to high doses of radiation. Congress says DOE has neither credible radiation-exposure records for 600,000 U.S. nuclear workers, nor adequate medical monitoring in 26 of its 33 types of facilities.[13] The result? Because of flawed record-keeping and safety violations, in 2000 U.S. president Clinton was forced to provide taxpayer-financed health care for all DOE nuclear workers, despite their employment as industry contractors.[14] Yet as early as 1991, the OTA had condemned DOE's regulatory capture and called for the abolition of DOE or its external regulation. Neither recommendation has been followed.[15]

Instead, despite 6 decades of repeated violations and criticism by government oversight agencies, nuclear-regulatory capture continues. Nuclear power continues to receive the vast majority (more than 60 percent cumulative) of U.S. government energy subsidies, but it supplies only about 19 percent of U.S. electricity. It provides a much smaller percentage in the rest of the world. Even if one excludes taxpayer subsidies, like those for permanent radioactive-waste storage and the Price-Anderson Act, nuclear energy is costly. After solar photovoltaic, DOE data show it remains the second-most expensive electricity source. That is why, except for countries seeking nuclear-weapons capability, the only nations with substantial atomic-energy programs are centrally planned and must subsidize them—as France does. Although nuclear power has not been able to survive in a free market, regulatory capture protects it, when economics cannot. Does this explain the summer-2005, billion-dollar handout from U.S. taxpayers to the U.S. nuclear industry? Consider a July 2005 analysis, in the business publication *The Economist*. It warned that nuclear costs, safety, and permanent waste storage make atomic energy "extremely risky." It noted that for decades bankers in London and New York have refused loans to nuclear industries. *The Economist* blames nuclear lobbyists and campaign contributors for the economically indefensible, billion-dollar, 2005 U.S. nuclear subsidies. A more economically efficient U.S. choice would have been squeezing "polluting activities" and "taxing the use of carbon . . . to encourage energy consumers to switch to other sources." Similar conclusions recently came from Massachusetts Institute of Technology (MIT) and European Union scientists who say problems with cost, safety, proliferation, terrorism, security, and permanent waste storage are major obstacles to using atomic power.[16]

Nuclear proponents, however, deny that regulatory capture has occurred. They defend massive U.S. nuclear subsidies by saying atomic energy will help reduce greenhouse gases. European Union and other scientists agree that atomic plants produce less global warming than do coal facilities. Yet they say the seven-stage nuclear fuel cycle (including mining, milling, enriching, and transporting uranium) emits three to four times more greenhouse gases than many other less expensive electricity sources—such as natural-gas-fired cogeneration, wind, and hydro. They also say that even a doubling of global nuclear plants—unlikely because of concerns about accidents, waste, proliferation, terrorism, and costs—would reduce greenhouse emissions by only 5 percent. Why? The largest chunk of global warming is caused by transportation (40 percent).[17]

Given the straight talk of *The Economist* and European Union scientists; nuclear bans by Sweden, Italy, Belgium, and Germany; and no approved U.S. facility for permanent nuclear-waste storage, the 2005 billion-dollar U.S. nuclear subsidies suggest regulatory capture. So does the 2005 revelation of falsified safety data at DOE's proposed waste-storage site, at Yucca Mountain, Nevada. Knowing DOE's problematic and "captured" history, cities and states are challenging proposals for hundreds of thousands of unguarded nuclear-waste shipments across U.S. interstates to the proposed Nevada dump. They call the transport "Mobile Chernobyl." Since the core melts at Three Mile Island, Pennsylvania, and at Chernobyl, critics also say that citizens will not accept atomic energy.[18]

Whether or not global warming argues for increased atomic energy, and whether or not increased nuclear subsidies are defensible, the main point here is ethical and democratic. Just as Congress, the GAO, and the OTA criticized U.S. nuclear-regulatory secrecy and deception, a NAS committee likewise concluded that "lack of trust in the DOE and its [nuclear-industry] site operators is a major impediment to radiation protection."[19] They all suggest that nuclear interests appear to have partially captured both DOE and even nuclear-related studies done by health-related agencies like the National Cancer Institute (NCI). In 1982, Congress told the NCI to assess fallout-related health effects from the 200-plus above-ground, U.S. nuclear-weapons tests that were conducted during the 1950s and 1960s. The NCI did one part of the study but buried the results for more than a decade. After repeated pressure from Congress and the Department of Health and Human Services, NCI finally released part of the report in 1997.[20] It said bomb-related iodine-131 fallout would cause up to 214,000 premature U.S. thyroid cancers—apart from additional cancers caused by other fallout radionu-clides.[21] Although the U.S. NAS and independent scientific associations criticized NCI estimates as possibly too low,[22] again the crucial question was ethical. Why did government delay releasing the report? Because of the NCI delay, the statute of limitations has kept thousands of fallout victims from claiming government-guaranteed compensation for 13 different types of radiation-related cancers, especially leukemias. Although Congress called for fallout-dose assessment in 1982, and the full report on effects of all radionu-clides was due in 2000, government still has not released it. One hypothesis for this delay is that the results could damage commercial and government nuclear interests.[23] Providing further evidence of nuclear regulatory capture and resulting threats to life and to human rights, a presidential commission warned that additional radiation experimentation and civilian harm from ra-dioactive pollution was possible. Why? The commission cited "serious defi-ciencies" in government radiation protection and oversight.[24]

Other Health-Related Regulatory Capture

If the nuclear case is typical, capture of U.S. federal-regulatory agencies may be one reason citizens have been misled about pollution hazards, like those surveyed in the previous chapter. How might citizens discover other possible cases of regulatory capture? One way is to "follow the money."

What industries receive massive government handouts, even when econo-mists and health experts cry foul, as with nuclear power? Some of the largest taxpayer subsidies have gone to the pharmaceutical industry. As analyses by former *New England Journal of Medicine* editors show, many of the top-selling drugs, like Taxol, Epogen, Procrit, and Neuprogen, were developed largely with taxpayer funding from the National Institutes of Health (NIH). NIH funds tens of thousands of studies at about 4,000 institutions, and it spends more than $20 billion annually on medical research, much of which is drug related. Yet the medical editors say that, since 1995, NIH has not ensured that the health needs of the public are served by public investments in pharmaceutical research. Instead public investments frequently contribute to private profits. Since 1995, NIH has not required reasonable pricing for drugs developed largely with government funds. As a consequence, the medical editors say the public has massively subsidized the pharmaceutical industry, giving it tax breaks, freedom from price regulation, and long periods of exclusive marketing rights.[25]

If a 2005 study by the former editor of the *New England Journal of Medicine* is correct, three facts suggest these handouts are undeserved—perhaps evidence of regulatory capture. (1) The pharmaceutical industry is not as innovative as it claims to be. During 1998–2004, the Food and Drug Administration (FDA) says only 22 percent of new drugs offered improvements over those already on the market to treat the same condition. Most were not made by major U.S. drug companies; 78 percent were merely higher priced (but no better) versions of old drugs, often those on which industry patents had run out. To obtain new patents and profits, the editor charges that industry mainly reinvents old drugs, misleadingly advertises them, but ignores their unimproved quality. (2) Drug companies make massively higher profits than other Fortune-500 companies. 2004 median drug-industry profits were 16 percent of sales; median profits for nondrug, Fortune-500 companies were 5 percent. (3) Despite claims to the contrary, most drug-company monies are spent on advertising and marketing, not research. The largest U.S. drug company, Pfizer, is typical. In 2004, Pfizer's profit margin was 22 percent of sales ($53 billion). It spent 32 percent of sales on marketing/administration but 15 percent on research and development (R & D). Typical U.S.-drug-industry expenditures on advertising and marketing are more than double expenditures on R & D. Yet, despite little innovation, disproportionate profits, and little research, federal regulators allow the United States to remain the only developed nation that does not regulate drug prices. Partly as a result, U.S. citizens pay higher prices than those in other nations who buy the same drugs. Consider 2004 prices for the name-brand drugs that are most prescribed for senior citizens: they rose twice as fast as inflation. Or consider the U.S. president's 2003 Medicare drug-coverage plan. He claimed in 2002 that it would cost $400 billion over 10 years. By 2005, the White House admitted the cost was $1.2 trillion. The reason for the increase? Medical-journal editors say federal regulators were captured by drug-industry lobbyists—the largest Washington lobby group. As a result, the 2003 bill prohibited taxpayer-funded Medicare from using its large purchasing power to negotiate drug prices.[26]

Regulatory capture does not merely raise consumer prices, encourage health-information suppression, and condone conflicts of interest. It also can lead to lax regulations that allow people to die. Consider 17-year-old Jesse Gelsinger. He died during University of Pennsylvania experiments. With a rare genetic disorder, Gelsinger was stable and able to lead a normal life, thanks to medication and a low-protein diet. He volunteered for experimental drug "treatment" only because Penn physicians told him it might help him and others. They did not tell him there was no evidence whatsoever, from earlier animal and human experiments, that the "treatment" helped. Scientists told him neither that the "treatment" had caused primates to die from organ failure, nor that they and the university owned stocks in the company hoping to market the "treatment." Gelsinger died of massive lung, liver, and kidney failures, 4 days after the first "treatment." Distinguished scientists (like former editor of the *New England Journal of Medicine*, Jerome Kassirer, MD) say Gelsinger died partly because, at industry behest, the Office for Human Research Protection (OHRP) and other regulators have been massively underfunded and understaffed. "Opposition from the pharmaceutical industry," says Kassirer, has kept OHRP from being effective. Even in 2002, 3 years after Gelsinger's death, OHRP had only $7 million to oversee tens of thousands of studies at more than 4,000 federally funded institutions. Not counting monies needed for regulators' office space, travel, and supplies, this prorated $7 million allowed oversight worth only several hundred dollars for any single project. This is not enough even for one scientist to review the documents and protocols in cases like Gelsinger's. On the one hand, scientists in the Gelsinger case deny that conflicts of interest caused their omissions. On the other hand, OHRP admits that it bows to drug-industry pressure; OHRP says it does not enforce its conflict-of-interest guidelines, violated in Gelsinger's case, because this would be "hindering academic innovation."[27]

Other evidence of how U.S. health-regulatory agencies may be captured arises from examining membership on 900 topic-specific federal science-advisory committees. Government recruits more than 41,000 nongovernmental expert-advisors to help draft regulations. Yet the Ethics in Government Act requires agencies to disclose publicly neither the principal employment, nor paid consulting, nor financial investments of these 41,000 committee members. As a result, often they work for the same industries they help regulate, as is illustrated by the recent Vioxx case. Because patients took the pain medication Vioxx, a FDA-led study showed that between 88,000 and 141,000 of them had heart attacks, of whom about 61,000 died. However, FDA officials suppressed this study, and its FDA-scientist-author (David Graham, MD, MPH) charged that FDA retaliated against him for trying to publish it. Under pressure, in 2004 FDA finally made a damning admission. No clinical trials had ever shown that Vioxx (made by Merck) and Bextra (made by Pfizer) were better painkillers than a dozen older, cheaper, and safer pain remedies like ibuprofen. Whistleblowers showed that Merck knew for years about the dangers of Vioxx. They also showed that Merck used research grants as bribes to pressure physicians, universities, and top medical schools like Stanford to withhold damaging Vioxx information from patients.[28] As a result, the FDA was finally forced to investigate. Yet in 2005, the FDA voted not to take Bextra and Vioxx off the market. Puzzled, *New York Times* investigative reporters discovered conflicts of interest. At least one-third of the FDA committee members, who voted on the drugs, had obvious financial ties to the affected drug companies. Yet because of the secrecy allowed by the Ethics in Government Act, reporters said those with financial ties probably were more than one-third of the committee. Of the one-third of the committee with obvious financial ties to the affected companies, 90 percent voted to continue marketing Bextra and Vioxx. Of the two-thirds of the committee whose ties were unknown, only 33 percent voted to continue marketing both drugs.

Known industry scientists were thus three times more likely to vote for keeping the drugs than those with no (or unknown) ties. If only those scientists without obvious conflicts of interest had voted, both drugs would have been pulled from the market.[29]

How widespread is such regulatory capture? Consider all 18 FDA expert-advisory committees that evaluate new drugs. A 2000 investigative report found that 92 percent of federal committees had members with financial stakes in the topics being assessed. In addition, since at least 2000, the U.S. president has made scientific-advisory-committee appointments without seeking recommendations from the NAS. Instead, often those named have been industry lobbyists and lawyers. In 2001, for example, the U.S. president dismissed most members of the committee assessing health effects of low-dose toxic chemicals. It included mainly scientists from leading medical schools, like Johns Hopkins and Harvard. In their places, he appointed people like Denis Paustenbach, the chemical-industry attorney who represented Pacific Gas and Electric, the California polluter in the Erin Brokovitch case.[30]

The puzzling thing is that industry capture of drug regulators often succeeds, despite citizen desires for strong regulation. In 1937, the first U.S. FDA poll showed that 88 percent of Americans wanted government food-and-drug regulation. Since then, public support for FDA's strict standards has never fallen below 75 percent. One reason is that, for decades, the FDA worked more effectively than comparable regulatory agencies in other nations. Analyzing all drugs marketed in Britain, France, Germany, and the United States between 1970 and 1992, physicians showed that the U.S. agency was most protective of public health. Because of serious injury or death to patients, France, Germany, and Britain, respectively, were forced to withdraw 31, 30, and 23 approved drugs, while the United States had to withdraw only 9. According to *New York Times* health journalist Philip Hilts, however, this has all changed in the last 15 years. The U.S. pharmaceutical industry has used its multimillion-dollar advertising programs and campaign donations to claim that FDA "red tape" is keeping Americans from getting the drugs they need. In 1996, he says the drug industry almost succeeded in dismantling and privatizing the FDA. The attack failed, but Hilts says much of the agency has been captured.[31]

Regulatory capture has become so extreme in the administration of U.S. president George W. Bush that, beginning in 2004, many NAS members and more than 7,000 eminent scientists (including 48 Nobel laureates and scores of U.S. Medal of Science winners) signed a statement criticizing the administration for "misrepresenting and suppressing scientific knowledge" so as to serve its special-interest donors. Claiming the administration loads federal science-advisory panels with political supporters, not experts, the scientists claimed that "the pervasive, systematic nature of these practices is unprecedented" in history. Prominent professional journals like *Science*, *Nature*, and *Lancet* said the same. *Nature* claimed, for instance, that President Bush violated global scientific consensus in denying climate change, in implementing a costly and unworkable missile-defense system, in setting flawed rules for stem-cell research, in weakening mercury-pollution rules, and in suppressing EPA evidence that 8 percent of U.S. women have blood-mercury levels able to cause harm to unborn children. In response, the Bush administration ignored scientists' charges of regulatory capture but hired a PR firm—Wexler & Walker—to "handle" the problem.[32]

Regulatory capture continues partly because some of the behaviors that produce it are not illegal. For instance, as later sections will show, the sheer economic power of special interests frequently enables them to use advertising and PR to control what people know about polluting activities. This economic power also enables them simply to out-spend regulators. Consider what happened when overworked, modestly paid government employees tried to counter the $5,000-per-hour, utility-industry attorneys who were hired to weaken the Clean Air Act. The act was weakened.[33]

Revolving Doors and Conflicts of Interest

Even when underpaid federal regulators do their best, politically appointed agency officials sometimes can undercut both regulation and citizens' health information because of "revolving doors" between government and industry. "Revolving doors" refers to the phenomenon of industry executives' often being appointed as federal regulators for the very industries from which they come, and federal regulators' often leaving government service to work for the industries they used to regulate. While in itself there is nothing wrong with revolving doors, since industry experts obviously may have significant expertise, later paragraphs show how revolving doors often create ethically questionable conflicts of interest. Tracking government officials who left public service in a single year, one citizens' group said that over half moved to Washington, D.C., lobbying and PR firms. The two major PR firms—Hill and Knowlton, and Burson-Marsteller—are full of former U.S. government officials and regulators. The head of Hill and Knowlton's Washington office was appointed to government office by U.S. president Bill Clinton. The person who took his place at Hill and Knowlton was a former aide to Clinton.[34]

More than any other U.S. president, George W. Bush has been criticized for using revolving doors to staff regulatory agencies with those from the regulated industries. In 1999, he chose Dick Cheney, former head of Halliburton oil-services company, as vice-president. As vice-president, Cheney continues to receive $300,000 annually in deferred compensation from Halliburton, to whom the government gave billions of dollars in U.S. contracts for post-invasion oil-related work in Iraq—without even asking for any open, competitive bids from any companies other than Halliburton. President Bush also appointed Gale Norton, cofounder of an antiregulatory chemical-and-mining-industry lobby group, as secretary of the interior. James Connaughton, a lobbyist for mining and chemicals industries, was appointed chair of the White House Council on Environmental Quality. Don Evans, CEO of an oil and gas company, was appointed secretary of commerce. Automobile-industry lobbyist Andrew Card was appointed White House chief of staff. Calgene biotech company official Ann Veneman was appointed secretary of agriculture. Former coal-, gas-, and oil-industry lobbyist Steve Griles was appointed deputy secretary of the interior. Griles continues to be paid $300,000 annually by his former lobbying firm; he wrote the proposal allowing coal companies to dump mining waste in streams instead of cleaning it up. Former Monsanto lobbyist Linda Fisher was appointed deputy director of the EPA. Former timber-industry lobbyist Mark Rey was made undersecretary of agriculture. Former coal-industry lobbyist Tom Sansonetti was appointed assistant attorney general for environment and resources. Former timber-industry and mining-industry lawyer Rebecca Watson was made assistant secretary of the interior. Former auto-industry lobbyist Camden Toohey was appointed special assistant for Alaska, Department of the Interior. Former General Electric vice-president Francis Blake was appointed deputy secretary of energy. Former energy-industry lobbyist Deborah Daniels was appointed assistant attorney general. Former chemical-industry lawyer Jeffrey Holmstead was appointed EPA assistant administrator—to name only a few. The problem with such revolving doors is not that industry employees cannot be trusted. Often they are decent, ethical people. Rather, "revolving doors" often create conflicts of interest that ought to be avoided. As defined by *New England Journal of Medicine* authors and editors, a conflict of interest occurs when an individual's or group's "professional judgment concerning a primary interest tends to be unduly influenced by a secondary interest, such as financial gain." Conflicts of interest thus signal no overt corruption, fraud, or kickbacks. Instead they are like "institutional weeds" that take root below the surface of an organization and can compromise its integrity and objectivity. Such conflicts are subtle, outside, or personal interests that can wrongly influence duty. Sometimes these conflicts are financial, as when federal-advisory-committee members also are paid consultants to the industries they help to regulate. As a consequence of these conflicts, special interests often capture regulators, induce public servants to follow special-interest ethics, or give government officials financial incentives to behave so that they receive future jobs with the companies they regulate. The alternative is to reveal, in public, all such conflicts of interest and to avoid them. Instead, however, many federal regulatory agencies allow the conflicts, claiming they need the expertise of the experts with ties to special interests. Revolving doors and conflicts of interest also can enable political appointees to punish honest public servants who try to follow the law. Since 2000, hundreds of federal scientists have filed lawsuits claiming they were penalized merely for doing their jobs, releasing information, or enforcing the law. When EPA ombudsman Robert Martin tried to enforce the Superfund Law, he was reassigned and then demoted. When atmospheric scientist Robert Watson chaired a prestigious international climate-change panel that proposed limiting greenhouse emissions, contrary to the administration position, the White House replaced him with an economist. When Martha Hahn, director of the Bureau of Land Management, Montana, reduced cattle grazing on some ecologically fragile federal land, and when Tim Salt, bureau desert director, protected endangered species on bureau desert lands in California, they were reassigned and demoted. When Brad Powell, regional head of the U.S. Forest Service, tried to limit logging, grazing, and off-road vehicles in national forests, he was demoted and reassigned—and so on. Chapter 4 tells of Adam Finkel, an Occupational Safety and Health Administration (OSHA) regional director, who was demoted and reassigned when he tried to protect people from workplace beryllium exposures. The result of these silencings? Citizens have less health information and less environmental-health protection and thus are less able to fulfill their rights to know and to consent to risks.[35]

White-Collar Health Crime and Information Suppression

Regulatory capture, conflicts of interest, and revolving doors also can encourage white-collar environmental crimes such as fraud or suppression of pollution data. Just as great profits and regulatory weaknesses encouraged fraud in the U.S. accounting, banking, energy, and telecommunications industries, early in this century, they also can encourage fraud among polluters. In 2003, the bankruptcy of WorldCom exposed the fact that its founder and chair, Bernard Ebbers, perpetrated an $11-billion fraud that destroyed his telecommunications company and caused millions of people to lose money. Kenneth Lay, the largest campaign donor to the incoming 2000 U.S. president, did something similar at the energy giant Enron. His fraud caused the largest bankruptcy in U.S. history. Millions of investors lost billions of dollars, and Enron's 21,000 employees lost their pensions. Are U.S. crimes like those of Ebbers and Lay typical? Ranking 145 nations, in 2004 *The Economist* evaluated countries in terms of their being plagued by corruption. Not surprisingly, nations like Bangladesh, Nigeria, Indonesia, and Argentina were among the lowest ranked and apparently the most corrupt. The United States, however, was ranked seventeenth from the top. Democracies like Finland (alleged to be the least corrupt), New Zealand, Britain, and Germany were far ahead of the United States. Yet they subscribe to roughly the same capitalist, market-based economic theories as the United States.[36]

The Economist suggests that poor regulation, not the market, may encourage U.S. corruption, and the encouragement may extend into pollution- and health-related areas. Special-interest capture of federal agencies like the DOE and NCI is one indicator. Other indicators are government-industry suppression of information about pollution. Consider the case of dioxin. Created when chlorine is brought together with organic matter at high temperatures, dioxins are a family of about 75 different chemicals. Processes like chemical manufacturing, waste incineration, and pulp and paper bleaching all create dioxins as an unintended byproduct. Chemical companies like Dow and Monsanto produce tens of millions of tons of chlorine annually, in addition to tons of dioxin-containing compounds like the herbicide Agent Orange. To see how dioxin information has been suppressed, recall what happened when Agent Orange was used in Vietnam. It caused cancer, birth

defects, infertility, hormone disruption, immune suppression, and other problems in more than 200,000 Vietnam veterans. As a result, veterans or their
survivors filed lawsuits and received hundreds of millions of dollars from Dow
and other chemical producers. Both a U.S. congressional inquiry and a NAS
report, however, established that federal agencies did not help protect victims.
Instead congressional hearings revealed that the CDC had suppressed dioxin
data—to protect Dow and other chemical companies from lawsuits. Again to
protect the industry, Congress said the CDC ignored or misused abundant
data and did dioxin assessments that were "flawed and perhaps designed to
fail." Similar problems occurred with U.S. EPA dioxin studies. The EPA's own
records, obtained through lawsuits and Freedom of Information Act requests,
implicated EPA in helping the chlorine industry minimize dioxin hazards and
delay regulation. EPA chief Anne Burford and her assistant, Rita Lavelle, were
fired because of their roles in the dioxin coverup, and Burford's successor,
John Hernandez, resigned in disgrace after Congress investigated his altering
an EPA report on dioxin. Contrary to the CDC and EPA coverup, repeated
1991 *New England Journal of Medicine* studies showed that dioxins are
"extremely potent" carcinogens, "perhaps the most potent ever tested."
Refereed scientific journals showed that only a billionth of an ounce of dioxin
is sufficient to cause serious human-health problems, that dioxin is easily
taken up by the body, and that it persists essentially forever. In 1993 the
10,000-member American Public Health Association reinforced these medical
findings. It called for phasing out virtually all U.S. use of chlorine, except for
water treatment and pharmaceuticals. The International Joint Commission,
the California Medical Association, and other health groups did the same.
Years later in 1995, however, the U.S. House of Representatives Committee
on Commerce continued the questionable behavior of the CDC and EPA when
it allowed a Dow-funded lobbyist to plan House opposition to EPA chlorine
and dioxin regulations.[37]

How was this dioxin coverup possible? Why can polluters get away with
suppressing information and blocking regulation? One reason is that polluters make their victims agree to gag orders, in exchange for lawsuit-ordered
financial awards. The Dow case is typical. Although it has paid millions of
dollars in dioxin–lawsuit damages, Dow denies that dioxin causes any health
problems except severe acne. If victims contradict this denial, the polluters can
sue to recover their damage awards. This has happened repeatedly, as in the
famous Ford Pinto case. As a condition of financial settlements in wrongful-
death lawsuits filed by families of Pinto owners, Ford used gag orders. This
allowed "business as usual," future deaths, and even crime to continue. Despite repeated lawsuits, Ford continued making defective Pintos until the
government stopped it. The reason? Ford had carefully calculated two things.
Gag orders would protect it, and Pinto profits would outstrip the costs of its
court settlements to victims.[38]

As the next chapter will discuss in more detail, polluter suppression of
information also takes the form of scientific fraud. In the dioxin case, three
Monsanto studies, exonerating dioxin, appeared or were reported in *Science,*

the *Journal of the American Medical Association,* and *Scientific American.* Yet later in lawsuit hearings, the Monsanto medical director was forced to admit, under oath, that these studies were fraudulent. He said Monsanto "had knowingly omitted" many dioxin deaths of its workers and had "re-classified four exposed workers as unexposed." The director also admitted that the number of dioxin-related deaths among Monsanto workers had actually been double what Monsanto had reported in the scientific journals. As a result of Monsanto's fraud, the *Journal of the American Medical Association* and other scientific reviewers had been unable to detect flaws in the published studies.[39]

Environmental-health crimes and information suppression, like Monsanto's, may be more common than people realize. A number of scientists, physicians, and attorneys have made, for instance, the following claims.

- The American Chemistry Council and the vinyl-chloride industry, including Dow and others, knowingly suppressed data on the toxicity and carcinogenicity of vinyl chloride.

- Dow suppressed risk data on its genetically engineered milk hormone as well as its own occupational-risk data on carcinogens such as benzene.

- Rohm and Haas suppressed carcinogenicity data on its chlorine compound bischloromethylether.

- Allied Chemical suppressed carcinogenicity data on its pesticide Kepone.

- Velsicol Chemical suppressed data on toxic effects of its pesticides chlordane and heptachlor.

- Eli Lilly suppressed evidence of ovarian cancer caused by its drug Evista.

- Despite controversy over the health effects of breast implants, Dow-Corning, Bristol-Myers-Squibb, and other manufacturers suppressed evidence of cancer risks from some types of silicone breast implants.

- Monsanto marketed acrylonitrile plastic Coca-Cola bottles prior to any carcinogenicity testing.

- Dupont deliberately destroyed its own epidemiological data on its occupational carcinogens.

- Hazleton Labs, under contract to Searle, falsified test data on the drugs aldactone and the artificial sweetener aspartame.[40]

In more recent times, tens of thousands of Americans have died because pharmaceutical companies suppressed information on drugs like Vioxx. Merck claimed Vioxx caused heart problems in only 0.5 percent of patients in its clinical trials. Yet Merck's own records showed 14.3 percent—30 times more patients—experienced problems.[41] And Guidant Corporation admitted it did not tell doctors for at least 3 years about the electrical flaws in one of its heart-defibrillator models. For years it kept selling older versions of the defibrillator and covering up its flaws, even after developing a version not subject to short-circuiting...and so on. Although such information-suppression in the drug industry may be better known, later paragraphs suggest that coverup of pollution information may affect more people. Obviously, most companies do not suppress information, but enough do so that citizens must be watchful.[42]

Even outside their own companies, polluters and manufacturers sometimes try to suppress information. Chemical manufacturer W. R. Grace tried to stop Tufts University research on its local toxic-waste pollution. Similarly, when Microfibres paid Brown University physician David Kern to study its employees' ailments, he discovered that company workplaces caused "flock workers' lung." Microfibres refused to allow Kern to publish the results, even after Kern said he would reveal neither the company's name nor its locations. One week after Kern presented his results at 1997 American Thoracic Society meetings, Brown University said his employment contract would not be renewed. And after scientist David Healy established that the drug Prozac was linked to higher teen-suicide rates, the University of Toronto withdrew his job offer, perhaps because Prozac's manufacturer, Eli Lilly, is a major donor to the university's medical school.[43]

Another well-known information-suppression case is that of physician-hematologist Nancy Olivieri at the University of Toronto. Working with the Canadian pharmaceutical company Apotex, Olivieri was investigating its drug deferiprone, used for blood-transfused children with hereditary blood diseases. After she discovered that the drug both lost its effectiveness and posed a risk to patients, she warned the company. Although she had no confidentiality agreement with Apotex, it said it would sue if she communicated any risks about its drug to anyone, including patients. When Olivieri presented her results at a scientific conference in 1997, she was fired. When Apotex sued her, and the university agreed in 1999 to pay her legal fees, Apotex withdrew a $13 million research donation to the university. Only in 2001 were faculty able to force Olivieri's reappointment.[44]

Olivieri's case, however, may not be typical of information-suppression problems. Often, special interests actually sometimes succeed in suppressing whatever results they wish. The reason? Tufts University researcher Sheldon Krimsky showed that more than a third of authors of medical-science publications have significant financial interests in their conclusions. The ethical situation worsens when major industries actually sponsor the research. Published in the Annals of Internal Medicine, a 1996 study showed that 98 percent of papers based on industry-sponsored research reflected favorably on the industry's products. It showed that half of industry-funded studies have missing or inconclusive statistics, yet peer-reviewed journals publish them anyway.[45] A Journal of the American Medical Association article concluded that industry-funded drug studies were eight times less likely to reach conclusions unfavorable to the drug than were nonprofit-funded studies. Polluter-funded studies of pollution are likely to reach similar conclusions.[46]

Several reasons suggest that information-suppression and white-collar crime may be more pervasive among polluters than within the drug industry. One reason is that polluter misbehavior often is easier to cover up. Pollution victims frequently are hard to identify, unlike those who take particular drugs in clinical trials. Another reason is that, to establish harm, pollution victims must be able to establish their pollutant exposure. This often is difficult, as the chapter-1 case of Emily Pearson showed. Yet drug exposure is rarely an issue, because researchers know who is in their pharmaceutical trials, and patients know what drugs they have taken. Still another contributor to pollution coverup is that although polluters must report some of their emissions to the government, government rarely checks their reports. And as the earlier Monsanto case showed, even when polluters lose lawsuits, they can use gag orders to suppress information, while drug companies often cannot. As a result, polluters frequently make production decisions based solely on market costs and benefits. They know that most ordinary people cannot afford to initiate a wrongful-death lawsuit against well funded corporations. They also know that top lawyers rarely take cases on contingency. In addition, polluters can promote information-suppression by suing thousands of legitimate critics, hammering them with multimillion-dollar SLAPPs, strategic lawsuits against public participation. Plaintiffs virtually never win such cases. Yet, as the Supreme Court noted, SLAPPs are powerful instruments of deterrence, harassment, intimidation, distraction, coercion, and retaliation. Forcing public-health whistleblowers to defend themselves in court, SLAPPs can drive honest citizens into bankruptcy. In the 1980s, the lead industry SLAPPed Dr. Herbert Needleman. It orchestrated false charges of scientific misconduct against him after he proved lead pollution harmed children. In the 1940s, when Harvard physician Randolph Byers showed lead paint was harming children, the lead industry SLAPPed him. When journal editors reported on Monsanto's falsification of its dioxin data, Monsanto SLAPPed them. Yet Monsanto scientists had already admitted the falsification in court, under oath. The editors merely reported it. When high-school science teachers urged rejection of mercury-spewing local waste incinerators, the polluters SLAPPed them. When ordinary citizens publicized the fact that its hamburgers are unhealthy, McDonald's SLAPPed them. In 1996, when a guest of TV host Oprah Winfrey warned about mad-cow disease, the beef industry SLAPPed her. By 2000, Winfrey had two beef-industry lawsuits dismissed, but only after she had paid millions of dollars in attorneys' fees.[47]

Even without SLAPPs, polluters often intimidate scientists whose results jeopardize their profits. Harvard-trained scientist Mary Amdur was repeatedly threatened not to reveal the hazards of acid aerosols. Polluters tried to destroy the career of Mario Molina after he revealed Mexico City air pollution and chlorofluorocarbon hazards. Molina was saved when he later won the Nobel Prize. When epidemiologist-physiologist Devra Lee Davis showed how chlorine compounds cause breast cancers, the Chlorine Chemistry Council called her a "junk scientist" and tried to destroy her career. When Arpad Pusztai did experiments showing that animals who ate genetically engineered potatoes exhibited heart, liver, brain, spleen, and thymus problems, biotech and chemical companies smeared him and claimed he was senile. After Ralph Nader reported on how unsafe automobiles annually killed thousands of Americans, General Motors hired teams of investigators to follow him and spy on him. Nader began his public-interest work with the court settlement he received when courts forced General Motors to admit its repeated violations of Nader's civil liberties. Spy cases like Nader's, however, are not the exception. Entire public-relations firms, like Mongoven, Biscoe, and Duchin, provide "corporate spy information." They claim to maintain "extensive files" on "public-interest groups, churches, unions, and/or academia." To obtain information, they also sometimes misrepresent themselves as journalists or interested citizens. Although Mongoven, Biscoe, and Duchin will not reveal its ongoing spy cases, its known clients are Monsanto, Dupont, Philip Morris, Shell Oil, the Chlorine Chemistry Council, and companies producing genetically engineered food. Companies typically pay Mongoven, Biscoe, and Duchin a retainer of $3,500 to $9,000 per month. In return, it infiltrates various public-health and consumer groups. Charging its corporate clients thousands of dollars for "reports" on these groups, it admits to monitoring groups working on clean air, clean water, Superfund, toxic waste, environmental justice, drinking water, risk assessment, children's health, incineration, dioxin, chlorine, pesticides, multiple chemical sensitivities, endocrine system disruption, biotechnology, and many other issues. The Mongove, Biscoe, and Duchin PR firm got its start in 1981 by defending Nestlé Corporation against those who criticized its Third-World marketing strategies. In developing nations, Nestlé gave away free infant formula, so that women's breast milk would dry up, and families would be forced to buy the formula. Nestlé also lied in poor nations, claiming that its infant formula was healthier for babies than breast-feeding. The company likewise withheld information. It never mentioned that its powdered formula could be fatal in countries without clean drinking water and sterilization facilities. As a result of Nestle's fraudulent infant-formula-marketing practices, the World Health Organization (WHO), UNICEF, and the APHA all charged Nestle with these deaths and called for a boycott of all Nestlé products. African pediatricians accused Nestlé of the "massacre of . . . infants by unsuitable feeding." They said Nestlé deserved "criminal" punishment for its infant-formula "propaganda"—which "should be regarded as murder." Defending Nestlé against the WHO, UNICEF, and the APHA, Mongoven, Biscoe, and Duchin responded by collecting dossiers on the church and citizen groups that protested Nestlé's Third-World marketing practices. It then supplied Nestlé with this information and mounted a campaign against the groups. It painted them as irrational radicals, guilty of an "attack on the free world's economic system." In the last 25 years, Mongoven, Biscoe, and Duchin has continued this "spy and smear" campaign, compiling dossiers on hundreds of public-health groups.[48]

Besides paying private PR firms like Mongoven, Biscoe, and Duchin to gather information on public-health groups, polluters also sometimes involve government in their information collection and suppression. Recall that in the Karen Silkwood case, Kerr-McGee worked with local police, the FBI, and the CIA to gather information against her, some from wiretapping. Yet when government gathers health or pollution information, it may be suppressed. In 2004 the National Highway Traffic and Safety Administration prohibited public release of taxpayer-funded data on unsafe motor vehicles. Directed by the Bush administration, the agency said that "publicizing the information would cause 'substantial competitive harm' to [auto] manufacturers." In August 2003, the administration also dropped a labeling requirement that food containing olestra, a fat substitute, warn of health risks. In June 2002, it likewise chose the weaker of two standards to warn drivers about underinflated tires. In August 2002, it said health-care providers need not obtain patients' informed consent before sharing their medical records with others . . . and so on. Often such cases of information-suppression extend to covering up the way captured regulators weaken public-health protections. For instance, in March 2003, federal regulatory agencies increased allowable levels of coal-mine dust. In April 2003, they increased the number of hours that truckers can drive in on-duty shifts. In September 2003, they reduced training requirements for workers who feed nursing-home patients, and so on. In each of these and other cases, the agencies retained federal *health laws* but covertly weakened the *compliance or enforcement rules* governing these laws. The changes are covert because government typically never widely publicizes weakened compliance rules. Instead it publishes them in the fine print of *The Federal Register*. Consider what happened in 2005, for instance, when U.S. president Bush proposed changing compliance rules regarding the Toxics Release Inventory, federal laws requiring polluters annually to report their volumes of toxic emissions. Bush claimed to support the Toxics Release Inventory yet reduced many requirements for how often and what releases needed to be reported. His rationale, repeatedly criticized by the APHA, was that this weakened reporting would ease the paperwork burden for polluting industries. As a result of such weakened compliance rules, fewer polluters can be said to violate federal law. Publicly, regulators, politicians, and polluters then claim to protect health and safety—by retaining federal laws like the Toxics Release Inventory. Privately, they can do the bidding of special interests and weaken health and safety—by weakening the compliance rules for those laws.[49]

Apart from their threats to life, two other things are ethically troubling about government's or special interests' sometimes covertly weakening health regulations through information suppression and manipulation. (1) They violate *rights to know*. For reasons just explained, most citizens probably do not realize when regulations are weakened. Frequently people are misled by the different private and public behavior of captured regulators and polluters. They often publicly preach concern for health—but privately undercut health regulations. The results of such behavior are clear from workplace-safety fatalities. Medical journals report that, for decades, at least 50,000 Americans have died annually from workplace-induced ailments, like cancers from exposure to toxic chemicals. However, few people know about these deaths—partly for reasons the next chapter will make clear. Citizens also do not know about these deaths because the Justice Department has prosecuted only a handful of employers for thousands of annual U.S. workplace-safety violations. Only one employer has gone to jail—for 45 days. Yet Congress cannot easily stop this weakening of compliance rules, because federal regulatory agencies are under the executive branch of government, outside the jurisdiction of the legislative branch. The result is that both public health and public-health information suffer.[50]

(2) Government and special interests also violate rights to *informed consent*, the second ethical casualty of information suppression and white-collar crime. All legitimate government, all legitimate risk imposition, and all medical ethics rest on the consent of subjects. To give genuine free informed consent, four classic conditions must be met. The risk must be disclosed, victims must understand it, they must voluntarily accept it, and they must be competent to give or withhold consent. Yet most people are unlikely to consent to weakened compliance or enforcement rules like those just illustrated. For one thing, they probably do not understand compliance rules. In addition, publishing rules in *The Federal Register* may not constitute adequate disclosure. Too few people know what it is or how to read it. After all, despite the controversy over genetically engineered food, as late as 1999 the majority of Americans surveyed did not know that it was being marketed. This is in part because regulatory agencies set compliance rules that do not require labeling of all genetically engineered foods. Yet this failure to label is questionable, even on the most conservative economic grounds. By definition, efficient market transactions require full information and free choice. Earlier examples, however, suggest that those buying genetically engineered food, tires, or olestra obviously have neither full information nor free choice. The point here is not to argue for some particular compliance rule. Rather, the issue is ethical. Full disclosure is *necessary* for ethical, medical, democratic, and economic legitimacy—even though disclosure alone often is not *sufficient* to achieve justice. Justice also frequently requires solutions like those offered in chapter 6. Nevertheless, full disclosure of pollutant or product risks, and recognizing rights to know and to give or withhold consent, are necessary first steps to justice. Did the pollutant risks, sketched in chapter 1, surprise readers? If they did, government may be ignoring these required first steps. It may not be meeting disclosure and consent conditions for the risks surveyed in chapter 1.[51]

Providing citizens with information, necessary for citizen consent, is even more difficult when government rewards environmental criminals. Consider the 12 U.S. companies—like Ford, General Motors, and Exxon Mobil—that cause the greatest volume of U.S. worker deaths, illegal acts, and multimillion-dollar, government safety penalties. Nearly all the major violators are from the oil and automobile industries. Yet partly because of covertly weakened enforcement and compliance rules, taxpayers are largely unaware of these companies' criminal activities. As a result, taxpayers continue to subsidize them and their threats to health and safety. How were compliance rules for these oil-and-auto-industry polluters weakened? Within months of taking office in 2000 and largely in secret, the U.S. president Bush rescinded the Corporate Responsibility Rule. This is the executive order making "persistent violators" of health, worker-safety, consumer-protection, environmental, tax, labor, and antitrust laws ineligible for government contracts. This order is consistent with laws prohibiting blue-collar criminals from profiting by their behavior. If blue-collar criminals are subject to this rule, why would someone revoke the Corporate Responsibility Rule, undercut disclosure of health and safety violations, and thus jeopardize consent? One possible reason is that these 12 worst environmental-health criminals represent mostly the oil and auto industries—two of the three largest corporate donors to the successful U.S. presidential campaigns of 1996 and 2000. Such data suggest that *The Economist*'s verdict on U.S. corruption may have been correct.[52]

In 1979, Congressman John Conyers, then chair of the House Judiciary Committee, introduced into Congress a bill requiring criminal penalties, including imprisonment, for white-collar crimes such as suppressing health threats posed by pollutants and consumer products. Scientific testimony on the proposed legislation claimed that

> the regulatory database of a wide range of consumer products and industrial chemicals... [reveals] a pattern of... gross negligence, manipulation, distortion, suppression and destruction of data, which are so frequent as to preclude their dismissal as exceptional aberrations.... Such constrained data are a complex of commercial testing and consulting laboratories and organizations and academic consultants, supported by a network of industry-front organizations and quasi-professional societies. Such constrained data have... resulted in a burgeoning toll of cancer and other preventable diseases.[53]

Conyers's bill was not passed. Nor were others like it. Aided by regulatory capture and information suppression, these repeated government failures suggest that wealthy polluters and white-collar criminals often are protected, while blue-collar criminals are not. "Jail for crime in the streets, bail for crime in the suites." This double standard—for white-collar and blue-collar criminals—may help explain citizen ignorance of health and pollution data like those presented in chapter 1.[54]

Whistle-Swallowing News Media

In a democracy, of course, news media can blow the whistle when wealthy white-collar environmental criminals get "bail for crime in the suites." Instead, why do media frequently swallow the whistle? One reason is that media ownership is becoming more concentrated, often in the hands of major polluters.

- In only 12 years, the number of corporations controlling all U.S. news media has gone from 46 to less than 20. In 98 percent of U.S. cities, there is only one newspaper and no competitor.[55]

- Only two cable companies, TCI and Time-Warner, control half of all U.S. cable systems.[56]

- Only three movie studios make 60 percent of all film profits.[57]

- Only three corporations control the major U.S. TV networks—NBC, CBS, and ABC. Yet most Americans get their news from television. For 81 percent of citizens, all their information about presidential candidates comes from television.[58]

Not surprisingly, media watchdog groups—like Fairness and Accuracy in Reporting (FAIR)—have repeatedly shown that concentrated corporate owners and advertisers can determine much of the news that most citizens receive or fail to receive.[59]

Consider the case of television. General Electric owns NBC, and Disney owns ABC. From 1995 to 2006, Westinghouse owned CBS. For more than a decade, this means that the two dominant U.S. nuclear corporations, General Electric and Westinghouse, controlled two of the three major TV networks. General Electric and Westinghouse have made tens of billions of dollars annually on commercial and military nuclear energy, including billions of dollars from U.S. nuclear-weapons contracts. In particular, General Electric has repeatedly been accused of bias in its NBC-TV nuclear coverage. Journalists say General Electric's NBC-TV gave a one-sided presentation in its 1993 news program on the U.S. Three Mile Island nuclear accident, *What Happened?* Three Mile Island residents claim their video interviews were skillfully edited and cut, so that NBC portrayed them as nuclear supporters, although they said the opposite. Even injured victims of Three Mile Island radiation releases, like Debbie Baker, say their quoted statements were cut and manipulated by NBC. Baker's son was born retarded shortly after the accident. As a result, she received a multimillion-dollar settlement. Although hundreds of Three Mile Island residents have received millions of dollars in accident settlements because of birth defects, retardation, cancer, and death suffered after the Three Mile Island core melt, the NBC news program mentioned none of this. It also included no nuclear critics, only proponents who kept claiming that Three Mile Island backup-nuclear-safety systems had "worked." The program did not explain why, if the systems worked, lethal radiation was released, and a core melt occurred. Critics say this case of Three Mile Island coverage is typical of General Electric. It also forced NBC to remove references to it in a TV special on substandard products. It likewise used NBC-TV news programs to repeatedly run promotional videos, presented as news, about its x-ray machines. Yet it did not tell the audience that it owns both NBC and the x-ray equipment, and other media did not find the x-ray equipment newsworthy. In a news program about consumer boycotts, journalists also say that General Electric forced NBC to delete all references to the company although, at the time, it was the subject of the largest U.S. consumer boycott. When NBC's *Today Show* did a story on defective bolts in bridges, planes, and nuclear plants, General Electric forced the network to delete references to its use of defective bolts. And although Australian physician Helen Caldicott had appeared on the *Today Show* and was scheduled for a future appearance, as soon as one of her books illustrated some of General Electric's nuclear and environmental damage, the show mysteriously canceled her scheduled appearance. News programs on NBC-TV have also been accused of failing to cover several French nuclear accidents—all reported by other news media. Yet the same NBC programs nevertheless broadcast so-called documentaries promoting nuclear power. Even when General Electric does not own media, it often uses its media donations to control news content. As a major donor to the U.S. Public Broadcasting Service, General Electric was able to stop scheduled PBS coverage of an Oscar-winning documentary on its environmental and nuclear violations. Critics also say General Electric has stopped multimillion-dollar funding of another PBS series that documented environmental damage—not done by General Electric. And immediately after one program illustrated environmental threats from U.S. logging, General Electric withdrew all its funding from the PBS program *The World of Audubon*. Obviously, General Electric should protect its interests, but neither funders nor advertisers should censor news information. Citizens need to expose polluter-media partnerships, to reject uncritical acceptance of so-called news programs, and to force government to try to prevent media censorship and monopolies. Without these and other reforms outlined in chapter 6, citizens are likely to continue to be surprised by pollution data like those presented in chapter 1.[60]

Advertising

Apart from powerful media *owners* like General Electric, wealthy media *advertisers* also influence news content, including health news. Although 9 out of 10 Americans say advertisers have too much influence over news content,[61] advertising influence continues to grow. Advertising revenues in the United States have doubled seven times since the 1950s. Hundreds of billions of advertising dollars are spent annually, half in the United States. Growing faster than the world economy and three times faster than population, advertising reaches the average American 3,000 different times each day.[62]

Advertisers can skew citizen perceptions of pollution threats in part because of lack of balance. Roughly three-quarters of all advertising is paid for by corporations. Often they try to convince people that environmental problems have been solved, that pollution has been cleaned up, or that certain products are safe. Advertisers also try to convince people that notoriously dirty corporations, like General Electric (see "Public Relations" later), are good environmental citizens. Frequently advertisers succeed in these messages because polluters control much of the multibillion-dollar advertising on which virtually all commercial TV and radio income is dependent. By 1981, three-quarters of all prime-time shows on PBS were subsidized solely by the oil industry. One result may be U.S. reliance mostly on foreign oil. Another result may be U.S. failure, for decades, to require improved corporate average fuel economy (CAFÉ) standards for automobiles. Corporate advertising is particularly dangerous because its TV and radio funding for U.S. PBS is increasing, while government PBS funding is decreasing. As a result, journalists say that even at PBS and U.S. National Public Radio (NPR), there are chronic funding shortages. They claim PBS and NPR news projects are unlikely to go forward unless they have corporate sponsors. Purely for economic reasons, they say corporate-funded projects are those most likely to be pursued. Even after news projects are completed, reporters claim, PBS and NPR must be careful not to anger their funders. Ford Motors withdrew its donation after PBS aired an Audubon Society documentary. Gulf and Western Oil withdrew funding after PBS aired a documentary on questionable activities of multi-national corporations in developing nations, and so on. Similar censorship occurs in newspapers. Partly because of declining readership, newspaper income depends mostly on advertisers, not readers. As a result, media surveys show that 90 percent of U.S. newspaper editors say advertisers have tried to interfere with newspaper content; 70 percent say advertisers have tried to stop news stories altogether; and 40 percent admit that advertisers actually influence news content. How do advertisers do it? After the medical reporter at KKTV-TV, in Colorado Springs, mentioned McDonald's in a story on health hazards of fast foods, the burger giant pulled its TV advertising for 3 months. Mercedes-Benz vowed to pull its ads from every magazine containing anything critical of the company. Even *New York Times* editors admit they must keep major advertisers, like the auto industry, from pulling their ads. Consumer groups also charge that advertisers even influence negative media coverage, as in *Forbes* magazine. Dependent on insurance advertising, *Forbes* ran articles criticizing personal-injury attorneys who won settlements from insurance companies.[63]

Advertisers' influence on citizens' health knowledge is powerful because it typically is subtle. Advertisers partly control not only *what* people hear about public health but also *how* it is presented. Knowing that news programs will be accused of bias unless they present "both sides," a media survey done by the American Society of Mechanical Engineers showed how advertisers try to appear fair when they are not. They ensure that their "side" is presented by people who appear professional, while the other side is represented by irrational or ill-informed laypeople. The result? Even when citizens' groups have articulate, professional spokespersons, FAIR has shown that news media edit and portray them as irrational. FAIR says Media news presentations almost never use independent scientists, such as those from universities, to present the health or environmental point of view. Advertisers also control *how many* experts represent a particular point of view. FAIR surveyed guests who appeared in the last 4 years on the ABC-TV news program *Nightline*. Sources representing corporate, professional (such as lawyers), and government officials constituted 80 percent of *Nightline* guests, while 5 percent were from public-interest groups. Less than 2 percent were from labor or ethnic groups—those most often and most severely harmed by pollution. All of the four most-frequent guests on *Nightline*, FAIR said, were conservative icons, like Henry Kissinger and Jerry Falwell. Even on PBS, surveys show that 18 percent of the experts used are corporate representatives, while 6 percent are consumer representatives of some kind, while about 3 percent are environmentalists.[64]

The point is not that advertisers should be censored, but that most citizens probably do not realize how advertisers sometimes influence what appear to be news presentations—even about public health. As a result, many citizens are probably misled. Consider news coverage of public-health information about the dangers of tobacco, alcohol, and illegal drugs. Apart from their lobbying expenditures, the U.S. tobacco and alcoholic-beverage industries annually spend $6 billion and $1.3 billion, respectively, on advertising. Although the tobacco and alcohol industries cost the nation nearly 100 times those amounts—from death, injury, and law enforcement—their advertising dollars help ensure reduced news coverage of their products' risks. A *New England Journal of Medicine* article found "strong statistical evidence that cigarette advertising in magazines is associated with diminished coverage of the hazards of smoking." As a result, the authors showed that "Americans substantially underestimate the dangers of smoking as compared with other risks to health." The problems are not just that image-conscious adolescents are vulnerable to alcohol and tobacco ads; nor that, within only three years after the "Joe Camel" ads began, Camel's share of the U.S. under-age-18 cigarette market grew from 1 percent to 33 percent; nor that U.S. children recognize Joe Camel as often as they recognize Mickey Mouse. Rather, the problem is that people do not realize how alcohol and tobacco advertisers influence both news coverage and citizens' misinformation about these health threats. University of California studies showed that tobacco kills about 400,000 Americans annually; alcohol kills about 100,000; and illicit drugs kill about 20,000. Yet network news coverage of these three hazards is not proportionate to the deaths they cause. Each year, tobacco kills 20 times more people than illegal drugs, and alcohol kills 5 times more people than illegal drugs. Yet 77 percent of all news coverage—on tobacco, alcohol, and drug risks—is on illegal drugs. Tobacco, the biggest killer and the biggest advertiser, receives 10 percent of this risk-related TV news coverage. Alcohol, the second-largest killer and the second-largest advertiser, receives 14 percent of coverage. Of course, illegal drugs may be of greater news interest, just because they are illegal. Nevertheless, it is curious that the ratio of deaths caused by tobacco compared to alcohol, compared to illegal drugs, is 20:5:1—*directly proportional to the advertising spent on each*. Both the numbers of these *deaths* and their *advertising expenditures* are inversely proportional to *news coverage* of tobacco, alcohol, and drug deaths—10:14:77. The same University of California studies showed that, although alcohol is associated with 50–66 percent of all homicides, 20–30 percent of all suicides, and more than 50 percent of all domestic violence, news coverage of these incidents virtually never mentions alcohol. Perhaps because of advertisers' influence? To help counter all these advertising abuses, the APHA has called for strict curbs on health-related advertising, especially alcohol- and tobacco-related advertising to children.[65]

Targeted advertising makes children particularly vulnerable to misinformation and resulting health threats. Some of the largest advertisers to school children are the chemical, nuclear, petroleum, mining, coal, and logging industries. They produce and distribute, free of charge, millions of copies of environmental-education materials for American schoolchildren—including videos, games, booklets, and teacher lesson plans. By 1993, corporations like AstraZeneca-Imperial Chemicals, McDonald's, Proctor and Gamble, and Shell already were spending $400 million annually on free "educational" materials for U.S. schools. In addition, 350 different corporate groups pay corporate-owned Lifelong Learning Systems to create school materials to promote their interests. This company says it reaches 100 percent of all U.S. schools. One of its industry clients is the American Nuclear Society, a group of U.S. commercial atomic-power generators who want to promote nuclear energy. Many teachers accept these corporate materials because they save them work. Yet virtually all of these materials promote corporate opinions as facts. They cite only industry-funded studies, but without saying who funded them. They also include infomercial "test" questions such as "Taco Bell has [blank] and burritos."[66]

Underfunded schools bear the brunt of in-class corporate advertising and misleading health information. Knowing poor schools typically have no video, TV, or satellite equipment, "Channel One" offers schools this equipment "in exchange for students' minds for 12 minutes each day." Corporate marketers then provide mandatory infomercials that 40 percent of all U.S. classrooms and 8 million schoolchildren see daily. Their content is partly determined by corporations like Phillips Petroleum. While teachers can emphasize good health habits, for 12 minutes daily they and children frequently must watch the opposite on Channel One, including ads for fast and junk foods. Teachers say they need the corporate-provided school equipment. University researchers say the children, especially in the younger grades, believe the advertising because it is presented during school, with teachers present.[67]

Public Relations

Although school-based educational programs are less transparent ways to shape health perceptions, special interests also hire PR firms directly, usually to "greenwash" their public images. Using selective facts and emotional appeals, PR firms attempt first to deny pollution problems. When they cannot be denied, the PR firms try to show either that pollution produces compensating benefits, or that it cannot be stopped. To disseminate these messages, PR firms produce corporate speeches, soundbites, opinion pieces for newspapers, and

TV and radio "news" videos to be used on national news programs. The secret of this or any PR or propaganda? As Hitler lieutenant Joseph Goebbels said in 1933, people must be "persuaded... without ever noticing it." Media scholars say that when people see TV news or read the newspaper, they never realize that at least 40 percent of news comes "virtually unedited from public-relations offices." Reporters use it partly because it saves them so much time.[68]

Such PR is most dangerous, however, when it selectively uses facts and misleading labels—"doublespeak"—to promote particular agendas. In the Reagan administration, "taxes" became "revenue enhancements." Gambling casinos call themselves the "gaming industry." Corporations say their failed business ventures are "nonperforming assets." The military calls civilian deaths "collateral damage." In 2001–2002, the presidential administration used the rhetorically powerful term "death tax." Crafted to drum up support for repealing the inheritance tax on estates of the very wealthiest Americans, this PR-produced label conjures images of grief-stricken family members, forced into poverty to pay the tax on their tiny homestead, after the father of the family has died. Although the PR label appeals to populist, tax-cut rhetoric, repealing this inheritance tax is hardly populist. The administration rejected taxes even on estates worth more than $5million. Princeton economists say PR "sob stories," promoting the "death-tax-repeal" campaign, were merely "sustained, lavishly financed propaganda—of... fake populists." The results? The economists say this PR propaganda—rather than either sound economics or ethics—helped allow the wealthiest 1 percent of the population to receive more than 40 percent of the supposedly populist 2001 U.S. tax cuts, and the wealthiest 3 percent to get 75 percent of the cuts. Each of only 3,300 families was able to collect its full $16-million inheritance rather than a mere $10-million after-tax inheritance.[69]

Similar use of scientifically misleading PR was evident when, on Earth Day 2002, the U.S. president Bush touted his air-pollution plan as the "Clear Skies Initiative." Yet the plan doubles total allowable pollution and triples allowable mercury pollution. Even more appalling PR was behind the same administration's education proposal, entitled "No Child Left Behind," which pledged to use testing and funding to ensure improved school performance. While claiming credit for this apparently populist program, the presidential PR neglected to mention that the federal government would supply only about 62 percent of the billions of dollars needed to fund it; that the economically and educationally poorest states did not have the remaining 38 percent; and consequently that many poor states were suing the federal government for requiring them to implement the plan. Still another example of skillful PR (and data manipulation or misrepresentation) is U.S. president Bush's 2002 promise to reduce "greenhouse-gas intensity" by 18 percent. Yet greenhouse-gas intensity is the volume of greenhouse gases divided by the GDP. In an expanding economy, greenhouse-gas intensity decreases, even if greenhouse gases themselves increase substantially. In developed nations, because greenhouse-gas intensity falls naturally over time, it is a completely worthless measure of greenhouse-gas reduction. The term represents merely a clever PR move.[70]

When he appealed to his reduction of "greenhouse-gas intensity," President Bush used the well-known propaganda technique of "transfer"—using public support for one thing (reducing global warming) to gain support for another thing (his own policies). Other basic propaganda techniques include "name-calling," as occurred in the earlier death-tax example, and "glittering generalities," illustrated by the No Child Left Behind example. The Clear Skies label is an example of the "euphemism" technique. Still other PR or propaganda strategies include "testimonial," gaining the support of a respected third party, and "plain folks," illustrated when President Bush took on a Southern accent and pretended to eat pork rinds. The "bandwagon" technique suggests that everyone supports something. "Fear" warns of dire consequences unless people accept something, such as threats to national security unless civil liberties are reduced. Using such techniques, propaganda about public-health threats has become so sophisticated that industry consultants like Peter Sandman have developed PR rules to follow. He says polluters should always describe corporate behavior in terms of the first, rather than the second, terms in the following pairs.[71]

voluntary versus *coerced*
natural versus *industrial*
familiar versus *exotic*
not memorable versus *memorable*
not dreaded versus *dreaded*
chronic versus *catastrophic*
knowable versus *unknowable*
individually controlled versus *controlled by others*
fair versus *unfair*
morally irrelevant versus *morally relevant*
trustworthy versus *untrustworthy*
responsive versus *unresponsive*

Such PR often is effective precisely because it appeals to emotion and uses facts selectively. For instance, when U.S. vice-president Cheney called for oil drilling in the Arctic wilderness, he used PR to claim that energy conservation was merely a "personal virtue." Cheney neglected to tell his audience that the five top U.S. national laboratories showed that energy-efficiency programs could immediately, cost-effectively, reduce electricity demand by 20–47 percent. Nor did he reveal that Arctic drilling would benefit Halliburton, the company of which, as mentioned earlier, he was CEO and from which he continues to receive $300,000 annually in "deferred compensation." Cheney's PR also avoided mentioning that raising CAFÉ standards gradually over 13 years would save more oil (2.5 million barrels daily) than the Arctic wilderness contains. Perhaps as a result, in 2005 Congress voted for billions of dollars of oil-industry subsidies–and against improved CAFÉ standards.[72]

Public relations succeeds partly because citizens cannot be well educated on every issue. Consequently, they must trust government and media to help inform them. Yet both often betray this citizen trust. In 2005, the U.S. GAO issued a "blistering" indictment of the Bush administration for using $1.6 billion in taxpayer money to fund "covert propaganda" for its proposed policies. The GAO said the administration "violated the law" by paying newspaper and TV commentators, reporters, and video producers billions of taxpayer dollars for covert PR praising Bush's policies.[73]

"Covert propaganda" or PR is dangerous because it turns facts into market commodities. Millenia ago, people sold what they grew or gathered. Centuries ago, they began selling what they made. Now people often sell what they know— or what they can convince people to believe—PR. This is partly because manufacturers, to sell what they make, must control what people believe about their companies and products. As a result, U.S. revenues for the top 25 PR companies are about $4 billion annually and increase as much as 42 percent annually. The U.S. Bureau of Labor Statistics says PR is the fastest-growing occupation in the nation. Every 3 years, PR revenues double. Two of the top PR firms, Hill and Knowlton and Burson-Marsteller, each employs thousands of people and has about 80 offices in 35 countries. Their work? Surveys of U.S. executives show their top PR concern is environmental—finding ways to "green" their companies' images. Polls show that 75 percent of Americans consider themselves environmentalists and tend to invest only in companies with good environmental reputations. As a result, PR firms brag that they can control citizens' perceptions of pollution. "Spin doctors" like Hill and Knowlton, the world's largest PR firm, literally create those perceptions. For the last 50 years, a major chunk of tobacco lobby money has gone to Hill and Knowlton. The purpose? To use flawed science and front groups to create, for the tobacco industry, what *Public Relations Journal* calls one of the "most formidable public relations/lobbying machines in history." The company also uses pricey "facilitators" and interactive CD-ROMs. They train polluters to manage crises, control public opinion, "ward off the media," and create a "virtual reality" about their questionable actions. Thus, despite hundreds of thousands of tobacco-related U.S. deaths annually, for 50 years Hill and Knowlton enabled Philip Morris to deny the hazards of smoking. Despite record-breaking oil-industry profits, Hill and Knowlton also helped the American Petroleum Institute keep taxes low on gasoline. After people discovered that Kathie Lee Gifford's brand of clothing was manufactured by child laborers in sweatshops abroad, Rubenstein Associates told her what to say and do to reduce public outcry. After the Bhopal chemical catastrophe, Burson-Marsteller helped Union Carbide resurrect its image. After Shell Oil contributed to the murder of nonviolent Nigerian playwright and activist Ken Saro-Wiwa and others, Peter Sandman; Mongoven, Biscoe, and Duchin; and many other PR groups helped Shell. They defused outrage against the oil giant for destroying the homelands of Saro-Wiwa's Ogoni people and for using African oil-drilling practices that fail to control pollution. In the face of such PR commodification and manipulation of information, citizen understanding of pollution risks is frequently a casualty.[74]

The U.S. Council on Economic Priorities says that poor public-health information is also a result of the fact that many corporations "are using 'green' PR as a pro-environment smokescreen while they continue to pollute." Consistently on the council's annual list as one of the eight-worst toxic polluters in the United States, General Electric, the owner of NBC, is a case in point. Although it sells pollution-control equipment, General Electric is the responsible party at more Superfund sites (70-plus) than any other company. Its fines for PCB-related health and environmental threats are among the highest ever levied by EPA. General Electric also falsely advertises being "green." It said its refrigerators were free of chlorofluorocarbons and ozone safe, when they were not. And attorneys general in 32 states forced General Electric to change its false claims about its supposedly energy-efficient "Energy Choice" light bulbs. Fines of General Electric for violations of worker health and safety regulations are also 150 percent higher than those of any other company in the electronics industry. Yet, thanks to millions of dollars spent on PR, General Electric is consistently rated in Roper polls as one of the top 10 companies regarding environmental reputation. Working with Dow, Dupont, Union Carbide, Monsanto, and other major polluters in an industry-funded front group—the Conservation Foundation—General Electric is spending millions of dollars to defeat U.S. Superfund legislation. Yet its PR claims it is an environmentally sensitive company. Dow Chemical and other corporations do the same thing. Dow created an onslaught of favorable publicity from a wetlands project at its Michigan plant. Continuing to pollute, it suppressed the findings of scientists who showed that downstream of the Michigan plant, birds had deformities caused by Dow's releases of dioxin. Likewise 3M, the thirteenth-worst U.S. corporation in terms of its volume of toxic-chemical releases, does something similar. Its PR firm brags about creating and publicizing 3M's "Pollution-Prevention Pays" program, which has "softened" regulators, saved 3M hundreds of millions of dollars on pollution control, and kept customers happy. Similarly, British Nuclear Fuels misleadingly advertises that 97 percent of highly radioactive atomic-reactor fuels can be recycled "into clean uranium and plutonium for reuse." Saab advertises that because its tailpipe emissions of hydrocarbons are at levels lower than in some London air, therefore Saab "cars actually clean the air." The underlying rationale for such false claims? Polluters' "green" PR is cheaper than reducing pollution. What is important in PR is not what the truth is, but what people believe is true. Consequently, polluters may ask two questions. What is the minimum amount that must be spent on PR, to convince the public that some product or pollutant is safe? Is this amount less than the costs of controlling pollution? Often it is.[75]

A common polluter-PR strategy is organizing phony "grassroots" (or "astroturf") front groups. In fact, 80 percent of corporations pay PR firms to create such astroturf groups, whose hired employees pose as ordinary citizens. In 1993, tobacco company Philip Morris paid PR firm Burson-Marsteller to create the astroturf group, the National Smokers Alliance. Burson-Marsteller paid smokers to pose as citizen activists, to disseminate pro-smoking messages, and to claim that their "rights" were violated by anti-smoking laws. Burson-Marsteller also created the astroturf group, the Foundation for Clean Air Progress. Funded by the energy, manufacturing, and transportation industries, this front group's goal is to weaken the Clean Air Act. And millions of dollars of corporate-organized, astroturf PR has been spent to promote what is called "free-market environmentalism."[76]

Free-market environmentalism is the view that pollution ought to be controlled by the market, not regulations, and that pollution ought to be allowed whenever it is not cost-effective for polluters to reduce it. Touted by fake grassroots groups who demand "rational" policymaking, free-market environmentalism takes no account of who causes the pollution, why it is caused, who benefits, or who suffers from it. Nor does it recognize any ethical constraints such as not harming people, ensuring consumer consent, whether the pollution is equitably distributed, whether people are compensated for it, whether a polluter is negligent, and so on. Instead, the PR ideology of free-market environmentalism counts only overall market costs and benefits associated with pollution. Whenever PR is genuinely cheaper for the polluter than reducing pollution, free-market environmentalism dictates using PR. Whenever using SLAPPs, court-mandated gag orders, and financial settlements with pollution victims is genuinely cheaper for the polluter than reducing pollution, free-market environmentalism dictates using these three strategies instead.

The free-market-environmentalism stance on air pollution provides a dramatic illustration of how the combination of free-market environmentalism and PR can harm health. More than a quarter of a century ago, U.S. Congress ordered cleanup of coal plants' health-damaging smog and acid rain. Instead of requiring individual plants to install pollution controls, as Congress desired, President Bush appealed to free-market environmentalism. His 2005 scheme "would allow some of the dirtiest plants to buy their way out of their obligation to reduce emissions," just as he proposed doing for dangerous mercury emissions.[77] Both proposals permit any polluting facilities to "buy their way out of obeying the law" by purchasing "pollution credits" from cleaner facilities far away. The result? Pollution "hot spots" where those most victimized by air pollution, like children, would be forced to breathe even dirtier air. The alleged rationale underlying free-market environmentalism is that pollution laws need not provide everyone with equal treatment or individual rights to life. Instead, free-market environmentalism defines two types of "rational" behavior, depending on pollution laws. If pollution laws exist, free-market environmentalism says polluters may break health laws, provided they are able to pay for pollution credits from other regions. If pollution laws do not exist, then even when pollution is seriously harmful, victims must either bear it or pay polluters to reduce it. The ideology of free-market-environmentalism thus assumes that polluters, not the people, have property rights over common resources, such as air and water. Following this assumption elsewhere, however, could lead to deadly consequences. Anyone anywhere—including murderers—could "pay" to avoid following the law. Victims of injustice could have no rights. Victims could have only duties to pay others not to harm them.

On the one hand, proponents of free-market environmentalism are right to follow classical economists who say that financially independent, informed consumers will not support products, manufacturers, or pollutants that harm them. They also are right that consumers should make their own decisions, through the market. On the other hand, this chapter suggests that otherwise-reliable market processes have been subverted because many people have neither financial independence nor accurate information about dangerous products and pollutants. Information is lacking partly because of polluter misrepresentations. In the face of such information-suppression, free-market environmentalism thus has neither economic nor ethical justification, both of which require full information and voluntary choices. *In theory*, free-market environmentalism could control pollution—provided these two economic requirements were met. *In practice*, however, free-market environmentalism makes neither economic nor ethical sense because these conditions are rarely met. Nevertheless, although free-market environmentalism cannot be justified economically, it often succeeds as PR—and enables polluters to avoid regulation.

Health Tracking and Polluter Self-Policing

Citizen understanding of pollution threats likewise would improve if government collected all relevant health data. Yet it does not. Special-interest lobbyists have kept the U.S. Congress from passing the National Health Tracking Act of 2002. Providing geographical epidemiological data showing locations of clusters of specific diseases, this act would enable regulators to detect local-pollution "hot spots." It would make it more difficult for companies to deny the hazards of their pollution, to falsify their Toxics Release Inventory reports, and to commit white-collar crimes. In fact, if the nation had used health tracking, it could have exposed the causal connection between nuclear testing and subsequent deaths, and between the Three Mile Island nuclear accident and later cancers and genetic deformities. As it was, independent university scientists, working on their own time, eventually revealed the fallout and Three Mile Island deaths—but decades after many victims already had suffered and died.[78]

Without government health-tracking data, citizens frequently are forced to rely on polluters' PR claims about their releases and their effects. As already mentioned, the Toxics Release Inventory requires polluters to report releases of about 60 industrial chemicals. But government has tested only about 1 percent of the 80,000 chemicals used in industry, and it does not check the accuracy of the Toxics Release Inventory. As a result, polluters have financial incentives (avoiding fines) not to report illegal releases. As the last chapter noted, even government reports say the inventory sometimes underestimates pollution by a factor of up to 14. Besides, as late as 1995, only 66 percent of the industries, that are required to report inventory data, even did so.[79]

As the tobacco case suggests, relying on polluters to police themselves, through means like the Toxics Release Inventory, can be dangerous to both public health and health information. For half a century after epidemiologists confirmed high mortality from cigarette smoking, tobacco companies falsified research and misled the public. They deliberately and secretly made cigarettes addictive and targeted underage smokers—so they would have lifetime customers. After scientific journals confirmed epidemiological evidence of tobacco hazards, the United States took 40 years to require warning labels on cigarette packages. It took even longer for victims of nicotine addiction to win court settlements from tobacco interests. Yet because polluters control most pollution records, because there are tens of thousands of different pollutants, and because hazardous materials are released to air and water, not just in particular products, uncovering pollution hazards may be more difficult than uncovering tobacco hazards. To address these difficulties, some physicians have proposed an international public-health crimes tribunal that would be analogous to the International War Crimes Tribunal. As a further incentive to polluters' providing full information and accurate self-policing, the state of California in 1986 passed laws allowing citizen-victims to recover damages from a percentage of company profits on carcinogenic consumer products.[80]

Campaign Contributions and Lobbying

Health experts obviously want more public-health information, including a National Health Tracking Act. Why has it not been passed? A July 2001 cartoon in USA Today may have the answer. It was published soon after Congress passed U.S. president Bush's tax breaks, 40 percent of which went to the 1-percent-wealthiest Americans, and 75 percent of which went to the 3-percent-wealthiest. The cartoon's caption was "Things You Can Buy with Your Tax-Rebate Check. The cartoon depicted several items: a DVD player, clothing, a bicycle, and a congressman (shown ripping up a piece of paper on which were written the words "Campaign Finance Reform").[81]

The cartoon may be correct, at least if one recalls The Economist's analysis and earlier examples of the U.S. nuclear, pharmaceutical, and chemical industries. As already mentioned, the former editor of the New England Journal of Medicine says the drug industry does little that is innovative, spends most of its money on advertising, and enjoys profits that are three times those of Fortune-500 companies. By 2002, the drug industry was spending more than $91 million annually to pay its 675 registered lobbyists (even more were not registered) from 138 Washington lobbying firms. This is more than one drug lobbyist for every person in Congress. Besides having the largest single group of lobbyists in

Washington, the drug industry typically gives $85 million annually in campaign contributions, 80 percent to Republicans. Three likely results of these campaign donations? The United States has higher drug prices than anywhere in the world. The United States is the only developed nation not to regulate drug prices. Of 143 countries in 2006, the United States is the only nation that opposes drug-patent relaxation in order to help HIV/AIDS victims in the Third World.[82]

Campaign contributions and lobbying have given many polluters, as well as drug companies, regulatory protection and information suppression. About 2,500 firms have lobbyists in Washington. The purpose of more than a third of lobbying work is to minimize public-health and environmental threats from corporate products and pollution. Among the largest companies, three-quarters have senior executives responsible for "grassroots organizing" of astroturf groups opposing environmental-health regulations. Companies like Chevron, Exxon, and Dow Chemical, for example, each give millions of dollars annually to create and support both astroturf groups and anti-regulatory political candidates and think tanks.[83]

Lobbying and campaign contributions are probably the main reason that, even after the hazards of smoking were clear, for decades legislators defeated bills to ban smoking in restaurants and public places. Instead, officials claimed that health effects of cigarettes were controversial. As the former editor of the *New England Journal of Medicine* has warned, campaign contributions are a key reason that prices of prescription drugs are much higher in the United States than anywhere in the world, and part of the reason that costs for phone, cable, food, and health care all rose dramatically after these industries made large campaign contributions in the 2000 U.S. presidential election. Something similar may have happened with regulation of alcohol. In the last 15 years, the alcohol industry alone has given more than $26 million in campaign contributions to federal political candidates. Perhaps as a result, Congress has enacted neither tough drunk-driving standards nor tough taxes on beer, wine, and hard liquor. Yet, as mentioned earlier, U.S. alcohol-related deaths number 100,000 annually, not counting alcohol involvement in a majority of all U.S. homicides. Surveys conducted in 2001 by U.S. Republican congressman Dick Armey show 67,062 business lobbyists in the capitol—not counting lawyers, PR employees, and journalists hired by special interests. This represents nearly an eightfold increase in 20 years; an annual increase of between 2,000 and 4,000 lobbyists; and 13 percent annual growth in dollars spent on lobbying. In 1999, just the 20,000 Washington lobbyists who were formally registered cost their funders $1.5 billion. By 2004, this number rose to 34,000. The total number of Washington lobbyists (registered and unregistered) may be over 100,000—and they may cost their industry funders more than $5 billion annually.[84]

What have lobbying and campaign expenditures bought? One example comes from a 2005 report in the *New York Times*. Omar Bongo, president of the small African nation of Gabon, paid Republican lobbyist Jack Abramoff $9 million in "lobbying fees" in exchange for a meeting with U.S. president Bush.

Yet Gabon has a government that is "regularly accused by the United States of human rights abuses." Besides access to government officials, empirical studies uncontroversially show that lobbying dollars and corporate campaign contributions have statistically significant effects on legislative voting, access to officials, and citizen information. Corporate donations have "a great deal of influence on political outcomes." They create conflicts of interest, affect votes, and influence public-health policies. If their dollars did not have these effects, special interests probably would not spend them. Earlier examples—of failed national health-tracking acts and of suppressing information about harmful products and pollutants like dioxin—illustrate the power of campaign contributions. Yet from a purely economic and free-market-environmentalism point of view, campaign contributions represent an efficient investment of special-interest dollars. Most Americans make little on their saving deposits. Even a mutual fund rarely goes above a 20 percent dividend. Yet consumer groups charge that campaign donors can engage in "legalized bribery" and make as much as 5,725 percent on their campaign investments. By investing only $8 million in federal campaign contributions to preserve the logging-road subsidy, the timber industry received a return of $458 million in taxpayer subsidies. By spending only $1.2 million on campaign contributions designed to promote patent extension for its drug Zantac, pharmaceutical giant Glaxo-Wellcome gained $1 billion—an 83,333 percent return on its initial legislative investment. In one recent election cycle, the tobacco industry spent $30 million in campaign contributions and received tax breaks worth $50 billion. Its return was 167,000 percent. The broadcast industry spent $5 million in campaign contributions to avoid paying for digital-TV licenses, but it received a $70 billion return on its investment.[85]

Campaign contributions are part of a vicious cycle in which most members of Congress must rely on wealthy corporate donors in order to get elected, then must "pay back" these donations—sometimes in ways that harm public health. In the last 25 years, campaign expenditures of incumbent U.S.-Senate winners have gone from $610,000 to $4,400,000—an increase of more than 700 percent. Because primary elections are often "wealth primaries," campaign funding can be an accurate predictor of ultimate election winners. U.S. Republican senator John McCain says the current U.S. campaign financing by wealthy special interests is "an elaborate influence-peddling scheme by which both parties conspire to stay in office by selling the country to the highest bidder." The largest donor to the U.S. president's successful 2000 campaign was Enron Corporation. As already mentioned, Enron fraud caused millions of people to lose their pensions and savings in the largest bankruptcy in U.S. corporate history. Likewise, the major mercury polluters—the electric-utility, oil, mining, timber, and chemical industries—together gave $44 million to the president's 2000 campaign. In return, he promoted his "Clear Skies" air-pollution plan, which allows 3 times more mercury emissions and 50 percent more sulfur dioxide emissions. The president also reassigned (to non-environmental work) 40 percent of the EPA staff that enforces criminal violations of environmental laws. One result? President Bush annually refers 80 percent fewer criminal violations under the Toxic Substances Control Act than President Clinton did.

Under Bush, the EPA halved the number of Superfund sites scheduled for cleanup, then shifted the worst costs of cleanup from the industries responsible to the taxpayers.[86]

While everyone has rights to lobby and to donate to political campaigns, the obvious problem is that those with more money ought not be able to buy votes, delay environmental cleanup, or suppress health information. Financial imbalance in donations is a special problem for public health because not all lobbyists and campaign contributors have equal economic power and thus equal opportunity to threaten citizen health. Public-interest or consumer groups virtually never have, or make, large contributions to political campaigns, and labor unions gave only 1 percent of donations in the 2004 U.S. presidential elections. Corporations gave about 80 percent.[87] This means consumer and public-health groups are competing on a legislative and economic playing field that is heavily tilted against them. One result? An "information playing field" that also is frequently tilted against public-health disclosures.

Conclusion

This chapter suggests that at least 10 special-interest or government behaviors—from advertising and lobbying to white-collar crime and information-suppression—sometimes can enable private-interest polluters to subvert the public interest. As a result, polluters can "corner the market" in public-health information, fail to disclose risks to citizens, and threaten their health. When relevant risks are not disclosed, citizens are unable to fulfill their rights to know, to give or withhold consent to the risks, and to receive equal protection. What ought citizens do to protect their rights? Instead of condemning all private interests—interests that are essential to economic prosperity—citizens ought to follow the suggestions of chapter 1. They ought to use the tools of deliberative democracy to educate themselves and others, to help prevent conflicts of interest, and to ensure that government regulators and oversight agencies behave as they should.

Government reform, however, is not alone sufficient to protect public health. Ultimately, health threats do not arise merely because of ineffective regulators or a few corporations who behave unethically. They arise because people themselves do not play the role in democracy that they ought to play. Instead, many people live in a world that Plato described in his allegory of the cave, already mentioned in chapter 1.[88]

Plato believes that most people are like prisoners, chained in a dark cave where they fail to see and to understand things as they are. Manipulative lobbyists, campaign donors, and PR experts are like the cleverest cave dwellers. They receive money and honor for their skills at manipulating shadows and understanding cave life. Because the prisoner-citizens cannot easily escape from the cave, they are influenced by those who manipulate in darkness. Besides, most people cannot even envision a world outside the cave. Assuming Plato's analogy is correct on all these points, regulating the most manipulative lobbyists and advertisers is not sufficient to produce full information and more ethical public-health behavior. What is needed is not only better health *information*, in part obtained through regulations promoting disclosure and consent. What also is needed is better health *action*, in part by convincing people who escape from the cave to return to it, to help the prisoners there.

Who escapes from the cave? Anyone who uses factual information, logical analysis, and ethical scrutiny to counter the false claims that are rampant in the cave world. One problem is that many of those who could counter these false claims have been coopted by the cave controllers—by those who pay for special-interest public-health research, PR, advertising, and campaign donations. As a result, many experts do "science in the private interest" of the cave controllers, not science in the public interest. One of the engines that drives the cave system, private science is both better funded and easier to obtain than science funded by independent federal agencies, like the U.S. National Institutes of Health. Without their private-interest science, private-interest law, private-interest education, private-interest lobbying, and so on, the cave controllers could not so easily promote a cave view of reality. Countering their false claims thus requires countering their private-interest science, private lobbying, private ethics, and so on. The next chapter begins this task. It exposes private-interest science as neither scientific nor ethical.

Private Science, Public Injury

Built like a linebacker, Reason Warehime was eager to help the United States win World War II. When he enlisted in 1942, he told the recruiter he was 18—that his birth certificate had been destroyed. He was only 16. Soon Warehime was fighting in the famous battle at Saipan. In all, he was wounded three times in the Pacific. After the United States dropped the atomic bombs, he was sent as part of the occupation in Japan. On Nagasaki streets and walls, Warehime says he saw shadows of people and animals, vaporized by the bomb. Eight years later, he was assigned to Camp Desert Rock, in Nevada. There he participated in "Shot Simon" atomic test. He and his men witnessed the nuclear explosion from a foxhole 300 yards away. Immediately after detonation, Warehime says he and his platoon were marched to ground zero, into even higher levels of radiation. Some of the sand had melted into smooth brown glass. When the men held up their hands and arms, they could see their bones, as in x-rays. "Then we got a kind of sunburn," Warehime says. "All the guys started throwing up, sick as dogs, all of them.... Nobody out there knew what he was doing."[1]

Reason Warehime and Private-Interest Science

The bomb was supposed to be 23 kilotons, twice the size of the one at Hiroshima. Instead it was nearly four times larger. Its fallout spread quickly, all the way to the East Coast. Although military and government leaders denied it, within hours the Nevada cloud killed cows in Idaho. Students at Rensselaer Polytechnic Institute in Troy, New York, noticed their Geiger counters were clicking wildly. Radioactivity in their tap water was 2,630 times higher than normal. Undeveloped film at Kodak, in upstate New York, was ruined by fallout. Yet officials said the radiation was harmless. Meanwhile, back in Nevada, weeks after Shot Simon, Warehime says his hair fell out. He became sterile. Later, all his teeth turned black and had to be pulled. By age 30, he had developed radiation-induced cataracts, osteoporosis on the side of his body facing the bomb, and muscle deterioration. Three years later, at age 33, his health problems became so severe that Warehime was forced to retire after 17 years of military service. A decade later, in 1982, Veterans Administration doctors diagnosed him with lung cancer. They denied that radiation exposures had caused any of his health problems except sterility. Warehime says their denial was based on the government's hiring consultants to estimate radiation doses to the soldiers, then giving the consultants false exposure information. The soldiers' actual radiation exposures and closeness to ground zero, claims Warehime, were many times greater than the government admitted. As a consequence, the consultants badly underestimated the risk. They concluded that Shot Simon soldiers had received only low doses of radiation—not enough to cause the health ailments they all shared.[2]

The Veterans Administration repeatedly denied Warehime and other test victims medical benefits for their cancers and radiation-induced bone loss. He believes the government did not want to pay claims to nearly half a million "atomic veterans." He also discovered something strange about thousands of soldiers, from all over the nation, who had been assigned to Camp Desert Rock. For each of approximately 200 above-ground nuclear tests, the army had assigned no two men from the same platoon. The reason? Warehime says this assignment made it more difficult for soldiers to contact each other and to compare their shared radiation-induced ailments. Nevertheless, through years of public-records requests and informal meetings, Warehime and other soldiers tracked down many atomic veterans or their widows. They discovered they all shared the same fallout-induced illnesses, like leukemia and bone cancer. They also discovered their military-service medical records had been falsified, to underestimate their radiation doses. Again and again, the Veterans Administration denied that radiation caused their common health problems, then rejected their benefits claims. Warehime and other atomic veterans responded by founding the National Association of Radiation Survivors (NARS). Continuing to work for NARS, Warehime earned his GED and college degree on the GI Bill. To learn better how to fight for Veterans Administration disability benefits for himself and other soldiers, he took law courses at night, assembling his own law library. At the same time, Warehime's wartime experiences and Veterans Administration mistreatment led this tough, straight-talking veteran to study religion. For several years, he worked as an ordained minister. But ministry was not his calling. A "soldier's soldier," Warehime claims he did not have the temperament for church work. His pro-military and pro-government views disturbed his congregations. Instead, using skills learned partly from his military service, he became a private investigator. For decades, he also used these skills to track down atomic veterans and unearth evidence of government nuclear coverup and falsification of military records.[3]

By the mid-1980s, Warehime had painstakingly assembled, for NARS, the only nonconfidential (nongovernmental) database of atomic veterans. It was on his home computer. However, when he and his wife returned to their California trailer-home one day, it had been ransacked. Their belongings had been thrown outside. Nothing was missing except copies of the NARS database. Yet Warehime and NARS members kept working. After another decade, government finally admitted its weapons-test coverup. It offered fallout-related benefits to atomic veterans or their survivors. But Warehime claims the conditions for qualifying for these benefits remain too strict—on purpose, he says. The conditions rely on the same flawed science and falsified exposure records that the Veterans Administration used earlier to deny claims. As a result, almost no atomic veterans have received radiation-related health awards. Warehime's only such benefit is $75 per month, for having been made sterile.[4]

Today Reason Warehime lives in a modest manufactured home in Gibsonton, Florida. He moved there after the mysterious California robbery. His wife of 40 years died in the late 1990s, and a niece now helps care for him. Of thousands of soldiers at Shot Simon, he is the sole survivor. Using his phone and computer from his wheelchair, he is still helping injured soldiers with their claims, still fighting for recognition of his other radiation-related ailments. Despite repeated cancers, pain medication helps him continue his unpaid work for veterans. Often he is on the road, testifying in Washington. Intensely patriotic and proud to be a veteran, Warehime says he is not a hero, only a good citizen. He also claims that specific people—officers and scientists—could have stopped the fallout coverup, but they chose not to do so. The task was left to Warehime, a high-school dropout with a keen sense of justice.[5]

Why did government deny atomic veterans' radiation-induced health problems? Warehime says one reason is "fixed" science, or private-interest science—science manipulated and misused to serve the agenda of the funder. Without adequate oversight from independent investigators, the army, the Veterans Administration, and their consulting scientists used private-interest science to "blame the victims" for their health problems. This blaming was occurring as late as 1999, when Sergeant Warehime gave an ROTC talk at the University of Notre Dame. Two university physicists, formerly on the government's nuclear-testing payroll, challenged this decorated, three-time Purple Heart winner. They knew the government had admitted that nuclear tests had sterilized Warehime. Yet in public they claimed that his hair, teeth, and bone losses were probably caused by his "poor hygiene," not radiation.[6]

Chapter Overview

Chapter 1 summarized many pollution-related health problems, and chapter 2 began to explain why so few people are aware of these threats. Special interests often have captured regulators and suppressed public-health information. Special interests would not be able to capture regulators and media, however, unless they could sometimes control pollution-related science. How do they do so?

In answering this question, the chapter first explains *why* the complexity of health-related science often makes it susceptible to manipulation. Second, it shows *what* some special interests do when they literally "buy" private-interest science through front groups, think tanks, and "hire education." ("Hire education" refers to industry funding of academic research that serves its corporate goals. As a result, instead of standard university education, students and professors are influenced by education whose content is partly driven by outside interests.) Third, the chapter surveys *how* private-interest science is done—with incomplete data, contraindicated models, inadequately sensitive tests of pollution damage, and so on. Fourth, using the debate over causes of cancer, the chapter illustrates *who* funds and *who* does private-interest science. The chapter closes by showing *how* and *why* private-interest science often leads to death, injury, and flawed ethics. These flawed ethics include committing the naturalistic fallacy; ignoring conflicts of interest; confusing the absence of evidence (for pollutant harm) with evidence for the absence (of harm); and ignoring rights to life, to know, and to consent.

Statistical Casualties and Invisible Bullets

Not all ignorance of environmental-health risks, however, arises from flawed science or ethics. Often the complexity and uncertainty of pollutant threats cause them to be misunderstood. As already mentioned, the U.S. National Academy of Sciences (NAS) admits that causes for half of all cancers are unknown. As a result, different scientists often explain these unknown causes differently. Experts on various sides sometimes overstate the merits of their own positions. Pollution-related health effects also are frequently neither immediate nor obvious, particularly for low-dose exposures to multiple chemical or radioactive releases. Blue-collar crimes like murder have direct and immediate impacts, therefore direct and immediate publicity, even if the perpetrators are not found. White-collar crimes, like falsifying pesticide data, however, can cause more harm. Yet their effects are often indirect, not immediate, and not easily attributable to someone. As a result, only rarely are they publicized and stopped. They are known mainly statistically, as spikes in curves that track numbers of deaths. The FBI collects no data on white-collar crime, and cancers do not wear tags saying they were caused by releases from Monsanto or Ferro Chemical.

Given no national health-tracking act (see chapter 2), often scientists must do costly studies even to discover that some area or occupation has higher rates of death or disease. Yet to avoid damning data, polluters sometimes try to keep the relevant research from being done. In the early pollution coverups, like Union Carbide's famous Hawk's Nest silicosis tragedy of the 1930s, coverup was cruder. Thousands of West Virginia workers died in this worst industrial disaster in U.S. history. Yet for years Union Carbide avoided scrutiny by hiring mostly minorities, keeping few records, and burying victims in unmarked graves. Company executives knew that prosecuting them required records of death and disease—just as murder trials typically require bodies. Their solution was to try to leave no evidence. Even today, when government has evidence, often it is incomplete. When pollution-related epidemiological studies are done, they typically reveal only "statistical casualties." These are fatalities identified only as population-level increases in the percentage or number of deaths. Statistical casualties alone do not enable scientists to know which particular people have been killed by some pollutant. They show only that some percentage of deaths is above average, or only that some percentage of people will die after exposure to some toxin. Yet identifying these victims is difficult. Often toxins cause different symptoms in different people. Except at very high doses, effects typically occur probabilistically, in only some people. Frequently pollutants are tasteless, odorless, and unseen. As a result, people's senses may mislead them. They confuse aesthetics with environmental health—wrongly assuming that what looks healthy is healthy. Because air in most cities is not filled with coal soot, as it often was a century ago, people may not realize that they are at risk from unseen threats like dioxins, PCBs, and ionizing radiation. They may not realize they are living in a complex "soup" of chemicals whose multiplicity and ubiquity make it difficult to distinguish specific environmental causes of different diseases. The contaminants sometimes can make it difficult for scientists to find an uncontaminated control group for testing. Besides, almost all exposures are to combinations of hazards, yet virtually no data exist on effects of multiple exposures. Given the different combinations of 2 or 3 or 400 different toxins—of the 80,000 human-made chemicals to which people are exposed—millions of combinations need to be tested. Yet only about 1 percent of all chemicals has been tested individually. Virtually no combinations have been tested. And most pollution victims do not have measurements of their various exposures, over time. Only costly individual testing may reveal who has been harmed by some exposure. For all these reasons, polluters often can deny that some chemical caused an individual's death or injury—just as they did in Emily Pearson's case (chapter 1). The result? Many pollution threats go unrecognized or are blamed on something else. As the U.S. Centers for Disease Control (CDC), the International Commission on Radiological Protection, and most scientists confirm, illnesses occurring after years of exposure to low-level pollutants typically are not detectable—until it is too late. Cancers may be dormant, latent, or unnoticed for 10 to 40 years—long after people remember what exposures they had. Instead, low-level pollutants bioaccumulate until their effects are obvious, and people become ill or die. They are like slow-acting "invisible bullets," harming people who often cannot even prove they were "shot."[7]

AIDS provides a good analogy for the difficulty of pinpointing the causes of many environmental-health effects. As early as 1978, AIDS probably entered the blood supply. But it was seven years before health professionals knew what caused AIDS and how to screen for it. When cases were first discovered, it took another three years until the virus was identified. Yet AIDS seems easier to track than most pollution-induced sickness. People know their sexual and drug habits. They are less likely to know all the chemicals or radiation to which they have been exposed. AIDS also has several classic symptoms. Yet the same contaminant can induce different diseases, depending on individuals' different vulnerabilities. Even physicians may not see a pattern. Trained to discover diseases caused by identifiable organisms or physiological conditions, physicians often have little education in environmental disease, occupational disease, or public health. Also, most dangerous contaminants came into use only 50 years ago, and special interests have sometimes covered up their effects. Unless physicians see obvious trends of illness in particular groups whom they treat, they may not suspect pollution-induced health problems.

Front Groups and Think Tanks

The complexities associated with statistical casualties illustrate why some polluters can easily deny pollution-induced disease, particularly when there is no national health tracking. This denial is particularly easy because polluters can create front groups to do private-interest science and to deny their responsibility for harm. In July 2000, the World Health Organization (WHO), a UN group, issued a report on industry-funded, scientific front groups that spend billions of dollars annually to generate misleading, antiregulatory health-related research.[8]

Arguing that such front groups compromise both scientific information and public health, the WHO showed that polluters like tobacco companies "use" them to mislead people. Because the groups are given scientific names, citizens erroneously think they are professional groups, like the American Public Health Association. Thus the "the American Chemistry Council," formerly "the Association of Chemical Manufacturers," is an anti-regulatory group, funded by the chemical industry. It spends more than $4 million annually in U.S. lobbying and scientific writing against regulation of industrial chemicals. The American Crop Protection Association, funded by pesticide manufacturers, does science and lobbying to block regulation of pesticides by the U.S. Environmental Protection Agency (EPA). The Global Climate Coalition, funded by the oil and automobile industries, opposes global-warming regulations. The Advancement of Sound Science Coalition (TASSC), funded by the tobacco and chemical industries, argues for the health and safety of tobacco smoke, fast food, saccharin, pesticides, and growth hormones in cattle. Responsible Industry for a Sound Environment, also pesticide-industry–funded, opposes right-to-know provisions in pesticide regulations. Keep America Beautiful, funded by the bottling and plastics industry, opposes bottle-deposit legislation. The National Wetlands Coalition, funded by the oil and gas industry, has a logo that shows a duck flying over a wetland. It lobbies for wetlands oil and gas drilling. Citizens for Better Medicare, supposedly a coalition of senior-citizens' groups, is funded by the pharmaceutical industry to fight regulation of drug prices. In the 2000 U.S. elections, it spent $65 million on this goal. One result? The United States is the only nation in the developed world that does not regulate drug prices.[9]

Such front groups are particularly misleading when they circulate alleged informational materials to health professionals, students, and other citizens. Recall the discussion in chapter 2 of how special-interest front groups and advertisers provide supposed educational materials that reach every U.S. school child. Nearly the same is true in medicine. In 2002, for instance, many U.S. cardiologists received a 450-page book on blood coagulation. *Quick Consult: Guide to Clinical Trials in Thrombosis Management* was totally funded by Aventis Pharmaceuticals. Physicians say the book is "a thinly veiled advertisement for Lovenox," an Aventis blood thinner. They also charge that non-Lovenox treatments for thrombosis "are given short shrift"; that most of the book is non-refereed, unpublished testimonials on managing thrombosis; and that most of the book's authors have conflicts of interest—financial ties to Aventis. Drug companies also create product-promoting front groups, like the National Initiative in Sepsis Education. (Sepsis is a type of bacterial infection.) Founded and funded by Lilly Drug company, this front group promotes the use of the company's expensive ($7,000 per treatment) drug, Drotrecogin Alfa, for sepsis. Yet most of the front group's board members have financial ties to Lilly and hence conflicts of interest. Other companies do the same. Using "editors" and "faculty" who all have financial ties to Pfizer, the *Lipid Letter* and the front group "Emerging Science of Lipid Management" are totally funded by Pfizer drug company to promote its statin drugs for treating lipid abnormalities (fat disturbances in blood). In all, there are three different "statin-education" groups that are funded, respectively, by Pfizer, Merck, and AstraZeneca to promote their company's products. While many charge these industry consultants with "financial conflicts of interest," the physicians involved respond that they are merely trying to "exploit a corrupt system in a way that benefits patients." They may be right. However, if they believe that "the end justifies the means," the physicians' corporate ties may be questionable. Obviously, such industry educational activities do much good, are essential to product promotion, and are not all suspect. The clear conflicts of interest, however, require citizens and especially physicians to be both well informed and on guard for biased science or private-interest science.[10]

Front groups are especially effective in promoting special interests because their goals and funding sources are not transparent and because they often dominate news media. Front-group employees typically appear to be merely independent experts, and few citizens realize their special-interest ties. As a result, media watchdog groups say that such front groups supply 28 percent of the experts on television news. Academics—less likely to have a particular commercial agenda—supply only 10 percent. Mostly journalists and politicians supply the remainder. One reason for the nearly three-to-one imbalance is that academics are busy teaching and doing research for peer-reviewed scientific publications. However, some companies pay front-group or think-tank employees extraordinarily well to do mainly media and promotional work, like PR pieces and TV "sound bites." In 2005, the business journal, *The Economist*, analyzed the top 10 companies (by revenues) in different developed nations.

In the United States, the top 10, Fortune-500 companies were Wal-Mart, Exxon-Mobil, General Motors, Ford Motors, General Electric, Chevron Texaco, ConocoPhillips, Citigroup, AIG, and IBM. Ranking the transparency of the business practices of the top 10 companies by nation, *The Economist* said the companies of Germany were most transparent, followed by those of France, then Britain. The United States was second to last, ahead of only Japan. The poor transparency among top U.S. corporations is explained partly by questionable U.S. accounting practices (like those that brought down Enron and WorldCom) and partly by the nontransparent front groups (like TASSC) that are covertly funded by many top U.S. companies. A 2002 *Harvard Business Review* article and the statistics in chapter 2 both suggest that special-interest funding virtually determines the conclusions reached by the scientific-sounding front groups. The result? Citizens probably have more difficulty fulfilling their rights to know and to consent to risks associated with the pollutants or products of companies such as Exxon, Ford, and General Electric.[11]

Besides front groups, misleading scientific or pollution-related information also sometimes comes from two other main sources: political-action committees and think tanks. Front groups and think tanks mainly produce agenda-driven research. Because political-action committees use this research to promote favored political candidates, they have government restrictions on donations. Front groups and think thanks are private and tax-exempt, like universities, but without students. They differ mainly in their types of research. Front groups do science favorable to the particular industry sponsoring them. Think tanks, however, do broader research designed to influence policy and to benefit many different groups, usually all from industry. Much think-tank research has been promoting free-market environmentalism, discussed in chapter 2. The Heritage Foundation, one of more than 100 Washington D.C. think tanks, is the wealthiest. With an annual budget of about $30 million, its research promotes industry deregulation, unrestrained markets, privatization of all government services, and selling off public lands, especially to oil and mining interests. Other prominent industry think tanks include the Cato Institute, the Reason Institute, and the American Enterprise Institute—all with this same agenda. As already mentioned, most think tanks represent industry, their major funder. Partly as a result, U.S. media surveys found that among newspaper, TV, and radio references to think tanks, those representing industry viewpoints were cited three times more often than were progressive or centrist groups.[12]

This is not to argue for censorship of front groups or think tanks. Rather, the point is lack of transparency and the need for supposed experts to clearly identify who pays them. When citizens hear these individuals on the evening news, they assume their views are representative and balanced by the views of other experts. Often, however, they are not. This lack of transparency is particularly acute when industry-funded think tanks sponsor research done by university professors who fail to report their industry ties. Since at least 1999, for example, University of Chicago attorney Cass Sunstein has written about 20 "working papers" for the industry-funded American Enterprise Institute.

Relying often on nonrefereed, industry-funded studies, Sunstein's articles promote the industry stances of free-market environmentalism, "the cost-benefit state," weakened environmental-health standards, and victims' being "willing to pay" for protection against pollution. Although these American Enterprise Institute articles appear in his books, Sunstein virtually never identifies his ties to the institute and his industry funding. Because he presents himself as merely a university professor, people likely are misled about his conflicts of interest and may give his views more credence than they deserve.[13]

While think tanks and other groups are important contributors to diversity of opinion, and while healthy democracies require such groups, Sunstein's case illustrates important ethical worries about conflicts of interest, lack of transparency, and resulting threats to rights to know and to consent. These threats are serious because the so-called scientific reports of front groups rarely meet strict university research and tenure requirements, ethical and scientific guidelines for federal grants, and standards for pre-publication scientific peer review. Think-tank and front-group research is thus often manipulated and agenda driven, but the public is mostly none the wiser.[14]

What is the solution? Full and clear identification of media experts' major funding sources, whenever they are cited or interviewed; active citizen education; deliberative democracy; and implementing reforms, like those discussed in chapter 6.

Capturing Private Charities

Health-related information can be manipulated in particularly subtle ways when special interests use their donations to influence private charities and professional health groups. Even medical organizations often are dependent on industry dollars to fund conferences, awards, and grants. In return, the companies receive advertising, information about society members, and special access to them.

- In behavior typical of many medical groups, the Society of Critical Care Medicine offers companies opportunities to pay for "sponsorship" of various society events like symposia. They also can put their logo on society tote bags, pens, lanyards, and so on.

- In exchange for a large financial payment to the American Academy of Pediatrics, the academy allowed the infant-formula manufacturer, Ross, to display its logo on the academy's pamphlet about breastfeeding. Physician-authors of the pamphlet argued that the academy had "sold itself to the highest bidder."

- When the American Gastroenterological Association produced an official pamphlet on heartburn, a majority of the authors were industry consultants for Wyeth Pharmaceuticals, a major manufacturer of gastroenterological drugs.

Similar conflicts of interest occur routinely with groups such as the American Heart Association; the American College of Cardiology; American Thoracic Society; the American Academy of Allergy, Asthma, and Immunology; the American College of Allergy, Asthma, and Immunology; the Endocrine Society; the American Society of Nephrology; and the American Psychiatric Association. In 2001, the American Medical Association recommended that physicians not accept gifts from any pharmaceutical companies. Physicians, however, mostly have not followed the AMA advice.[15]

Even when well-intentioned professionals begin health-related charities, sometimes they can be co-opted by special interests. Consider the International Foundation for Gastrointestinal Diseases, founded by patients to raise monies for gastrointestinal-disease research. Today, more than 90 percent of this foundation's income comes from 18 pharmaceutical companies, and a majority of the physicians planning foundation meetings have ties to drug companies producing gastrointestinal-disease products. Something similar happened with the American Obesity Association, a group founded by a University of Wisconsin researcher, Dr. Richard Atkinson. Today virtually all funding of this organization comes from diet-pill companies. One result? Instead of obesity prevention, Atkinson and the association now claim that diet drugs are needed because "diet, exercise, and behavior modification just don't work" to control obesity.[16]

In the area of pollution-induced disease, something similar has happened with the American Cancer Society (ACS). The society is a private charity, not to be confused with the National Cancer Institute (NCI), which is funded by taxpayers. As a private charity, the ACS has followed a path similar to that of the American Obesity Association. Now dependent on funding from the petrochemical industries, the ACS touts mainly drug treatment for cancer, not prevention. Partly as a result, physicians, the *Chronicle of Philanthropy*, and the *Wall Street Journal* criticize the ACS for being more interested in "accumulating wealth . . . than in saving lives." They claim that the ACS spends 52 percent of its national budget on executives' salaries, benefits, travel, and overhead; 32 percent on cancer-treatment drugs and research; and 16 percent on cancer services like taking patients to doctors.[17] In 10 states, including California, they claim the ACS spends 90 percent of its revenues on executives' salaries, benefits, and travel, but only 10 percent on cancer-related services. Critics say the ACS has been coopted, but donors do not realize it.[18]

These critics also say that the policy influence of ACS special-interest donors, like the tobacco industry, is even more worrisome. They claim that tobacco donors forced the ACS to downplay cigarette risks on at least two occasions. The ACS hired tobacco-related PR firms both to rewrite the ACS version of the National Cancer Act and to handle ACS voter-education campaigns in the 2000 U.S. presidential elections.[19] Critics also claim that large pharmaceutical, oil, and chemical-company donors—like Dupont and Conoco—each gives ACS hundreds of thousands of dollars annually, with similar effects on ACS cancer recommendations.[20] For instance, contrary to the chlorine warnings of the American Public Health Association, in 1992 the ACS and the chemical industry's Chlorine Institute issued a joint statement. It supported continued use of organochlorine pesticides, despite their long history of causing cancer. Critics also say the ACS used press releases, crafted by agrichemical-company experts, to downplay risks of food-borne pesticides. The director of the Agriculture Board of the NAS called this joint ACS–chemical-industry press release "unconscionable," a "conflict of interest."[21] Physicians likewise claim that for years, the ACS refused to join the March of Dimes, American Heart Association, and American Lung Association in supporting the Clean Air Act. Instead, they say, the ACS contradicts the WHO, NAS, NCI, and scientific consensus by calling risks from dietary pesticides, toxic-waste dumps, and ionizing radiation "negligible."[22]

Regarding foods and pharmaceuticals, physician-critics claim that the ACS

- Opposed the U.S. Food and Drug Administration (FDA) ban on saccharin and even advocates some saccharin use by infants and nursing mothers.

- Refused to testify at U.S. congressional hearings on banning the drug diethylstilbestrol or DES, even after its carcinogenicity was confirmed.

- Pressured the FDA to ease regulations on silicone-gel breast implants.

- Failed to follow U.S. Office of Technology Assessment directives to pursue information on 200 non-chemical treatments for cancer.

- Has issued many statements hostile to regulation of pollutants; has campaigned against the Delaney Amendment, which prohibits addition of carcinogens to food; and has opposed regulations on hair dyes known to cause liver and breast cancers.

- Has rejected laboratory tests and data on animal carcinogenicity, as sufficient for chemical regulation, and has demanded human studies; yet most human experiments are unethical, and many animal experiments accurately predict human risk.

- Allocates less than one-tenth of 1 percent of its approximately $700 million in revenues to addressing environmental carcinogenesis, yet claims to allocate four times as much.

- Largely ignores occupational and environmentally induced cancers.

- Claims that higher cancer rates among blacks are caused by poor diets and smoking, yet ignores the well-known fact that blacks have much higher pollution exposures.

Are these criticisms of the ACS merited? On the one hand, there is evidence that at least some of the criticized ACS policies have changed, as when it joined the American Lung Association in 2003 to promote a California tax on cigarettes. On the other hand, the criticisms have some plausibility because of their independent confirmation by individuals like those from NAS and because of ACS dependence on industry donors. Money talks. The criticisms also are consistent with earlier accounts of pharmaceutical-industry capture of private charities. The upshot? The ACS obviously does much good through its cancer services and research funding. But whenever wealthy polluters are major contributors to health-information groups, like the ACS, there is a potential for bias, in part because the public often is unaware of such funding and its potential significance.[23]

Hire Education and the Best Science Money Can Buy

One reason that polluters often fund private charities and university researchers is that they hope to gain something from them. Obviously, whenever their investments do not pay off, they do not continue funding. A typical example is tobacco-industry research. Multiple logistic-regression analyses (that control for article quality, peer-review status, topic, year, and so on) have conclusively shown its bias. The only factor associated with a scientific author's concluding that passive smoking is *not* harmful is affiliation with the tobacco industry. Something similar occurs in pollution-related research. After all, the vast majority of U.S. science is funded by special interests, often as "hire education" in which industry funds university research that both serves its corporate goals and influences the content of education. In 2003, the American Association for the Advancement of Science reported that roughly 75 percent of all U.S. scientific work is funded by industry ($300 billion). About 25 percent is funded by government, some of which also goes to universities. Because more than half of government science funding is military, for every $6 that private interests spend on science, the U.S. government spends about $1 for nonmilitary science. The American Association for the Advancement of Science estimates that for every $100 that industry spends on its science, environmental-health groups spend about $1. The result? Sometimes, it is the best science money can buy.[24]

Despite peer review, repeated instances show that private-interest science, often funded by "hire education," has found its way even into medical-science journals.

- In 1994, claiming the postpartum drug Parlodel caused strokes, the U.S.Food and Drug Administration (FDA) forced the drug company Sandoz (now Novartis) to recall it. Novartis, however, paid Dr. Baha Sabai of the University of Cincinnati about $20,000 per year to challenge the FDA findings. In lawsuits filed by patients, he repeatedly testified for Novartis. Even 5 years after the FDA ban, Sabai succeeded in publishing an article in the *American Journal of Obstetrics and Gynecology* in which he withheld information about his Novartis funding and used incomplete, nonreproducible, and purely "recollected" data, yet concluded that Parlodel did not cause postpartum strokes.[25]

- In 1994, Wyeth Pharmaceuticals paid a New Jersey firm $180,000 to write a scientific article promoting one of its drugs, to place it in a leading medical journal, and to get an academic author to put his name on it. The freelancer who wrote the article received $5,000. The university scientist, whose name appeared on the article, received $1,500.

- In 2002, medical researchers reported that the "going rate," for British psychiatrists to sign ghostwritten articles, was $2,000. For American psychiatrists it was $3,000–$10,000.

- One researcher found that, over a 5-year period, 50 percent of the medical-journal articles on the antidepressant Zoloft were ghostwritten.

- When there have been neither clinical trials nor FDA permission for new uses of existing drugs, pharmaceutical companies often avoid doing the costly trials. Instead, they pay physicians to sign their names to industry-ghostwritten articles that provide anecdotal evidence for "off-label" use of the drugs (for non-FDA-approved uses). Because the FDA allows doctors to prescribe off-label uses, this anecdotal evidence is used to encourage it.

- Warner-Lambert, later acquired by Pfizer, hired two marketing firms to ghostwrite articles alleging beneficial effects of off-label use of Neurontin, an epilepsy drug. Each firm received $12,000 per article. The doctors signing them each received $1,000. Yet no clinical trials were ever done. In May 2004, after pleading guilty to Medicaid fraud for paying tens of thousands of dollars to physicians to promote off-label use of Neurontin, Pfizer was forced to pay a fine of $430 million.

- Provigil is one prominent drug whose "off-label" use is currently being promoted. The FDA approved it only to treat narcolepsy. Yet without clinical trials, its manufacturer, Cephalon, is promoting it for a variety of psychiatric effects and simply for those who want something like amphetamines.

- Neurontin and Provigil are not isolated cases. A 1998 review in the *Journal of the American Medical Association* found that 30 percent of all articles in the six leading medical journals were either ghostwritten or had "honorary" authors—many to promote off-label use.

How can such private-interest science so dominate medical publications? The case of Regent Hospital Products' employee, Margaret Fay, provides an illustration. For decades, Fay helped design research protocols and edit Regent-funded research by university scientists. She also ghostwrote articles that she paid university scientists to sign. As late as 1999, Regent was still claiming that Fay held a doctorate from the University of Minnesota, a postdoc from Cornell University, a surgery professorship at the University of Virginia, and membership in the NAS and the American Academy of Sciences. By 2002, all of these claims had been proved false. One way to police ghostwriting and hire education, like the Fay case, is for journals to adopt guidelines requiring that authors disclose their funding sources and whether they materially participated in research bearing their names. As of 2006, however, most scientific and medical journals have not done so.[26]

Results of biased and agenda-driven science also sometimes appear in respected publications because the relevant research is done abroad, outside normal channels of scrutiny. Chemical companies, for instance, pay for drug and pesticide experiments in developing nations when they would not be allowed in the United States. Even in the United States, similar experiments may occur. The reason? Whenever special interests receive no federal-research funding, they are required to follow neither government medical-ethics requirements nor typical scientific peer review. As a result, polluters routinely use scientifically flawed, inadequately sensitive tests for environmentally induced harm. These are designed to produce false-negative results, conclusions that some pollutant is not harmful. In 2000, for instance, when the U.S. EPA Science Advisory Board analyzed pesticide-industry studies, it found all of them used too-small experimental samples, mostly under 50. Yet, as the board notes, a sample of 50 has only about a 4 percent chance of detecting some harmful effect. The board confirms that sample sizes should be at least 2,500. Even when these flawed studies do not survive peer review for good journals, why are they often used for industry PR and for determining regulations? One reason is that in 2000, U.S. president Bush reversed past precedents. He began allowing regulators to accept non-refereed, unpublished, small-sample, polluter-funded studies on humans. Examples include pesticide studies criticized by the 2000 EPA and Dow's dioxin experiments on prisoners in Pennsylvania. As late as 2005, companies like Dow were experimenting in California—paying college students to ingest chemical-warfare agents, used as pesticides, every day for 28 days. These flawed polluter studies are the analogue of anecdotal claims supporting off-label drug use. Both are paradigm cases of private-interest science.[27]

In part because of the 2005 California experiments by Dow, the U.S. Congress recently called for a moratorium on using ethically and scientifically questionable studies in government regulation. Nevertheless, biased private-interest science continues, partly because special interests want its results for PR. Polluters have been particularly successful at producing health-related promotional videos—used as news segments for TV. Typically, they pay others to claim these videos as their own, so no one knows their source. As a result, the vast majority of TV news stations in the United States—80 percent—cut reporting costs by using these special-interest clips as "news." While the Federal Communications Commission in 2005 required media owners to reveal the sources of their news clips, transparency remains a problem. Because the video clips are laundered and circulated via front groups, audiences rarely realize who produced the prepackaged "news" they present.[28]

Agenda-driven private-interest science also influences scientific and health-related higher education. After World War II, America built the world's greatest system of public higher education. Yet from 1991 to 2004, average taxpayer support for higher education declined from 74 percent to 64 percent. Since 2001, taxpayer support for public universities has declined more precipitously than at any time in the previous two decades. Experts warn that universities are being "privatized." At the University of Virginia, state taxpayers provide only about 8 percent of funding for higher education. At the University of Michigan, only 18 percent, and at the University of Illinois, only 25 percent. Instead, much university support now comes from corporate hire education and from universities themselves, setting up private companies to make profits on faculty discoveries. As of 2005, more than 100 U.S. medical schools and universities had set up their own internal "companies." The result? The public has lost some control over public education, public information, and public health.[29]

Hire education through corporation-university contracts began in earnest in 1974. Monsanto gave Harvard a hefty donation in exchange for some future patent rights and control over research. For providing only a few million dollars to one department at University of California, Berkeley, Novartis Pharmaceuticals gained control of all that department's patents. Hoecht Pharmaceuticals did the same in one department at Harvard. All these companies gained patent rights to at least some work funded only by taxpayers. At Duke, 31 percent of the research budget is from industry. At Georgia Tech and MIT, the figures are 21 and 20 percent, respectively. Even at lesser schools, similar effects are occurring. By 2000, 48 and 32 percent, respectively, of research budgets at Alfred University and the University of Tulsa were from outside industries. At Eastern Virginia Medical School and Lehigh University, the respective percentages were 24 and 22 percent. While such funding should not be abandoned, it requires ongoing ethical scrutiny. For one thing, hire education can coopt university researchers, the most likely group to challenge poor science done at the behest of special interests. After all, Gwen Pearson's comments in chapter 1 suggest that local universities did not criticize the flawed U.S. ATSDR and Indiana Department of Health studies because the professors had financial relationships with local polluters. Hire education also can threaten the open inquiry that is essential to scientific progress and to citizens' rights to know. Even important health-related information, generated in part by taxpayer dollars, can become part of "trade secrets." Consider that 92 percent of all biotech companies have financial relationships with university scientists, from whom 41 percent have gained trade secrets. In addition, 82 percent of companies have confidentiality requirements for professors, and 88 percent, for students. As chapter 2 illustrated, even deaths may result from these so-called trade secrets about pollutants and pharmaceuticals. Industry dollars also can turn university research toward private profits and away from student needs. They increase the probability that graduate students do research that funders want, not research that society, science, or their own training requires. The result? Hire education gives private interests partial control of public resources—resources needed to address public problems. As a consequence citizens often receive less environmental-health information than they need to protect themselves. Critics like Harvard's Richard Lewontin charge that hire education amounts to selling universities, society's intellectual capital, to the highest bidder. They say it amounts to a privatization of public resources.[30]

Even if Lewontin is wrong, hire education can manipulate the free flow of knowledge and therefore jeopardize both health and citizen consent to health risks. Consider what happened after a 1997 U.S. NCI study and a 2004 *Science* article showed that benzene causes much higher-than-recognized rates of cancer and other diseases, even at exposures below what is allowed. The industry-funded American Petroleum Institute immediately sprang into action. To challenge these prestigious results, the institute allocated $27 million for studies to be completed in 2007. Yet university scientists who accept this funding may not be doing purely disinterested science or serving public health. Instead, they are likely to be pursuing private-interest science. The institute says the research will be independent, but two factors suggest it may not be. One is the confidentiality agreement the institute requires. The other factor is that the oversight committee, required to approve all scientific-research protocols or methods, includes only oil-industry employees.[31]

Agenda-driven private-interest science also occurs in more subtle ways. Chemical companies often cultivate scientists and physicians with extravagant gifts, or with meals and vacations that are touted as educational seminars but are really advertisements for company products like drugs or pesticides. Scientists who cooperate with such tactics can receive lavish vacations and hefty "speaking fees" for touting company products or condoning company pollutants. And private-interest science often influences even the way many physicians learn about new drugs. Every year 87,000 scientifically untrained, U.S. pharmaceutical representatives visit doctors' offices to promote company drugs. Such arrangements have at least the appearance of conflicts of interest.[32]

Of course, ethical conflicts do not occur only among scientists and physicians who are paid by drug or chemical companies. Sometimes experts are paid by attorneys representing plaintiffs in class-action suits. When patients sued Wyeth Pharmaceuticals for heart damage from its drugs Pondimin and Redux, their law firm paid cardiologists to examine the plaintiffs' echocardiograms and to estimate heart-valve damage. Yet the pay of these consulting physicians was based on the level of damage they found. Not surprisingly, courts established that the physicians made unreasonable medical judgments. Recall the journal statistics mentioned in this chapter and chapter 2. They showed that, simply on the basis of who pays for a study, researchers typically can predict whether or not it finds particular drugs or products harmful.[33]

Obviously, abuses like private-interest science occur wherever great profits are at stake—for polluters or for the personal-injury attorneys who battle them. Merely because drug and chemical companies usually control far more money than personal-injury attorneys, however, their potential for scientific abuse appears greater. As chapter 2 revealed, these companies are among the highest-spending lobbyists in Washington, D.C. They also spend far more on campaign contributions and so-called educational programs than do attorneys.

Private-Interest Science

What do polluters want when they fund private-interest science, research designed to arrive at predetermined conclusions? Typically they want two things.

One is "false negatives"—conclusions that some pollutant is not harmful or is less harmful than thought. This is what the American Petroleum Institute research on benzene seeks. The other private-interest-science goal is to stigmatize public-health scientists who show that some pollutant is harmful.

The attack mode of private-interest science is typified by TASSC, the scientific front group, mentioned earlier, created and funded mainly by Philip Morris. This organization attacks what it calls "junk science"—which is defined not by its methods but by its conclusions. Studies alleging that tobacco smoke, pesticides, toxic chemicals, automobile emissions, asbestos, dioxin, or ionizing radiation are risky to health are called "junk science." Whenever *Science, Nature, Lancet*, the *Journal of the American Medical Association*, or other distinguished sources establish some health threat from pollutants like these, TASSC and the "junk science" lobbyists attack the science and the scientists. Yet they know they usually cannot debate the science and win. Instead, TASSC and its executive director, Steven Milloy, use two main PR strategies. Although they are industry funded, they use "plain folks" PR and claim to be a grassroots group that challenges "elitist" scientists. Using Milloy's "junk science" home page, rather than journals, they also employ the PR strategy (mentioned in chapter 2) of name-calling. Distinguished scientists are labeled "wackos," "blowhards," "food police," and so on. While such tactics may seem simplistic, they often succeed as PR. Partly this is because of polluter media influence. They also succeed because Milloy and TASSC help control powerful industry-funded front groups like the Cato Institute. Anyone who doubts the power of tobacco- and polluter-funded private-interest-science groups, like TASSC, should consider a 2005 article in the British medical journal, *Lancet*. It analyzes tobacco-industry research published as late as 2000 in the journal *Mutagenesis*. Lancet notes that in 1996, a landmark NCI study showed why cigarette smoke causes cells to grow into tumors. It damages p53, the tumor-suppressor gene whose injury has been implicated in more than 50 percent of all cancers. Denying this molecular and genetic confirmation, the tobacco industry claims the relationship between smoking and cancer is "just a statistical association." It also pays researchers, like David Cooper and Thilo Paschke, to challenge the NCI results. Cooper has received 5 years of tobacco-industry monies, and Paschke is a longtime tobacco-institute employee. They published their articles in *Mutagenesis* in 1998 and 2000. Unknown to readers, however, *Mutagenesis* was edited by a scientist, James Perry, whom the tobacco industry had funded for 15 years. Yet none of the three scientists disclosed their industry funding. It was unearthed only years later. While some scientific journals, like *Nature*, now require authors to reveal their sources of funding, as already mentioned, most journals do not. This laxness makes the 2005 *Lancet* case worrisome for several reasons. (1) The three scientists' conflicts of interest were discovered by accident, long after publication. (2), The $206-billion 1998 master-settlement of tobacco lawsuits, brought by 46 states to pay the costs of smoking-related health care, has not taught tobacco companies their lesson. They continue to fund private-interest science. (3) Because conflicts of interest are typical wherever great profits are at stake, some other wealthy polluters also produce private-interest science. (4) While 85 percent of *British Medical Journal* readers say universities should not accept tobacco-industry research monies, because the sole purpose of such research is to confuse and to delay "bad news," most universities still do so. As already mentioned, the authors of one-third of refereed medical publications have financial stakes in their results, and one-third are ghostwritten. Three-fourths of science generally is agenda driven and funded by private interests. As much as 60 percent of research funding at some universities, like Carnegie-Mellon, comes from outside groups—many of whom want specific scientific conclusions. As the authors of the 2005 *Lancet* article warned, polluting industries often use private-interest-science funding "to promote confusion rather than enlightenment." The result? Citizens are less likely to recognize threats to their health and to their rights to know.[34]

Most citizens know that one ought not use a flashlight to look for electrons. They are less able to recognize typical private-interest-science bias or misuse of scientific methods. One typical polluter bias is using the wrong tests, models, or data—so as to underestimate harmful effects of some product or pollutant. Another bias is using small samples or short-term studies, both of which produce scientific tests that typically are not sensitive enough to detect some harmful effect. A third private-interest-science strategy is relying on theoretical estimates of harm instead of actually measuring harmful effects. A fourth bias is failing to do uncertainty analyses of one's results—tests that would reveal their degree of reliability. A fifth common strategy is to demand human experiments, as a precondition for regulating pollutants, although such studies often are prohibited on ethical grounds. As a result, polluters can avoid regulations by alleging that no human data (only animal and other laboratory studies) show their pollutants are harmful.

Illustrating the first private-interest-science bias, chapter 1 began with the story of tragic childhood cancer cases in Hammond, Indiana. Because government and company toxicologists used the wrong data and methods, they drew false-negative conclusions. Their data were from nonresidential areas, upwind of the polluting facility. Their flawed methods also diluted local pollutant effects by analyzing only average cancer incidences and county-wide data. Similar private-interest-science biases occurred when U.S. Department of Energy (DOE) contractors assessed the proposed Yucca Mountain, Nevada, site for nuclear-waste storage. Scientists agree that the main route of radioactive leakage from the site will be through groundwater. Yet when DOE contractors predicted groundwater flow, they underestimated resulting radioactive contamination because they used the wrong models—porous-media models. These models give reliable results only when a site has uniform geological strata, no water flow through fractures, no springs, and no perched groundwater. None of these conditions is met at Yucca Mountain. As a result, DOE incorrectly predicted that the Nevada dump would be safe for the million years required by federal law.[35]

A second common private-interest-science bias is using small sample sizes (or what statisticians call "low-power" studies) or only short-term studies. To see why this strategy virtually guarantees underestimates of harmful effects, suppose a particular dose of a pollutant causes one additional cancer every 3 years, per 1,000 people exposed. If scientists conduct only a year-long test on 50 people, obviously not all damaging effects will appear. As the earlier discussion revealed, the U.S. EPA says such short-term, small-sample studies are typical of chemical-industry–funded studies of pesticide harm. These "sample sizes of 7–50 subjects" have only a "3–4 percent chance of finding any [negative] effect." Small samples also are one reason that private-interest science, done to investigate damage from the 1986 Chernobyl nuclear accident, underestimated health effects. The International Atomic Energy Agency initially conducted a study only several months long, in only several very mildly contaminated villages, chosen by the Soviet leaders. As a result, the agency said the accident caused no known cancers, but some thyroid cancers might appear in the future. Yet radiobiologists know that cancers can take up to 40 years to appear; that dozens of cancers—from bone cancers to leukemias—are caused by radiation; and that short-term, small-sample studies of mildly contaminated villages allowed no reliable conclusions. Yet the International Atomic Energy Agency mentioned none of these facts. As happened in Hammond, Indiana, the agency confused the *absence of evidence* (for harm) with *evidence for the absence* (of harm). This also is what Dupont did, when it sought to profit by avoiding regulation of formaldehyde. Using too-small samples, Dupont erroneously concluded that formaldehyde was harmless. Even if formaldehyde actually caused a doubling of some cancer rates, Dupont knew that its too-small sample sizes offered only an absence of evidence. They had only a 4 percent chance of detecting this doubling.[36]

A third private-interest-science tactic is using purely theoretical models or estimates, rather than empirical data, to support some claim, and then presenting these estimates as science. A relevant example is the 2005 recommendations of the International Commission on Radiological Protection. As its sole basis for (non-human) environmental-radiation protection, the commission endorses a two-step monitoring method. First, although it admits radiation-dose effects are unknown for most species, and all species' internal doses are unknown, the commission bases environmental monitoring solely on estimated radiation doses to several self-chosen "reference species." Providing neither a list nor a definition of reference species, instead the commission claims they should have "political significance." Second, the commission tells scientists to use these estimated reference-species doses to estimate radiation doses for all other species. As such, these two-step recommendations are arbitrary and susceptible to manipulation by the very groups—radioactive polluters—who do virtually all radiation monitoring. Instead of relying on direct, easy, reliable, and inexpensive *measurements* of air and water contamination—the early warning system for radioactive contamination—the commission recommends indirect, unreliable biotic *estimates* of dose. Instead of relying on dose estimates for known species, the commission recommends using only some, arbitrarily chosen, reference species. Yet radiation-dose effects can vary among species by three orders of magnitude. Instead of recommending ecosystem monitoring, the commission ignores ecosystem contamination. Instead of relying on scientific journals to defend its recommendations, the commission relies on "gray" science (unpublished work done by special interests). The result of all these private-interest-science flaws? The commission recommendations promote radiation protection based on arbitrary dose estimates, not actual exposure measurements. They make it easier for polluters to use estimates to cover up health threats, to thwart risk disclosure, and to jeopardize citizens' rights to give or withhold consent. Not surprisingly, the past president of the commission admitted that desires to reduce nuclear-cleanup costs, not science, were driving the 2005 estimate-, rather-than-measurement-, based radiation protections.[37]

Of course, in some scientific applications—like predicting the safety of million-year, hazardous-waste disposal—complete measurements are not possible. Here scientists must use estimates. They do so in scientifically credible ways when they check their estimates through uncertainty analysis. (As used here, "uncertainty" is a parameter that is associated with the result of some measurement and that characterizes the different values that could reasonably be attributed to what is measured. "Uncertainty analysis" refers to a set of systematic procedures—descriptive and inferential statistics—to determine and to estimate quantitatively the uncertainty introduced into the results of some mathematical model as a result of the cumulative effects of data variability and uncertainties in the input data. Uncertainty analysis tries to account for both random error and bias in the measurement process.) In a nutshell, uncertainty analysis provides credible limits to the accuracy of some reported value or model result. Proponents of private-interest science, however, typically neglect uncertainty analysis and thus fall into a fourth bias. The 2005 report of the International Commission on Radiological Protection, just discussed, recommends no uncertainty analyses. Indeed, when I (as the U.S. representative on the commission's seven-person international committee responsible for recommending environmental-radiation standards) asked that the document recommend performing uncertainty analysis, my proposal was rejected. Instead, the committee chair simply removed the document's admission that radiation-dose estimates need include no uncertainty analyses.[38]

This fourth private-interest-science problem—failing to do uncertainty analyses or to check one's estimates against actual empirical data—occurs even in pollution-related research done at premier institutions. For instance, MIT scientists relied on their largely theoretical nuclear-accident calculations, ignored relevant government nuclear-accident data, and then erroneously concluded nuclear risks were low. Their biased and largely theoretical nuclear risk assessment (the Rasmussen Report, also known as WASH 1400), funded by the U.S. government, is significant for three reasons. (1) It undergirds all U.S. claims of nuclear-reactor safety and thus has massive policy implications. (As mentioned in chapter 2, its predicted lifetime-core-melt probability for all U.S. nuclear reactors is about one in five. Indeed, a U.S. core melt has already occurred, in the 1979 Three Mile Island nuclear accident.) (2) The American Physical Society has suggested that this largely theoretical MIT report may have underestimated nuclear-accident probabilities and resulting deaths. These underestimates would have been less likely if the authors had not ignored nuclear-accident data from actual operating experience of U.S. reactors. (3) Because this MIT report ignored relevant empirical data, Dutch researchers have shown that it has massive overconfidence biases. That is, it underestimates nuclear risks and overestimates nuclear safety. It has the hall-marks of private-interest science. The Dutch obtained U.S.-reactor accident data and compared them with the MIT study's theoretical predictions of the same events. The Dutch conclusion? Actual occurrence rates—of *all* seven types of nuclear accidents studied—were outside the 90 percent confidence bands predicted by the MIT study. That is, for all the types of U.S. nuclear accidents that have already occurred, the MIT authors said they had only a 10 percent chance of happening. Funded by supporters of the technol-ogy being assessed, the MIT study exhibits typical biases of private-interest science. Such risk assessments routinely underestimate risk by four-to-six orders of magnitude. One culprit behind such underestimates? Failure to use either empirical data or uncertainty analyses to check theoretical estimates.[39]

Despite the obvious and elementary errors arising from not checking theoretical estimates either against the facts or through uncertainty analysis, this fourth bias of private-interest science continues. Consider the science used by the U.S. government, in perhaps the most ambitious and potentially dan-gerous nuclear project ever undertaken. This is the attempt to store lethal radioactive wastes underground for the next million years at Yucca Moun-tain, Nevada. Obviously, there are no million-year safety data for such a project. Consequently the DOE endorses largely theoretical radiation-risk calculations. Yet the DOE has failed both to perform uncertainty analyses on its estimates and to reveal that it has not performed them. Instead, DOE continues to make optimistic safety predictions about the dump. In 2001, when an international group of nuclear-industry representatives, from the International Atomic Energy Agency, used DOE's own dose numbers, from DOE's own reports, to check their reliability through uncertainty analyses, the results were damning. The agency said DOE's estimates of radiation doses were uncertain by 9 to 12 orders of magnitude—uncertain by a factor of up to a trillion. Yet even if DOE's *radiation-worker* dose estimates were only 100 (not a trillion) times too low, these doses would be enough to kill people. If DOE's *public*-dose estimates were only 1,000 (not a trillion) times too low, they also could kill people. Unfortunately, as this and the preceding chapter revealed, this DOE use of misleading, nonempirical methods may be typical. As noted earlier, DOE has falsified Yucca Mountain data. Its con-tractors also have repeatedly claimed to have "verified" and "validated" their low-risk conclusions about Yucca Mountain. They say "evidence indicates that the Yucca Mountain repository site would be in compliance with reg-ulatory requirements." But DOE's so-called verification and validation is merely using unchecked estimates, just as it did in the International Atomic Energy Agency fiasco. By "verification" and "validation," DOE scientists mean only that their theoretical computer models of the site are internally consistent. They mean neither that uncertainty analyses confirm their results, nor that empirical data show them to be factually accurate. The result? Such private-interest science can put citizens' lives and human rights at risk.[40]

Private-Interest Science: Diverting Attention from Pollution

Particularly in evaluating health effects of dangerous chemicals, private-interest science often falls victim to a fifth biased strategy, a diversionary tactic employed by many industry front groups and typified by the work of University of California geneticist Bruce Ames. Ames and many industry-funded scientists like Elizabeth Whelan—president of the industry front group, the American Council on Science and Health—employ this tactic. They say that animal testing of pollutants often is unreliable, that many foods are naturally carcinogenic, that people cause many of their own cancers through behaviors like smoking, and that human epidemiological data on cancers is limited. Consequently, they claim, human-caused pollution should not be regulated more strictly.[41] As even the statement of this four-part argument reveals, it is more rhetoric than logic. The remainder of this chapter addresses each part of this private-interest-science argument, showing how it errs.

Consider first the claim that because animal studies for assessing carcinogenicity are merely "speculative," regulators should use "epidemiological evidence in humans."[42] *On the positive side,* Ames and front-group scientists like Whelan are partly right. Correctly performed, human epidemiological studies rarely go wrong. In a world in which delayed regulations never imposed health costs on innocent people, one could always wait for human epidemiological studies before regulating pollutants. *On the negative side,* Ames and others are partly wrong. They demand human epidemiological data before regulating, but ignore the fact that delayed regulations can harm people. Recall the example in chapter 1 of how the WHO says that delaying air-pollution regulations for 50 years has annually caused hundreds of thousands of avoidable deaths. The WHO claim suggests that, at worst, demanding human studies, prior to regulation, is a very dangerous public-health position. At best, it is appropriate only for a perfect world where delay never kills people. But justice delayed is justice denied, especially when delay can kill people. Demanding human epidemiological studies before regulating some pollutant, even after animal studies show likely harm, also errs in at least six scientific and ethical ways. These private-interest-science errors rely on misunderstanding medical ethics, the burden of proof, ethical responsibility, harmful opportunity costs, practicality, and ethical reasonableness.

In claiming that human epidemiological tests are always essential to regulation of pollutants, the first, or *medical-ethics,* error demands human guinea pigs. Yet most pollution experiments on humans would be condemned on grounds of medical ethics, just as Dow's 2005 pesticide experiments in California were condemned. It is unethical to deliberately expose people to substances known to be harmful. By assuming that pollution regulation requires

human experimentation, Ames and others thus presuppose an ethically questionable stance. They beg the question against regulation, both by requiring
evidence that often ought not be obtained, and by rejecting animal and laboratory evidence that has already been used to assess harm. They also ignore
the role of explanation in science. When scientists have experimentally established that a certain class of chemicals is of type X, they have explained
something. They know that because chemicals in class X have a certain structure, therefore those chemicals will have particular properties or effects.
Whenever they discover a new chemical in this same class X, they do not
assume they know nothing about it. Nor do they demand all new tests on this
new chemical, before drawing any conclusions or considering any regulations
about it. Instead, they rely on their earlier experimentally established explanations about the structure and effects of chemicals in this class, at least until
those earlier explanations are proved wrong. Those who require human studies
for all regulations are like those who require all new tests for some chemical
that already is known to be in class X. If they were right, science would be
reduced to case-by-case "bean counting," rather than principled explanation.
Medical ethics would be reduced to a guinea-pig approach, doing nothing
until dead bodies started to appear.[43]

Ames and others err in a second way in their private-interest-science demand for human studies for regulation. They assume that when harm from
pollutants is controversial, the most vulnerable people, like childhood victims
of pollution, should bear the burden of proof. Yet no reasonable ethics justifies
placing the burden of proof on innocent victims. Indeed, two basic ethical
principles are to take precautions and to protect the innocent and the vulnerable. To do anything else is merely expedient, not ethical. Virtue ethics, in
particular, recognizes that precaution, benevolence, and care are necessary
for being a moral person. It is not benevolent to claim polluters can pollute, to
ignore animal and laboratory evidence of harm, but then to place a heavy
evidentiary burden on pollution victims until harm to humans is obvious.
This stance would be like allowing hunters to shoot anywhere at will, without
reasonable assurance that no people were in their paths. If hunters ought not
ignore evidence for possible human harm, like movement in nearby brush,
polluters ought not ignore evidence like animal or laboratory data. Besides,
ignoring such data unfairly assumes that pollution victims must meet a scientific standard that polluters themselves never meet. Polluters have never funded
(or at least have never made public) a multiple-decades-long epidemiological
study, with thousands of human subjects, to assess full health effects of some
product or pollutant. Yet Ames and industry researchers require that unless
pollution victims do so, they ought not to seek protective regulations. They
also require the relevant human proof to be only the most difficult, long-term,
and costly kind—epidemiological proof. Yet pollution victims typically are
more vulnerable and have less knowledge, money, and political power than
polluters. Because of their vulnerability and the probable harm from pollutants, ethics requires both taking precautions and having the "deep-pocket"
polluters bear the heavier evidentiary burden.[44]

A third ethical problem with the private-interest-science demand for long-term, large-sample, human epidemiological data, before regulating, is that it ignores ethical responsibility. Polluters typically profit from polluting activities. Their *rights* to pollution-related economic *benefits*, however, presuppose their corresponding *responsibilities* for the pollution-related *costs* they impose on others. This rights-responsibilities principle is fundamental to all accounts of human rights, deontological (or duty-based) ethics, and contractarian ethics (ethics based on contracts, promises, and treating people consistently). All law likewise is premised on equal treatment, equal rights, and corresponding equal responsibilities. That is why people have rights to their property, for instance, provided they use it in responsible, rather than harmful, ways. Their property rights end where other people's equal rights to protection begin. Ignoring this rights-responsibilities principle, Ames and others forget that if animal data suggest that some pollutant is seriously harmful, scientists have ethical responsibilities not to ignore these data. They should either accept them and reduce pollutants or show why the animal data are wrong. To do anything else, as Ames proposes, is expedient rather than ethically responsible.[45]

A fourth ethical problem with demanding human data before regulating pollutants is that it could lead to harmful consequences. Even the most basic utilitarian ethics requires that people act so as to minimize the harmful, and maximize the beneficial, consequences of their actions. Therefore, if animal or laboratory evidence shows some pollutant is potentially harmful, even utilitarian ethics requires that this probability of harm be taken into account. Utilitarian ethics requires people to calculate the expected utility of their acts: the *magnitude* of harmful or beneficial consequences times the *probability* that each of those consequences may occur. In demanding human studies but rejecting animal and laboratory studies before regulating pollutants, Ames and others violate utilitarian ethics because they ignore the probabilities of human harm suggested by animal harm.[46]

When Ames and others require human epidemiological tests before regulating pollutants, they also err in economic and practical ways. They set the bar too high. Epidemiological testing is extraordinarily expensive and impractical, given the large sample sizes and long time periods required. This is why less than 1 percent of all hazardous substances has been tested epidemiologically. Instead, government relies mainly on controlled laboratory testing of animals. By demanding human tests, Ames uses economics in a way that again begs the ethical question against regulation.

A final problem with requiring human evidence of harm, before regulating some pollutant, is that it is unreasonable. Ethics requires only what reasonable people would agree to do. Although Ames and others assume that only human epidemiological evidence is adequate to justify regulation, reasonable people often make decisions based instead on the preponderance of evidence. They do not demand only the most difficult-to-obtain evidence. They do not wait for flawless evidence before acting. Reasonable people don't wait until they see flames to call the Fire Department. They call when they smell smoke.

Reasonable people don't go to the doctor only when they are ill. Instead they get annual checkups. Reasonable people don't carry umbrellas only when it is raining. Instead they carry them even when it looks like rain. Reasonable people do not do nothing, merely because their evidence is not infallible. When lives are at stake, they make the best decision they can, based on the preponderance of evidence. What does the preponderance of evidence say about animal tests for human carcinogenesis? As Princeton University risk assessor Adam Finkel, most biostatisticians, and repeated NAS panels point out, human and animal tests for carcinogenicity are "highly correlated." In fact, they say there are no legitimate scientific tests showing that rodent carcinogens are not also human carcinogens. Besides, tests used to deny human carcinogenicity all employ small samples from which no reliable conclusions can be drawn. If anything, says Finkel, animal tests sometimes may underestimate cancer risks to humans. Why? The tests are performed on adolescent to late-middle-age animals rather than on neonatal animals, which are far more sensitive to carcinogens. For all these reasons, reasonable people do not reject animal testing as inadequate for all public-health decision-making.[47]

Framing the Questions, Controlling the Answers

This reasonableness problem illustrates perhaps the worst ethical flaw in the arguments of those who demand human testing before regulating pollutants. They frame an ethical debate as if it were purely scientific. While claiming to do science, they propose a default rule for behavior under uncertainty. "When laboratory and animal data suggest harm, do not regulate to try to prevent harm, while doing further testing. Instead, avoid all regulations until human epidemiological testing is complete." Yet precisely because this rule dictates default behavior for situations of uncertainty, it is an ethical rule. The previous section suggests that it also is a flawed ethical rule. Nevertheless, scientists like Ames use their scientific authority as a bully pulpit from which to preach this ethical rule. They should be wary of doing so, particularly when they are untrained in ethics, when their ethics can have life-threatening consequences, and when their views may dominate something—ethical decisionmaking—that is mainly the prerogative of the people. Despite Ames's scientific brilliance, he appears to have used his considerable scientific stature outside his area of expertise, just as Nobel Prize–winner Richard Shockley has done. Using his scientific renown as inventor of the transistor, Shockley overstepped the limits of his scientific expertise when he claimed that blacks were deficient in intelligence. Both Shockley and Ames appear to confuse their own scientific prerogatives with other people's rights, particularly stakeholders' rights to consent to risks that others wish to impose on them.

The final sections of this chapter investigate four important ways in which Ames and private-interest-science proponents confuse science and ethics. Claiming to do science, they tacitly presuppose four questionable ethical "frames" for discussing pollution and public-health problems. (1) They commit the naturalistic fallacy by dismissing pollution risks as insignificant as compared to natural risks. (2) Ignoring conflicts of interest, they emphasize cancer cures rather than also prevention. (3) Confusing the absence of evidence (for harm) with evidence of absence (of harm), they frequently "blame the victim" for cancer. (4) Ignoring justice and human rights to life, they call for more analysis, rather than regulation of pollutants.

Ames, Natural Carcinogens, and the Naturalistic Fallacy

One of the most questionable ethical frames used by proponents of private-interest science is the naturalistic fallacy. Bruce Ames and industry front-group scientists like Elizabeth Whelan emphasize "natural" chemicals in food, like the mold in peanuts. Claiming that threats from natural carcinogens far outweigh those from synthetic ones, they argue against additional chemical regulation. Ames claims regulation "will not appreciably reduce cancer rates." His argument is the same one that appears in much industry-funded private-interest science, like the magazine *Priorities*. Funded by the chemical-industry front group, the American Council on Science and Health, *Priorities* claims that pollutants present "trivial" risks compared to higher-priority risks like "natural" carcinogens.[48] While Ames and industry-funded scientists are correct to emphasize natural carcinogens, they err ethically in drawing anti-regulatory conclusions from observations about these natural carcinogens. They commit the naturalistic fallacy, ignore fairness and human rights, and sanction utilitarianism.

What is the naturalistic fallacy? Labeled more than a century ago by British ethicist G. E. Moore, it consists of either of two main errors. The general error is attempting to reduce ethics to science. The more specific error is defining something as good because it is natural.[49] In Ames's case, he commits the fallacy in the first or more general sense. He attempts to reduce the *ethical* question, of equitable regulations for human-produced chemicals, to the *scientific* question of how many deaths arise from natural versus synthetic chemicals. He assumes that because foods have many dangerous natural pesticides, synthetic pesticide risks are not problematic. This is like saying that because so many people "naturally" die in automobile accidents, it is ethical to knowingly cause another death. Those who commit the naturalistic fallacy err partly because they assume that ethics is merely a "numbers game"— harming fewer people than are harmed naturally. Yet whatever is natural, like a deadly tornado or premature death from a genetic defect, is not necessarily desirable. If it were, there would be no ethics, only Social Darwinism. For people following a naturalistic numbers game, there would be rampant discrimination, what John Stuart Mill called "the tyranny of the majority." Instead, ethics demands equal treatment, not just what benefits the majority. In reducing fairness and human rights to a numbers game, Ames and others forget that ethics requires avoiding harm, especially easily preventable harm. Whenever one cannot avoid doing harm, fairness requires compensating victims. This is why neoclassical economics recognizes principles of compensation for risk. Adam Smith warned that risky jobs should be given to workers, for instance, only if they received additional "hazard pay." Otherwise, he emphasized that market transactions would not be efficient. Ames and front-group scientists, however, ignore all these foundational ethical and economic truths and instead resort to the rhetoric of mere numerical comparisons.

They also ignore the fact that, regardless of whether U.S. pollution-induced-cancer deaths are 10 percent of total cancer fatalities (60,000 annually) or not, ethics requires that people never consider any lives expendable. Consequently, it is ethically worse for polluters seeking profits to deliberately allow a few pollution victims to die than it is for many more people to die, simply because they chose to smoke or to use alcohol. The first case is worse because it involves known and deliberate imposition of harm; because it involves some people's harming others, not themselves; because that harm brings benefits mainly to polluters but not to their victims; and because the polluters themselves do not pay the full costs of their actions. Ignoring such basic ethical points of fairness reduces ethics to expediency.

In illegitimately comparing natural and synthetic carcinogens, Ames and front-group scientists like Whelan likewise err in ignoring the fundamental ethical principle of informed consent, discussed in chapter 2. Comparing apples to oranges, they assume that harms from *involuntarily imposed* or *societal* risks, like pollution, are no worse than harms from *voluntarily chosen* or *personal* risks, like failure to exercise. This is as ethically erroneous as reducing murder to manslaughter. Pollution and personal risks are ethically irreducible partly because of consent, the most fundamental principle of medical ethics and of democratic government. If people do not consent, pollution cannot be imposed on them just because its consequences are smaller than other risks they choose to bear and just because others benefit from this pollution. Otherwise, society could impose unfair burdens on people, so long as the imposed burdens were smaller than those borne naturally, or chosen because of their benefits. Otherwise, society could sanction environmental injustice—imposing pollutants on people for purely arbitrary reasons, such as where they live or the color of their skin. Such impositions also would violate distributive justice—justice in allotting common societal goods like clean air or risk protection. Why do Ames and others make all these ethical errors? In dismissing risks of synthetic chemicals, just because they supposedly cause fewer cancers than natural carcinogens, they forget that overall number of deaths is not the main issue. The main issue is not science, but justice—fairness in how those deaths are imposed, fairness in who receives benefits, and who bears burdens. As chapter 1 revealed, cancer incidence in children is rising annually at a rate 40 percent higher than for adults. Most physicians and health agencies say the culprit is environmental pollutants. Even if environmental cancers were small in numbers, their disproportionate imposition on children, minorities, and poor people—and on those whose rights to know and to consent have not been fulfilled—would demand their reduction.[50]

In framing the pollution debate with the naturalistic fallacy, Ames and others trivialize harmful actions (from which polluters benefit) and ignore classical ethical principles about what makes acts moral versus immoral. Previous paragraphs show that they ignore distinctions between unavoidable versus avoidable, compensated versus uncompensated, unintended versus intended, profit-neutral versus profit-generating, equitably versus inequitably distributed, voluntarily chosen versus involuntarily imposed, and adult-borne versus child-borne risks. Their version of the naturalistic fallacy attempts to reduce ethics to science, justice to mere body counts.

Conflicts of Interest, Ounces of Prevention

Another frame of private-interest science—one that also trivializes pollution risks—is emphasizing cancer "cures" while largely ignoring pollution prevention. Physicist Albert Einstein recognized the problem with this frame when he said that clever people solve problems, but wise people avoid them. Obviously diseases like cancer require cures, but the problem with this "cure" frame occurs when scientists ignore the massive environmental causes of cancer. Funded by polluters, some scientists who promote the "cure" frame also have obvious conflicts of interest. Their positions help generate both their own and their funders' profits.

Like the ACS, discussed earlier, AstraZeneca, the chemical-industry sponsor of Breast Cancer Awareness Month, touts the "cure" frame, in part because of its conflicts of interest.[51] Yet cancer is rarely "cured." More often, it is "in remission." Hidden behind the pink ribbons that accompany most Breast Cancer Awareness Month literature is a well-orchestrated PR program, begun in 1984, in which a major polluter has confused the public about cancer. The originator and sole funder of Breast Cancer Awareness Month is AstraZeneca. A subsidiary of Imperial Chemicals, a multinational manufacturer, AstraZeneca produces many chlorinated chemicals that cause breast cancer. Just from one of its carcinogenic herbicides, acetochlor, AstraZeneca makes hundreds of millions of dollars annually.[52] It also manufactures the world's top-selling anticancer and anti-breast-cancer drug, Tamoxifen. In addition, it promotes healthy women's taking Tamoxifen, which is highly carcinogenic itself, for supposed prevention of breast cancer. It thus profits from partly causing, treating, and allegedly preventing, breast cancer. By sponsoring Breast Cancer Awareness Month and controlling its copyright, AstraZeneca internationally promotes the "cure" frame and diverts attention from pollution prevention. It also controls all breast-cancer information used by groups that join Breast Cancer Awareness Month, sponsor related events, or distribute pink-ribbon literature. Dominating global breast-cancer information, AstraZeneca tells women their best cancer protection is mammography and funding research for a "cure." Its trademark slogan is "Early detection is your best prevention." Yet once cancer is detected, it is too late for prevention. All the program's promotional materials "studiously avoid any reference to the wealth of information on avoidable causes and prevention of cancer," except for promoting mammography. In particular, there is never any mention of chlorinated chemicals, like AstraZeneca's herbicides, that have been implicated since the 1960s in breast cancer.[53]

Even AstraZeneca's promoting mammography for cancer "prevention" involves financial conflicts of interest. AstraZeneca manages cancer centers in 11 U.S. hospitals, all of which do mammography. It owns a 50-percent stake in them, known collectively as Salick Health Care. And although mammography provides early cancer detection, it is controversial because radiation sometimes contributes to cancer yet provides little improvement in five-year survival, after cancer diagnosis. Some physicians also claim that chemotherapy like AstraZeneca's Tamoxifen saves only 2–3 percent of cancer victims.[54] Alleging that chemotherapy generally "has not had much overall effect" on cancer,[55] they are even more critical of using Tamoxifen as a breast-cancer preventive. The reason? Tamoxifen is chemically similar to the uterine carcinogen diethylstilbestrol (DES). AstraZeneca's own clinical trials on 16,000 healthy women show it is a uterine and liver carcinogen. Yet the consent form for healthy women, who are given Tamoxifen as a breast-cancer preventive, essentially says the drug is safe and even beneficial.[56] AstraZeneca says it prevents 17 breast cancers in every 1,000 healthy women who take it for 5 years. What AstraZeneca typically does not say is that for every 1,000 women who take it, Tamoxifen also causes an additional 8 uterine cancers, 2 liver cancers, 10 potentially fatal blood clots, and increased strokes and cataracts.[57]

The point here is not scientific. It is not whether mammography is beneficial or whether Tamoxifen helps treat or prevent cancer. The ethical point is that, despite the good accomplished by AstraZeneca and Breast Cancer Awareness Month, both are involved in major financial conflicts of interest of which the public is largely unaware. As a result, citizens likely are misled, both about some of the causes of cancer and about some of the most effective ways of preventing it, through pollution reduction. As a consequence of this misinformation, citizens are less likely to be able to fulfill their rights to know and to give or withhold consent to mammography, Tamoxifen, herbicide use, and the whole cure-rather-than-pollution-prevention cancer strategy. People need to know that Breast Cancer Awareness Month is more about chemical-industry PR than about accurate medical information. They need to be able to decide whether to wear pink ribbons and take part in a local "Race for the Cure," or to spend their time promoting a phase-out of chlorine chemicals, as the American Public Health Association (APHA) recommended. AstraZeneca does not give people full information about this choice because it does not fully disclose its conflicts of interest.

Although they do so less directly than sponsors of Breast Cancer Awareness Month, Oxford epidemiologists Richard Doll and Richard Peto likewise seem to promote the "cancer-cure" rather than also the "pollution-prevention" frame, perhaps because of their conflicts of interest. Both have been funded by U.S. and United Kingdom petrochemical companies like Dow and Monsanto, by General Motors, and by the leading United Kingdom asbestos corporation. Because both repeatedly deny evidence that pollutants like petrochemicals cause cancer, they indirectly promote a "cancer-cure" rather than also a "pollution-prevention" paradigm. Despite Doll's superb early research on smoking and carcinogenesis, critics say he has fallen into both conflicts of interest and scientific error. They claim that as a consultant to General Motors, he testified that exposure to lead from leaded gasoline was not harmful to children. As a consultant to the leading United Kingdom asbestos manufacturer, he testified that low-level exposure to asbestos was safe. Supporting Dow and Monsanto, he denied dioxin risks and testified in court against Vietnam veterans who claimed dioxin harm from Agent Orange. He rejected EPA, *New England Journal of Medicine,* and other studies claiming that dioxin is the most potent carcinogen ever evaluated. Doll also ignored NAS warnings about dioxin threats to veterans and the fact that industry itself paid Vietnam veterans hundreds of millions of dollars in settlements. Critics likewise say that, even after the NCI and NAS said the opposite, in 1998 Doll denied that above-ground U.S. nuclear-weapons tests had caused leukemias and bone cancers among atomic veterans. Speaking on behalf of the chemical industry, Doll denied massive scientific-journal evidence linking vinyl-chloride exposure and brain cancer, as occurred with Emily Pearson (chapter 1). He also claimed that U.S. occupationally induced cancers number only 4 percent (24,000 annual deaths) of total cancers. Yet even industry studies—by the Chemical Manufacturers Association and the American Industrial Health Council—have found they could be 20 percent of total cancers. Apart from whether Doll has erred scientifically, his acceptance of repeated payments from major polluters raises obvious questions about conflicts of interest. Touting positions from which they stand to gain financially is especially problematic for private-interest-science scientists like Doll and Peto because they mislead the public about potential cancer causes, and they minimize their funders' responsibility for harm. As a consequence, they indirectly encourage people to adopt a "cure" frame for cancer and to ignore pollution prevention.[58]

Another "cure" proponent, University of California geneticist Bruce Ames, has similar conflicts of interest, partly because of his patented nutritional supplement, Juvenon. In dismissing pollution prevention as a key to health, Ames has a conflict of interest in promoting another health strategy, Juvenon, from which he profits. It is peculiar that Ames dismisses massive scientific evidence for pollution-induced disease and aging yet, with much less evidence, touts his supplement to remedy disease and aging. No supplements, including his, have been evaluated by the FDA. This means that Ames demands the highest standards of proof (epidemiological tests on humans) from pollution victims, people harmed against their wills. Yet for Juvenon, he accepts far lower standards (animal data). If anything, ethics demands higher standards of proof when people may be harmed against their wills. Ames also touts Juvenon, saying it improved performance in the rats he tested. Yet, as discussed earlier, he rejects animal studies as sufficient for regulation of pollutants. Why are animal studies sufficient grounds for promoting a supplement from which he will profit but not sufficient grounds for promoting pollution prevention—regulations that might save the lives of pollution victims? Ames also has a conflict in using his name and university affiliation in Juvenon ads from which he will profit. In denying any significant pollution-related harm, yet promoting his Juvenon as a health aid, Ames directly promotes medicinal "cures" but indirectly denigrates pollution prevention. Dentists learned long ago to emphasize prevention, not just treatment. Conflicts of interest and private-interest science may be one reason that many cancer victims do not do the same.[59]

Appealing to Ignorance, Blaming the Victim

Besides emphasizing cures rather than prevention, those who do private-interest science also often "blame the victim" for most cancers. In particular, industry front groups claim most cancers are caused by personal choices like smoking, eating fats, and not controlling infections. They say ionizing radiation, toxic chemicals, and other pollutants play a negligible role.[60] Although these "blame proponents" have softened their position recently, they continue to cite Doll's and Peto's classic 1981 article. It attributes 95 percent of cancers to "personal lifestyle" and largely ignores polluted air, dirty water, and workplace contaminants. Citing this 1981 article decades later, Ames follows the language of industry-funded think tanks. He continues to say that harms from pollution and synthetic chemicals (like PCBs, DDT, and chlorinated hydrocarbons) are "trivial," are of "minimal concern," and cause only a "tiny" proportion of cancer.[61]

On the positive side, blame theorists like Ames, Doll, and Peto are correct to emphasize both the carcinogenic importance of lifestyle choices, like smoking, and the public's often-misguided fears of synthetic chemicals. They also correctly criticize cancer studies that rely only on linear extrapolation of cancer risks or fail to control for confounders arising from personal choices, like diet.

On the negative side, those who overemphasize personal blame for cancer fall into both scientific and ethical errors. On the *ethical* side, Ames and others make many erroneous inferences that rely on at least seven controversial ethical assumptions. One assumption is that stricter regulation of non-tobacco pollutants is not justified, if people's bad habits—like smoking—supposedly cause more cancers than environmental pollutants. In addition to the numbers-game errors already noted, this flawed inference falsely assumes that the groups of people harmed by tobacco and by synthetic chemicals are identical. Because they are not, it is irrational and unethical to say that children like Emily Pearson deserve no better regulation just because other people, more people, smoke. Ames and others compare apples and oranges. In blaming cancer victims, they also assume that they know who deserves blame. Ames's hasty generalization ignores the fact that even many lung-cancer victims are not smokers. They sometimes are victims of passive smoke, airborne industrial particulates, or genetic predisposition. Even when people's poor habits do cause their cancers, Ames and front-group scientists err in a third way. They assume that no smokers and drinkers are addicts and presuppose that they have freely chosen these risks. Yet the behavior of the tobacco industry, outlined earlier, suggests that continuing to smoke often is not a wholly free choice. Fourth, even if cancer victims freely chose to smoke, Ames and others forget that smokers receive some benefits from their habit. Smokers' putting themselves at risk, for their own benefit, does not give others the right to put them at further risk, in ways that benefit mainly the risk imposer, not them. As they did in using the naturalistic fallacy, Ames and front-group scientists thus err in a fifth way. They erroneously assume risk imposers may profit from the harm they cause others. They ignore who bears the costs of risks, who receives the benefits, and who ought to receive each. A sixth, ethically flawed, assumption they make is that people forfeit their human rights when they make mistakes that harm themselves. Ames and others assume that people lose their rights to give or withhold consent to pollution when they make poor health choices like smoking. As a result, they assume that polluters ought to be allowed to further victimize those who have already made poor choices. Yet human rights to personal autonomy and self-determination always allow people to choose their pleasures, provided their habits do not harm others. Otherwise, rights would not be inalienable and universal. Otherwise, most of us would lose our rights in one area simply because we made poor choices in another area. In thus ignoring human rights, Ames and others make a seventh ethically questionable assumption. They assume that others may do to me what I do to myself. Yet I have the right to accept personal sacrifices, precisely because I consent. Indeed, I often benefit from such sacrifices. I even have the right to choose an unhealthy goal—like staying slim by smoking. Others do not have the right to impose sacrifices on me, for their benefit, just because of my own poor choices. Otherwise, some of the most vulnerable people in our society could be most victimized by others. This would result in a society that was fundamentally antidemocratic, anti-egalitarian, anti-libertarian, and totalitarian. Apart from relying on the preceding seven assumptions, this private-interest-science strategy, blame-the-victim, errs ethically in encouraging people to have less sympathy for some cancer victims. It suggests these victims "got what they deserved." Even if they did get what they deserve—which is often doubtful—"blame" proponents have no obvious right to judge others when doing so promotes positions from which they profit financially, because of their conflicts of interest. Besides, virtuous people show compassion, reserve judgment, and assume they are not privy to all the factors responsible for wrong choices.[62]

Private-interest-science proponents who blame most cancer victims also rely on several questionable *scientific* assumptions. (1) Doll, Peto, and others frequently blame fatty diets for much cancer, ignore the fact that animal fats accumulate toxic chemicals, but then assume that the fats, not the synthetic chemicals in them, are the problem. (2) They blame natural estrogens for 20 percent of cancers, yet, contrary to the NAS and scientific consensus,[63] they assume no cancers are caused by millions of pounds of synthetic-estrogen pollutants (mainly chlorinated hydrocarbons, like pesticides). (3) Ignoring ionizing radiation, heavy metals, volatile organic compounds, particulates, and other air pollutants, Doll, Peto, Ames, and others repeatedly assume that 90–100 percent of lung cancer is caused by smoking. Yet in recent decades, lung cancer among nonsmokers has more than doubled. As chapter 1 showed, NAS and NCI data also show that air pollution causes many lung cancers, heart attacks, respiratory diseases, asthma, and allergies.[64] (4) Blame theorists likewise erroneously assume that increased 5-year-survival rates, of cancer victims, show that cancer is not mainly environmentally caused. Yet this private-interest-science emphasis on 5-year survival misses three key points, as chapter 1 noted. (a) These are that cancer incidence is increasing about five times faster than cancer survival; (b) that cancer-incidence rates are increasing much faster among children than adults; and (c) that increases in alleged 5-year-survival rates may be artifacts of earlier diagnosis. (5) Blame theorists also err scientifically because they claim that one-third of all cancers are caused by infectious disease, but, contrary to chapter 1, they assume pollutants' immunity-depressing effects play no role in these infection-related cancers. They likewise err in claiming that only tobacco-induced cancers are increasing. Yet the study by Doll and Peto, on which this claim relies, excludes cancer-incidence rates for both blacks and certain age groups, yet then assumes this exclusion has no scientific effects.[65] As chapter 1 showed, however, blacks generally face worse pollution than whites. Partly as a result, they have correspondingly higher cancer rates.

Apart from their problematic scientific and ethical claims, blame-the-victim researchers like Doll and Peto also make logical errors. For instance, they admit their cancer estimates could err by a factor of 10.[66] This means that, because they blame victims for most cancers but say 5 percent of cancers can be caused by pollutants, their own pollutant-cancer figure could be as high as 50 percent of all cancers. Yet they ignore this logical consequence of their own claims. Instead, they inconsistently continue to say that pollution-induced cancers are "tiny."[67] However, 50 percent—300,000 U.S. cancer deaths annually—is not "tiny." Even their admitted 5 percent (30,000 annual U.S. cancer deaths) is not tiny. Ames also commits an appeal to ignorance (a logical fallacy discussed in chapter 1) when he claims both that "current science does not have the ability" to estimate carcinogenic hazards, since half the causes are unknown, yet that pollutants "do not contribute significantly to cancer."[68] An appeal to ignorance is the error of assuming that an absence of evidence (e.g., for pollution-caused cancer) enables one to conclude that there is evidence for an absence (of pollution-caused cancer). If one is ignorant about the causes of half of cancers,[69] then Ames is inconsistent to claim that pollutants are not a significant contributor. Logically, pollutants could be responsible for the 50 percent of unknown cancer causes, in addition to those causes already known. In this case, he ought not blame victims for most cancers.

Apart from such logic problems, to claim that pollutants are not significant cancer contributors, and instead to blame the victim for most cancers, is far outside the scientific mainstream. As chapter 1 revealed, this position con- tradicts the findings of prestigious groups like the U.S. NAS, the WHO, and the APHA. Data published in 2005 by the NAS indicate that "toxic agents" appear to cause about 60,000 U.S. deaths each year—apart from those caused by other pollutants like particulates and ionizing radiation. The NAS says legally allowed, food-borne pesticides, alone, will cause 1 million pre- mature cancers over 75 years.[70] Yet Ames and others continue to say che- micals and food-borne pesticides cause only negligible amounts of cancer. Ames also vocally opposed Proposition 65, the California law that imposes tough financial penalties on industries that knowingly discharge carcinogens into drinking-water supplies.[71] Because blame-the-victim views, like those of Ames, contradict scientific consensus and may confuse the public, private- interest-science researchers arguably have ethical duties to examine their positions carefully. Otherwise, citizens probably will not know who to be- lieve about pollution-induced cancer. As a result, they likely will be less able to protect their rights to life, to know, and to consent.

Delaying Regulation, Denying Justice

What do many private-interest-science proponents do when they can no longer deny some harmful effect of their funders' pollutants or products? One strat- egy is to admit the harm but to attribute it to causes other than their funders' products or pollution. As mentioned earlier in this chapter, when two DOE- funded physicists questioned atomic-veteran Reason Warehime, they ignored his radiation-induced sterility. Instead they ascribed his cancer, hair loss, and teeth loss to another cause—poor hygiene.

Another common private-interest-science strategy is what the 2005 *Lancet* article, discussed earlier in this chapter, says the tobacco industry has done: It has created confusion. Claiming that the precise nature of health threats from tobacco is not clear, the cigarette industry uses private-interest science to argue that regulations are premature. Instead it calls for more analysis. To some degree, its "paralysis by analysis" strategy has succeeded, partly because sci- ence always exhibits some uncertainties about various mechanisms of harm. As a result, polluters can exploit these uncertainties as excuses to delay regulation. Their tactic is similar to that of anti-evolutionists. They use minor uncertainties in the theory of evolution to deny its status as science. Yet both groups who use this delaying tactic ignore fundamental ethical guidelines about placing the burden of proof, exercising precaution, protecting the vulnerable, considering probabilities of harm, and following the preponderance of evidence. In the case of evolution, paralysis-by-analysis proponents say it ought not be accepted merely because the *preponderance of scientific evidence* supports it. Instead, they demand *infallible scientific evidence*—something science never has. In the case of pollution, something similar happens. Paralysis proponents frequently say knowing *that* some pollutant causes harm is insufficient reason to regulate it. What is necessary, they say, is knowing completely and precisely *how* it causes harm—something scientists often do not know.

In particular, private-interest-science proponents often say mere epidemiological or *statistical* evidence *that* some pollutant is harmful is inadequate for regulating it. Instead, they claim that full *mechanistic* knowledge—of *how* this harm occurs—is necessary for regulation. This is exactly the "paralysis by analysis" tobacco strategy, discussed above. Claiming the harms associated with cigarettes are merely "statistical," tobacco companies suggest the damage is caused by some unique (perhaps genetic) vulnerabilities in *smokers*, rather than by *tobacco* itself. Again blaming the victim, they demand analysis to sort out the difference between alleged smoker-caused, versus tobacco-caused, harms. Regardless of the analysis demanded, a key goal of private-interest science is to delay regulation. As the industry-funded Heritage Foundation noted, in a slightly different vein, "the most promising short-term solution [to block regulation] is to use the appropriations process to restrict the use of government funds to pursue . . . regulations until a general overhaul [analysis] of the regulatory process can be achieved. Such riders . . . would cool the regulatory zeal of federal agencies."[72]

One common regulatory-delay tactic of polluters, defended through private-interest science, is demanding that all public-health regulations pass the test of cost-benefit analysis (CBA). Thus, the industry-funded Competitive Enterprise Institute argues for "an across-the-board requirement that the benefits of any rule be shown to exceed the risks [costs]." Since 1995, U.S. law has required this test for all regulations. *On the positive side*, this requirement is partly right. CBA often can contribute to rational and efficient policy. It also can sometimes enable government regulators to spend pollution-abatement dollars wisely. *On the negative side*, this requirement is often wrong because, as currently practiced, CBA is incomplete and ignores distributive inequities. Regarding incompleteness, if CBA practitioners understood "benefits" to include what promotes human rights, civil liberties, clean air, clean water, and so on, there would be few problems with requiring that benefits exceed costs. But "benefits" in contemporary CBA are incomplete. They include only narrow, market-traded commodities. As a result, requiring CBA for all regulations amounts to requiring a market test for social policy, for right and wrong. Yet obviously there ought be no market test for whether murder-for-hire, racial segregation, human-rights violations, or pollution-induced injury ought to be allowed. Why not? Some acts—like prohibiting murder—are right and ought to be required, even if their market costs exceed their market benefits. Likewise, some acts—like violating rights to life—are wrong and ought to be prohibited, even if their market benefits exceed their market costs. To require a market test for all regulations subjects human-rights protections to tests of market expediency. After all, the Bill of Rights does not require CBA. Otherwise, there would be no Bill of Rights. Likewise, CBA critics claim that if the 1995 CBA rule had been adopted years ago, the United States could neither have banned leaded gas and the use of DDT on crops, nor required automobile seat belts. CBA critics also say that requiring CBA for all health-related laws and regulations falls into the same ethical errors as free-market environmentalism, discussed in chapter 2. Both free-market environmentalism and CBA base decisions on aggregate market costs and benefits, but they ignore fairness, justice, and equal treatment. As a result, both can sanction distributive inequities, like the environmental injustice that jeopardizes the lives of poor people, minorities, and children. With its ethically questionable character, its incompleteness, and its distributive inequities, why was the 1995 CBA rule adopted? Critics claim that multimillion-dollar, industry-funded front groups promoted the CBA rule as the only "rational" way of regulating. Despite the fact that many studies show that the public is as rational as economic experts, once it has the facts, industry groups claimed CBA was needed as a corrective to public irrationality.[73]

Who is right? Is the CBA rule a polluter tactic to delay regulations? Or is it needed to correct public irrationality? The answer can be determined only on a case-by-case basis, since using it in some cases would provide important information, yet requiring CBA for all decisions would fall into ethical error. In addition to the preceding arguments against universal use of CBA-based decisions, two additional reasons suggest it often can be both irrational and unethical. One reason is that, as currently practiced, CBA presupposes that things have value only if people are *willing to pay* for them. This willingness-to-pay criterion errs ethically because it begs the question that pollution victims, rather than polluters, should pay for clean air and water. Why should polluters be assumed to have property rights to the commons? Willingness-to-pay also begs the question against poor people. They are less able to pay than are the rich. Why should poorer people have fewer rights to the commons, to clean air and water, merely because they are poorer? A second problem is that using the CBA rule to assess health regulations undervalues biological resources that are not traded on a market, yet are needed to support life and health. This is particularly the case for benefits like ecosystems services. These include natural processes like water purification, recharging groundwater, waste decomposition, nutrient recycling, climate regulation, maintenance of biodiversity, and flood-risk reduction. Because there are no well-developed economic techniques for costing these free, biological services, which are not traded on markets, CBA typically does not "count" them as benefits. As a 2005 U.S. NAS report warned, these biological necessities are "taken for granted, and overlooked in environmental decision-making."[74] Thus the 1995 CBA rule not only can create antiregulatory paralysis-through-analysis, but also can err ethically, underestimate the benefits of regulation, and overestimate its costs. Because the rule contributes to undervaluing clean air and water, it helps undervalue lives saved by clean air and water. On both grounds, it misinforms citizens, undercuts their rights to know, and jeopardizes their rights to give or withhold consent to health risks.

Conclusion

When polluters use either private-interest science or flawed ethics to manipulate information about pollution, they undercut citizens' human rights to know and to consent, and they ultimately cause more citizen deaths. They create a situation about which Abraham Lincoln warned. If only a few informed people realize the severity of some problem—in this case, pollution—they can appear mentally ill, while uninformed people can appear sane. Polluters' manipulation and misuse of scientific knowledge thus can give them the power to define who is sane and who is not, who will live and who will not, and who will fulfill their human rights and who will not. They prove that Francis Bacon was right: knowledge is power.[75]

How does one gain the knowledge of pollution and therefore the power to control it? Chapter 1 suggests that one way is to understand how pollution threatens life and health. Chapter 2 and this chapter suggest that another way is to uncover the social, political, and scientific factors that keep citizens from understanding these threats. While the evidence presented in these three chapters is not complete, it is sufficient to establish two *prima facie* principles. Dirty air and dirty water harm people, despite what special-interest PR and private-interest science say. Dirty air and dirty water also harm people in ways that often are preventable, inequitable, and threaten their rights to know, to consent, and to receive equal protection of life. The obvious question is what people should do about it. The remaining chapters begin to answer this question.

Human Rights and Duties Not to Harm

Adam Finkel was worried. His longtime employer, the U.S. Occupational Safety and Health Administration (OSHA), was charged with protecting citizens from workplace hazards. Yet it was not protecting thousands of its own inspectors who monitored U.S. manufacturing facilities—like those where beryllium alloys are used to make everything from golf clubs, cell phones, ceramics, and dental bridgework to lasers, satellites, and x-ray tubes. These current and former OSHA inspectors were not being told of their own workplace-induced beryllium risks. As former director of health standards for all of OSHA, Finkel knew these risks were significant. He also knew that beryllium is a toxic metal, able to cause both cancer and a fast-progressing, potentially fatal, lung disease. According to noted beryllium-disease physician Lee Newman, ounce for ounce, beryllium can be more toxic than plutonium. Newman says only a few millionths of a gram can trigger massive health problems.[1]

Whistleblower Adam Finkel

By 1999, OSHA had determined preliminary procedures for testing its inspectors for sensitization to beryllium. In 2001, draft plans for it were complete. Finkel assumed the testing would go forward. In April 2002, however, OSHA head John Henshaw put the testing "on hold." Finkel was disturbed. As OSHA administrator for the Rocky Mountain Region, he knew that OSHA inspectors already worked under difficult conditions. Delaying the beryllium testing only added to their health risks. In Montana, for instance, there were only eight OSHA inspectors to cover the 150,000 square miles of the state. The inspectors were constantly on the road, walking into very dangerous places, often facing hostile employers. For dozens of operations in many different types of industries, these public servants had to know the relevant pollutants and their specific means of control. Finkel says the inspectors are "consistently professional, fair and diligent...like New York's finest—the policemen and firemen who braved the World Trade Center towers on September 11, 2001, in order to protect the public." As protectors of U.S. workers, they "deserve especially good rather than especially bad treatment."[2]

Looking at about 500 exposure records, Finkel suspected that many inspectors were getting especially bad treatment. They had unknowingly been exposed to levels of beryllium up to hundreds of times what OSHA permitted. Yet even this OSHA standard, set in 1949, was far too lax. Newman and other scientists had shown that cumulative beryllium exposures 10,000 times lower (than what OSHA permits) can cause serious health problems. Other federal agencies, like the U.S. Department of Energy (DOE), already had beryllium regulations that were 10 times more protective than those of OSHA and were testing thousands of employees. Given such flawed standards, screening exposed OSHA inspectors for beryllium sensitization was doubly important. Besides, beryllium blood-screening costs only about $150 per person. Finkel knew that the 1,000 currently exposed inspectors could be tested for only $150,000. A federal watchdog group, Public Employees for Environmental Responsibility (PEER), estimated that OSHA likely paid out more in annual bonuses for its 20 senior executives than what was needed to test its own inspectors for beryllium.[3]

After 3 years of delaying the recommended blood screening, in April 2002 OSHA director John Henshaw made a startling announcement in an OSHA-executives-only meeting. Over Finkel's objections, Henshaw said that the testing was "not going to happen anytime soon." He also decided that retired inspectors "would not be informed" of their health risks. Yet Finkel knew that the sooner the inspectors were tested, the better were their chances of surviving any possible disease. Why was OSHA prepared to "let them twist in the wind for many years"? Perhaps the agency feared the lawsuits and public outcry that might accompany disclosure of any problems. By late 2002, Finkel had exhausted internal channels in his push for testing. He knew he had to do something else.[4]

In the fall of 2002, over lunch with a reporter from *Inside OSHA*, Finkel revealed the inspectors' beryllium exposures and OSHA's 3-year inaction to protect them. On the day the reporter's article appeared, Finkel was summoned to Washington by John Henshaw, who had been an executive at Monsanto for 30 years before President G. W. Bush appointed him to head OSHA. Although Finkel had not been identified as the source of the *Inside OSHA* information, Henshaw told Finkel he was going to strip him of his Denver regional directorship, claimed he was not doing a good job, and reassigned him to the National Safety Council in Washington. From supervising 150 OSHA employees, suddenly Finkel had to move his family East and begin work alone in a small office. Charging his OSHA bosses with retaliation, in January 2003, he filed a whistleblower complaint with the U.S. Office of Special Counsel (OSC). (The OSC hears all public-sector-employee whistleblower complaints). After OSC ruled against him in September 2003, Finkel appealed to a federal judge and to PEER, which agreed to defend him.

In October 2003, he filed a public disclosure, asking OSC to force OSHA to disclose the potential beryllium health problems and OSHA's failure to do testing. In January 2004, the OSC again ruled against him. It concluded that Finkel "had not presented facts about beryllium's dangers that merited any investigation." PEER, however, forced disclosure of damning emails that revealed OSHA's retaliation against Finkel. As a result, late in 2003 OSHA was forced to settle the retaliation claim. In return for Finkel's dropping his whistleblower-retaliation suit, OSHA gave him an undisclosed lump-sum settlement and 25 months of continued salary and benefits. This was enough to cover Finkel's expenses and additional damages.[5]

Finkel's attempt to force OSHA to disclose the beryllium threats and lack of testing, however, was less successful. In October 2003, OSHA administrator Henshaw sent an email to all employees, falsely claiming that beryllium-sensitization tests of its inspectors were "already underway." Yet 6 months later, *Chicago Tribune* reporter Sam Roe phoned OSHA and discovered that no testing had begun. Because OSHA did not want Roe to write about "the delay and past lies," in April 2004 the agency distributed brochures that offered its inspectors voluntary beryllium blood screening. Of the 1,200 inspectors contacted, 300 asked for screening. Even this offer, however, was not handled ethically. Because the inspectors' real risks were not disclosed to them, they could neither give nor withhold genuine informed consent to screening.[6] Yet full disclosure would have been easy. Because "OSHA has exhaustive data on the precise beryllium levels that every inspector encountered," it would only have had to add each person's doses, "to estimate lifetime exposures." OSHA was still denying the beryllium risks in spring 2004, as it began screening. Suddenly, in November 2004, Finkel said, *Chicago Tribune* reporter Sam Roe called him. Roe revealed that, after only just beginning the beryllium screening, OSHA already had proved that Finkel's concerns were completely justified because many inspectors already had tested positive. One month later, in December 2004, Henshaw and his deputy, R. Davis Layne, both retired. In January 2005, the *Chicago Tribune* reported that Finkel's health predictions had been confirmed. For the first time ever, on March 24, 2005, OSHA was forced to admit that its inspectors had been harmed by beryllium exposure. It admitted that 4 percent of its inspectors, tested so far, had beryllium sensitization—a figure nearly four times higher than Finkel's original estimate of 1–2 percent. Yet in 2003 the U.S. OSC had dismissed Finkel's estimate as an "exaggeration." Soon after OSHA's admission, PEER sent a letter to Elaine Chao, the secretary of labor, asking her to investigate OSHA inspectors' exposure levels, explain the four-year testing delay, and admit OSHA deception and coverup about beryllium. In addition, PEER requested that OSHA warn retired inspectors and revise its more than 50-year-old beryllium standard—to make it consistent both with current science and with standards for other federal agencies. Chao has addressed none of these requests. Instead, she has only responded that OSHA wants to protect its inspectors.[7]

Part of what is surprising about the Finkel case is that, as scientist and policy expert, Adam Finkel is far better educated and "better connected" than any of the whistleblowers discussed so far in this book. He had 10 years at OSHA, a senior management position, and the support of other independent scientists and physicians. Ironically, neither this experience nor his Harvard doctorate protected him from retaliation. A second irony is that OSHA, the U.S. worker-protection agency for 130 million private-sector workers, "turned its back on the several thousand workers under its wing, casting doubt on its will to protect anyone." Yet "through 17 statutes, Congress has assigned to OSHA the responsibility to impartially hear the cases of whistleblowers, including most environmental, airline, and now financial (Enron) cases." A third irony is that OSHA protected its own employees against neither job hazards nor retaliation. Indeed, in Finkel's case, OSHA was the retaliator. Only a lawsuit was able to protect Finkel and OSHA's own workers. A fourth irony is that OSHA not only failed to protect whistleblowers and its own employees but also engaged in "going after the whistleblowers with malice." Most worrisome, these ironies do not seem limited to OSHA. Examining the more than 1,000 whistleblower complaints brought to the OSC during 2004–2005, PEER found that virtually all have been rejected without even an investigation, many without even contacting the whistleblower. Jeff Ruch, executive director of PEER, says "We do not know of any whistleblower retaliation complaint, received during [Bush-appointed special counsel Scott] Bloch's tenure, that his office has ultimately upheld."[8]

What has happened to whistleblower Finkel? As of late 2006, he is a professor at the University of Medicine and Dentistry of New Jersey and a visiting professor at Princeton University. Continuing his battle to protect public health and reform OSHA, Finkel is trying to help inspectors who have not been tested. Repeatedly he has used the Freedom of Information Act to request OSHA beryllium-exposure records, but OSHA has continued to refuse these requests. In November 2005, he filed suit in federal court to force OSHA to comply with the Freedom of Information Act. Finkel says his struggle has only just begun. He now hopes to convince OSHA to test its former beryllium inspectors and to recommend screening in the 21 states that have their own workplace safety and health programs. Epidemiologist David Michaels says the battle will take time. Michaels, who is former assistant U.S. energy secretary and now professor at George Washington University, says OSHA is "abdicating its responsibility." Even the nation's largest beryllium-alloy producer, Brush Wellman in Cleveland, agrees; it says current OSHA beryllium standards are too lenient.[9]

Speaking of his OSHA ordeal, Finkel says: "Some days I feel like the character in *The Shawshank Redemption,* who crawled through a river of s— and came out clean on the other side." Finkel claims that 90 percent of the reason he went into government service was that he thought he could "do the most good there." The other 10 percent of his reason? He says he "wanted to be part of an organization where hard work, creativity, and honesty were appreciated, and for which one of the rewards would be the kind of career and geographic stability that a new husband and father needed." Instead, he says, he found himself "part of a paramilitary cult where loyalty was a one-way street and where senior managers had to spend more time looking over their shoulders at organizational psychodramas than looking outward to the mission of the agency." Several weeks before Henshaw told him he was being transferred from Denver to Washington, Henshaw specifically told Finkel and other OSHA employees that he did not want them "to put work ahead of family and faith." Yet OSHA's retaliation did exactly that. In transferring him, his bosses gave Finkel 60 days, at the beginning of a school year, to move his wife and family across the country.[10]

Lessons from the Finkel Case

To an outsider, Adam Finkel appears to have had the ideal situation from which to protect workers and promote public health. As an OSHA regional administrator, he had access to many relevant pollution-exposure records. He also had the opportunity, at least within the Rocky Mountain states, to promote deserving OSHA employees. He could reward them for their honesty, competence, and dedication to public service. Yet when Finkel sought to protect these very employees under him—safety inspectors—he ran into many of the problems already outlined in chapters 2 and 3.

Chapter 2 showed how special interests use strategies like revolving doors and regulatory capture to "orchestrate ignorance" about pollution. Finkel faced OSHA's attempts to "orchestrate ignorance" about inspectors' beryllium risks. He also faced revolving doors when President Bush appointed a 30-year Monsanto-Chemicals executive, John Henshaw, to lead OSHA. Typifying regulatory capture, Henshaw then suppressed information and used retaliation to promote whistle-swallowing. He limited full disclosure and rights to know.

As chapter 3 argued, regulatory capture is possible partly because special interests use devices like front groups and hire education to do private-interest science—not science at all. Finkel faced the blatantly flawed private-interest science of the U.S. OSC when it rejected his beryllium claims as "exaggerations." As chapter 3 showed, private-interest science is used not only to misrepresent regulatory-related science, but also to destroy the careers and misrepresent the work of scientists who warn of health threats. In Finkel's case, OSC attorneys claimed that the massive scientific literature, cited by Finkel to confirm beryllium risks, did not show that U.S. inspectors were at risk. Why not? They said the scientific analyses were about "different populations of workers than the one you are concerned about." They used what Finkel calls the "Thalidomide Argument." "Yes, European babies are being born without limbs, but how do we know Americans will react the same way?"[11]

Chapter Overview

If Finkel is right, that his efforts succeeded in correcting only about 10 percent of OSHA's beryllium problem,[12] two obvious questions remain. Who will help correct the rest of the problem? Why should they do so? This chapter begins to answer both questions. It builds on the earlier discussions of moral exemplars like Gwen Pearson, Kate Burns, Reason Warehime, and Adam Finkel. Chapter 1 outlined the severity of pollution threats to health. Chapter 2 showed why factors like regulatory capture and media concentration keep most citizens from recognizing and giving legitimate consent to these threats. Chapter 3 described the characteristics of private-interest science, showing how it is used to deny health threats, delay regulation, and thwart rights to life and to equal protection. Building on these earlier arguments, this chapter first answers the *who* question. It does so by defending the responsibility argument. What is this argument? To the degree that citizens have participated in, or derived benefits from, social institutions that have helped cause life-threatening or rights-threatening environmental injustice, they have *prima facie* duties either to stop their participation in these institutions or to compensate for it by helping to reform them. (Environmental injustice occurs whenever children, poor people, minorities, blue collar workers, or other subgroups bear disproportionate burdens of life-threatening or seriously harmful pollution. *Prima facie* duties are those that one has in the absence of specific arguments to the contrary.) Next, this chapter offers a preliminary answer to the earlier *why* question. In the face of grave social wrongs to which citizens have partly contributed, like the Holocaust, justice requires citizens to act—to work to stop these wrongs.

Almost nothing can compare to the horrors of the Holocaust. Nevertheless, citizens facing public-health threats—caused by and covered up by polluters or by government—are in some ways like 1940s Red Cross workers. Inspecting the Nazis' concentration camp at Dachau during World War II, these workers faced orchestrated ignorance. The Nazis kept inspectors away from the incinerators. They showed them the barracks only of better treated political prisoners. They even hanged baskets of flowers from the wooden posts that were normally used as gallows.[13] What are today's "flower baskets" in the fight against environmental injustice and health-related human-rights threats? They are the campaign contributions, PR, scientific front groups, and private-interest science all analyzed in chapters 2 and 3. Just as the Dachau flowers should have been obvious, for what they were, today's "flower baskets" should be equally obvious. So is the response demanded by justice. Citizens have duties to help stop threats to health and human rights, just as they had duties to help stop the Holocaust. Defending the responsibility argument, this chapter first outlines *why* such duties exist.

Justice, Not Charity

Why do all citizens have *prima facie* duties to stop life-threatening and rights-threatening pollution? The short answer, sketched in this chapter, is that because citizens have contributed to and benefited from these threats, they helped cause them. Consequently, they have an *ethical responsibility* to help stop them. Because they participate in nations and institutions that help cause these threats, they also have a *democratic responsibility* to help stop them. There are longer answers to this question, of course—answers that do not appeal to human rights, as this chapter does. These additional answers rely on virtue ethics, consequentialist ethics, and other moral theories. (According to consequentialism, acts are right whenever they lead to a preponderance of good consequences. They are wrong otherwise.) Indeed, the factual data outlined in chapter 1 could provide a starting point for consequentialist arguments to prevent deadly pollution. These could build on the work of distinguished scholars like Princeton University philosopher Peter Singer and New York University philosopher Peter Unger, who already have given superb consequentialist arguments for ending world hunger.[14] The strategy here, however, is slightly different. Using insights similar to those of Columbia University philosopher Thomas Pogge, this argument builds on the heavily and almost uniquely American emphasis on human rights, especially rights to life. In part, this argument provides the justification for many recommendations of the American Public Health Association (APHA), which says that human rights provide "the ethical framework for public health practice." Calling for a constitutional amendment that guarantees all Americans rights not to be harmed by pollutants, the APHA has provided a model for initiatives in 40 states to guarantee rights against environmental-health threats. Although this chapter does not provide the *legal* and political arguments required to implement such recommendations, it offers an initial *ethical* foundation for doing so. Chapter 6 suggests how this ethical argument might be put into practice. One way is by working with various non-governmental organizations, bottom-up, to reform laws, agencies, and institutions one by one. The other strategy is by working, top-down, to implement all the human-rights recommendations of the APHA.[15]

Using human-rights arguments, this chapter explains that charity ought not be the main response to the environmental-health problems outlined in chapters 1–3. Life-threatening and rights-threatening pollution, like the horrors of Dachau, demands justice. It demands stopping the deaths, not merely offering charity to victims. The reason? As already mentioned, justice requires virtually all citizens to help prevent pollution-related deaths and human-rights abuses because they *allow* them, *benefit from* them, and *participate in* institutions contributing to them. When people participate in institutions—like a government that suppresses health-related information or limits others' access to basic necessities, such as clean air and water—they are partly responsible for harm done by those institutions. The chapter shows that even if they intend no harm to anyone, citizens are partially causally responsible for pollution-caused injustice and human-rights violations.

Human Rights

As traditionally understood, human rights are a special class of moral protections with which compliance is mandatory, not discretionary. As philosopher

Ronald Dworkin puts it, human rights are "trumps." They are universal claims, in the sense that all humans have them simply by virtue of being human, independent of whether particular governments recognize or implement them. Protections against taking life or discrimination, human rights include protection of life and health, as in rights not to be tortured; protection of due process, as in rights to a fair trial; protection of political participation, as in rights to vote and to know; and protection of equal treatment, as in rights not to be discriminated against on grounds of race or gender. As such, human rights are negative protections. They represent minimal standards *for treatment of humans* that governments, societies, and individuals ought to respect. They also represent standards for social criticism and reform. Oppressed minorities can appeal to human rights, and civil disobedience is often justified as a way to stop threats to them. Because the concern here is narrow—public health, human rights, and environmental injustice—this book takes no stand on the question of who or what, beyond human beings, might be said to have rights. The author believes, however, that Peter Singer has the best treatment of this larger question.[16]

Although *legal* rights exist only because government has recognized them, as already noted, human rights exist prior to and independent of their legal recognition. If human rights did not exist independently, there would be no standard on the basis of which to criticize the atrocities of governments who do not recognize them. How, then, does one justify the existence of human rights? There are at least three main answers to this question.

(1) The first answer is negative. Some British utilitarian moral philosophers, like Jeremy Bentham, have doubted that human rights can be justified in any meaningful sense. For them, only legal rights exist. As a consequence, they have a difficult time justifying condemnations of human-rights abuses in nations that do not recognize these legal rights. (2) Illustrating the second sort of response to the justification question, some moral philosophers say that people have some special and equal capacity, like the ability to feel pain, that entitles them to rights. As a consequence, they say all beings (including other animals) that feel pain have rights to have their interests considered. According to moral philosophers in the tradition of Immanuel Kant, this rights-giving characteristic is the capacity to engage in rational choice. (3) Most moral philosophers, like Ronald Dworkin, however, accept a third answer to the question of justifying human rights. They say that, by definition, human rights belong at least to humans and that the characteristic by virtue of which humans have *prima facie* human rights, is procedural, not factual. They believe human rights are procedural in the sense that they depend on recognizing the fundamental moral requirement of consistent and equal processes. According to this moral requirement, humans have rights not because they are rational, or can exercise agency, but simply because they are human, and humans ought to be treated consistently or equally. Their claims for equal treatment are deserving of equal respect. As a result, they have equal human rights. Another way of formulating this procedural justification for human rights is to say that all humans (regardless of their

factual characteristics) are equal subjects of "moral value." Although they may differ in intelligence or physical strength, they are equally deserving of respect or consideration precisely because they are human. As a result, they have equal rights—that is, equal claims to have their basic interests or needs considered. Espousing this third or procedural position, most moral philosophers have two reasons for not basing human rights on some factual characteristic, like capacity for free choice. One reason is that many humans, like infants and comatose patients, seem to retain their rights but may not always possess this characteristic. Second, such a characteristic would not enable different people to resolve their conflicting rights claims in a reasonable way. Why not? No two people possess any factual characteristic in exactly the same way or can be treated in precisely the same way. Despite some shared factual characteristic, often there are legitimate moral grounds for discriminating against some people in some respect. That is, because different people merit/need/deserve different treatment, their rights may take precedence over the rights of others. Consequently many thinkers believe that such moral justifications (rather than merely justifications based on some shared factual characteristic) seem more reasonable ways to resolve rights conflicts. Besides, regardless of their factual differences, all people deserve just procedures and equal consideration of their interests—even if they do not always deserve the same treatment. But if they deserve this equal consideration, then they have equal human rights.[17]

The problem, of course, is how to ensure genuinely equal consideration of everyone, despite different people's conflicting rights claims. Most moral philosophers use one of at least three main strategies to handle rights conflicts and to try to ensure that everyone receives equal consideration. First, they build exceptions into human rights, so that virtually none is absolute. They might say, for instance, that if a patient tells his psychiatrist that he is going to shoot someone, the killer's rights to privacy end where another person's rights to bodily security begin. Second, sometimes ethicists distinguish different classes of rights, according to which some take precedence over others. Thus Dworkin distinguishes strong rights, like rights to life, from weak ones, like rights to property. Strong rights are strong precisely because they are essential to personhood and human autonomy. As a result, they ought never be overridden merely to serve community welfare. Weak rights are weak precisely because, while they benefit the holder, they are not essential to personhood or autonomy. As a consequence, weak rights may be overridden whenever community welfare requires it. Other ethicists provide ways of resolving rights conflicts by distinguishing the class of negative rights (not to be harmed, as through torture) from that of positive rights (to be benefited, as through health care). Consequently, they argue that negative rights take primacy over positive rights. Still other philosophers, like Henry Shue, argue that most rights have both positive and negative elements. As a result, they resolve conflicts by appealing to the primacy of different reasons for overriding some rights. Third, moral philosophers often avoid rights conflicts by distinguishing *prima facie* from *ultima facie* rights. *Prima facie* rights are those that all humans possess, in the absence of any specific arguments to the contrary. They essentially guarantee that anyone who challenges some rights claim bears the burden of proof. *Ultima facie* rights are those that rights-holders possess in the actual situation, once all relevant factual and moral details are considered. Because basic moral arguments must be applicable to a wide variety of situations, by definition they do not take into account case-specific or conflict-specific factual and moral considerations. As a result, virtually all human-rights arguments are for particular *prima facie* human rights. The rights specified in the 1948 United Nations Universal Declaration of Human Rights, for instance, are *prima facie* rights—as are the various rights to know, to consent, and so on that are specified in all codes of medical ethics.[18]

As thus understood, human rights do not protect against all abuses. Nor do they protect any beings other than humans, as already mentioned. Rather, they protect against threats to human welfare and agency that arise when social systems or individuals show "official disrespect" for members' basic needs and interests. Thus governments, educational institutions, labor unions, churches, or corporations might fail to respect human rights. Individuals alone rarely fail to do so, because their power to threaten rights typically comes from some institution, not from themselves alone. Governments often are the primary guardians of human rights, simply because they police other institutions. Ultimately, however, the people themselves are the final guardians of human rights. Why? At least in democratic societies, by definition, the people should control and reform the governments and social institutions on which they depend. People who assert their human rights to life thereby require all social systems to be organized so that all their members have equal and secure access to life and to what is necessary to protect it. Although people possess human rights, independent of such social systems, fulfilling those rights always takes place within the social institutions of which people are members. How are human rights fulfilled? By the many people who have causal influence over their recognition. "All humans in a position to [causally] effect" those rights must recognize them. What is recognized and fulfilled? People's basic needs and interests. Following the strong / weak characterization given earlier, the most basic or strong human right is the right to life or bodily security. Close behind in importance are strong human rights to know and to consent to whatever could threaten life. These two human rights are the most basic, after rights to life, because they protect human agency, the main way people protect their lives. As thus sketched, human rights are recognized by most countries, many international treaties, and the United Nations. The Nuremberg war trials after World War II confirmed them. Consequently, human rights are largely noncontroversial, except among a few philosophical specialists. People might debate whether some particular threats are genuinely human-rights threats. Nevertheless, this book presupposes that human rights, as such, are not controversial. Nor is it controversial that, at the peak of their powers, the Nazis disregarded human rights.[19]

The Responsibility Argument

The basic human-rights argument here, against life-threatening environmental injustice, is not directed at condemning every assault suffered by every person. Rather, the argument is that some "official" assaults seriously threaten people's personal security because their harm exceeds certain thresholds. Pollution that never causes anything worse than a simple cough, for instance, obviously does not exceed this threshold for a human-rights violation. What does exceed it? Many of the harms surveyed in chapter 1 do so—like those causing statistically significant increases in deaths or serious injuries—especially harms that are inequitably distributed. Obviously, however, the thresholds for human-rights violations are different depending on the different rights, people, situations, and circumstances involved. Human-rights threats of greater severity, probability, and immediacy have more stringent, more protective thresholds than threats whose severity, probability, and immediacy are lower. Likewise, the threshold for protecting children's rights to life is far more stringent than that for protecting rights of others. Children deserve more protection because they are less able to protect themselves. Using such agreed-on moral principles (which are far too numerous to be listed here) as well as the techniques of deliberative democracy, people must carefully evaluate the case-specific threshold for human-rights violations.[20]

According to chapters 1–3 and the preceding overview of human rights, one class of human-rights violations occurs when people participate in, or benefit from, social institutions that promote or allow life-threatening environmental injustice. As a consequence, these people bear partial responsibility for environmental injustice and thus should work to stop it. This argument can be formulated in five main premises, as follows.

1. If some institutional order, like government, displays radical inequality in the degree to which citizens' human rights are fulfilled, this order is *prima facie unjust*, and consequently the burden of proof is on its defenders.
2. If citizens (to varying degrees) regulate this *prima facie* unjust institutional order, elect its leaders, and cooperate socioeconomically in it, citizens are partly responsible for this *prima facie* injustice.
3. If premises 1 and 2 are true, citizens must either defend this *prima facie* unjust order, withdraw from it, or compensate for the benefits they gain from participation in it.
4. If withdrawal from this unjust order is unrealistic, citizens must either defend it or compensate for their benefits gained from it. To defend this order, at least one of the following three "excusing" claims must be true.
    4.1. The radically unequal human-rights condition came about through no injustice, but solely through some natural occurrence, for example, some genetic inheritance.

4.2. Victims of this radical inequality (e.g., environmental injustice) receive adequate compensation for threats to their human rights to life, to know, and to consent.

4.3. Alternatives to these radically unequal human-rights conditions would either fail to improve the situation or cannot be achieved, that is, are unworkable.

5. If premises 3 and 4 are true, and claims 4.1–4.3 are false, the *prima facie* unjust order cannot be defended. To compensate for their benefits from it, citizens should work to stop injustice in this order.[21]

How might one argue for each of the preceding premises and apply them to cases of environmental injustice? Building on earlier chapters, subsequent sections defend and apply each of these premises.

Premise 1: Pollution Threats to Human Rights

According to premise 1, institutional orders that display radical inequality in the fulfillment of human rights are *prima facie* unjust, and this *prima facie* injustice places the burden of proof on the order's defenders. Why do some instances of pollution cause environmental injustice and therefore radical inequality in the fulfillment of human rights? Two main factors do so: the *severity* of pollution-caused harms (their high probability of leading to serious disease or death), and the *inequality* with which they are imposed. With respect to the severity, any institutional assault having a high probability of causing death or serious disease obviously is a threat to rights to life. But what is a high probability? If something causes an annual probability of death higher than one in a million, the U.S. government considers this an unacceptably high probability and initiates regulation. In the case of pollution, recall from chapter 1 that industrial and agricultural toxins cause some annual threats whose probability of fatality is far higher than one in a million. For instance, cancer is the leading premature killer of Americans, and the National Cancer Institute (NCI) says at least 10 percent of all annual cancer deaths (60,000 out of 600,000) are caused by industrial and agricultural toxins. Some biologists even claim that environmental toxins are responsible for about 40 percent of all premature disease and death. The APHA says industrial and agricultural toxins threaten the health of millions of Americans, and that occupational exposures, alone, kill at least 100,000 workers annually.[22] Other data from chapter 1 also suggest that many pollutant releases meet the "severity standard" for a human-rights violation. That is, they have a high probability of causing serious threats to life. For example:

- A 2002 *New England Journal of Medicine* study of 90,000 people concluded that "the overwhelming contribution to the causation of cancer...was the environment," part of which includes pollution, and not genetics or infection.

- The Office of Technology Assessment says that up to 90 percent of all cancer is "environmentally induced and theoretically preventable."

- Current cancer incidence is increasing roughly five times faster than cancer mortality is decreasing. The average cancer victim dies 15 years prematurely.

- The 2003 NCI study of 500,000 Americans in cities throughout the United States showed that there is no safe level of air pollution. It annually causes between 50,000 and 100,000 U.S. deaths.

- The U.S. Environmental Protection Agency (EPA) says that 1 in 12 (and perhaps 1 in 5) U.S. women of childbearing age has blood levels of mercury (mainly from coal-fired plants) that can cause neurological and developmental impairment in their children.

- A 1996 U.S. National Academy of Sciences (NAS) study showed that 1 million Americans will die prematurely over the next 75 years from allowable pesticides on foods. Yet U.S. pesticide use has increased by 50 percent over the last three decades.

- The EPA says that 45 million U.S. citizens now drink water that does not meet the government's own safe-drinking-water standards.

- Just from arsenic alone, 35 million Americans drink water that (the state of California says) will cause 1 in every 100 of them to have bladder cancer.

The preceding statistics from chapter 1, all from reputable sources, are alone sufficient to show that at least some avoidable U.S. pollution threats are so severe that they constitute *prima facie* threats to citizens' rights to life. Recall that chapter 1 avoided taking a position on the precise percentage of U.S. cancer deaths (600,000 annually) that could be partly attributed to environmental toxins like industrial chemicals. For the argument here to succeed, likewise, it is not necessary to defend a precise threshold for severity—a specific probability of death at which any pollutant threatens rights to life. Why not? Given so many instances of pollutant-induced deaths, like those noted above, at least some serious harms obviously threaten rights to life because their probabilities are so high. Even if one of the lowest estimates for preventable, pollutant-induced cancer deaths is correct—60,000 annually, claimed by the NCI, U.S. Centers for Disease Control (CDC), and U.S. National Institutes of Health (NIH)—this obviously is a severe U.S. public-health and human-rights problem. Not only have victims' rights to life been jeopardized, but they probably never fulfilled their rights to know, to give or withhold consent to, or to receive due process regarding the bodily risks imposed on them.

The simple point here, about determining precise thresholds for all pollution-induced human-rights threats, is often used in other ethics cases. Confronted with examples of severe racism, like Ku Klux Klan lynching, one need not be able to specify all the border cases, or all the necessary and sufficient conditions for racism, in order to know that a particular case of lynching was racist. Some harms are such severe instances of obvious, *prima facie* racism that they are noncontroversial. So also for many pollutant-induced human-rights threats. Confronted with damning health statistics like those given earlier, one need not specify a precise threshold, for *all cases* of pollution that threaten life and rights. For now, it is enough to know that obviously there are *many cases.*

Pollutants threaten human rights to life and bodily security, however, not only because of the *severity* of their assaults, but also because of the radical *inequities* they impose on citizens. Recall some of the evidence of pollution-induced inequalities from chapter 1.

- U.S. children's cancers are increasing at a rate of 1.4 percent annually, while adult cancers are increasing at an annual rate of about 1 percent.

- The World Health Organization says that up to half of all childhood cancers are probably associated with air pollution alone.

- Cancer causes more deaths (about 6,000 annually) of U.S. children ages 1–15 than any other disease.

- Among pesticides listed as reproductive toxins by the state of California, two-thirds are still in use.

The CDC say 900,000 U.S. children have blood-lead levels, much of it from industrial pollutants like waste incinerators, levels that are able to cause irreversible neurological-developmental damage.

- Half of the U.S. pediatric asthma population lives in areas that violate EPA's ozone standards, and asthma has increased by 40 percent in the last decade.

- Particulate air pollution, alone, causes 6.4 percent of all annual U.S. deaths of infants ages 0–4.

- Forty-one nations have better infant-mortality rates than the United States.

- In the United States, black children ages 5–14 are four times more likely to die of asthma than white children.

- Only 5 percent of whites, but 10 percent of blacks, live in areas that violate all five EPA air-quality standards.

- Statistics of the CDC show that 8 percent of poverty-level children, but only 1 percent of above-poverty-level children, are lead poisoned.

- Statistics of the CDC show that 11 percent of black children, but only 2 percent of white children, are lead poisoned.

- Cancer incidence among black males is 50 percent higher than among white males. Cancer incidence for black females is 30 percent higher than for white females.

- The percentage of U.S. minorities, living in counties with commercial hazardous-waste facilities, is three times higher than the percentage living in counties without them.

The preceding statistics suggest that, largely because of morally irrelevant factors (like age, race, or income level), some people's interests may receive far less consideration than others. Yet the standard account of human rights (surveyed earlier) requires equal consideration of people's interests—procedural equality. Age, race, or income level, alone, obviously are not morally defensible grounds for treating people unequally with respect to their needs for clean air or clean water. Therefore, such seriously unequal treatment constitutes *prima facie* injustice, *prima facie* threats to human rights to life.

Just as with the *severity* of some pollution threats, the *inequality* displayed in the preceding instances of *prima facie* environmental injustice is extreme. As a result, these inequalities are evidence of *prima facie* violations of human rights. Recognizing these violations, however, requires determining no *a priori* threshold for inequality. Why not? At least some of the preceding inequalities are so serious and so obvious—for example, five times more black than white children who are lead poisoned—that they clearly violate human rights. Likewise, as already argued in chapter 1, if 2,600 U.S. children annually die from murder, and another 1,400 die from child abuse, people should be even more alarmed that 6,000 children annually die of cancer, most of which is preventable and environmentally induced. After such severe and inequitable harms are addressed, there will be time to debate secondary issues, like the precise thresholds for calling any harm a "human-rights violation." For now, enough evidence exists to show that, *prima facie*, at least some pollution is severe enough and unequal enough to threaten human rights to life.[23]

Premise 2: Citizen Responsibility for Pollution and Environmental Injustice

Despite the evidence of chapters 2–3, polluters alone are not responsible for pollution-related threats to life and human rights. In a complex and interdependent society, this responsibility for human-rights problems like environmental injustice is shared, but is different for different people in different situations. Polluters typically are most responsible because they directly cause many citizens' unequal access to clean air, clean water, and protection of life. Insofar as special interests fail to follow the law, ignore obvious risks, or suppress health-related information, for instance, they contribute to citizens' failures to fulfill their equal human rights to life, to know, and to give or withhold consent to pollution-related risks. To the degree that government officials do not stop these threats, they are next most responsible. Yet to the degree that citizens in a democracy are able to influence government, they too are responsible for these threats. As philosopher Thomas Pogge puts it, discussing global hunger, many harms are caused by "economic arrangements designed and imposed by our governments." Because "these governments are elected by us, responsible to our interests and preferences, [and] acting in our name in ways that benefit us," the "buck stops with us." Citizens thus bear partial *ethical responsibility* for pollution-induced health and human-rights threats because of *what disproportionate benefits* they derive from such pollution arrangements. They also bear *democratic* responsibility for them because of *who they elect* and *how they participate* in democratic self-government. If citizens did not bear democratic responsibility, it would make no sense to hold those in a democratic society more responsible than those in a totalitarian society. Because people do hold citizens in a democracy more responsible, citizens obviously have at least some accountability for injustices perpetrated by their governments and institutions.[24]

How do citizen failures in democratic responsibility for pollution occur? Consider three ways—use of automobiles, pesticides, and waste incineration—in which virtually all citizens gain economically or medically as a result of their imposing higher pollution burdens on the most vulnerable members of society, like children.

Statistics from chapter 1 and from this chapter's discussion (of premise 1 of the responsibility argument) showed that children are particularly at disproportionate risk from ozone and from airborne particulates. Who and what cause the ozone and particulates that are implicated in so much disproportionate harm to children? The U.S. Environmental Protection Agency says motor vehicles cause at least half of ozone pollution, mainly because automobiles release most of the nitrogen oxides and reactive hydrocarbons that combine to produce ozone.[25] Even in California, with the strictest U.S. automobile-pollution standards, per mile each vehicle emits, on average, 2.1 grams of nitrogen oxides and 1.6 grams of hydrocarbons, for an annual California total of 1.2 million tons of nitrogen oxides and hydrocarbons.[26] Similarly, in Europe roughly half of all nitrogen oxides,[27] and half of urban airborne particulates, are released by motor vehicles.[28] This suggests that, to varying degrees, virtually everyone who drives an automobile is partly ethically responsible for the deaths resulting from ozone and particulates. People are more responsible by failing to purchase the most efficient, lowest-polluting, or zero-emission cars. They also are more responsible by failing to drive less, to carpool, to walk or ride a bike when possible, to shop by phone or mail, to ride public transit, to telecommute, to accelerate gradually, to use cruise control, to obey the speed limit, to combine errands into one trip, to keep cars tuned, to replace air filters frequently, to keep tires properly inflated, and so on.[29] By not driving lower-emissions cars (which the California Air Resources Board says would add about $1,000 in per-car costs, once all proposed California regulations were phased in), drivers save this $1,000;[30] impose much of their car's higher air-pollution risks on others, especially children; and thus fail to bear the full costs of their driving an automobile. As a consequence, they are responsible for some auto-related environmental injustice. As the chapter later mentions, they also are responsible for environmental injustice to indigenous people whose rights are violated because of questionable oil-extraction practices. Failure to control both auto emissions and locally harmful oil-extraction practices save money for oil and auto companies and therefore for their customers. Yet if consumers gain financially from oil-related environmental injustice, they arguable have some duties to help end the harm, to compensate those harmed, to pay the full costs of their own petroleum and auto use—and not to impose these costs on unwilling others.

Similar environmental injustices occur because of pesticide use, injustices whose death tolls were outlined in chapter 1 and in the earlier discussion of premise 1 of the responsibility argument. As these data showed, a disproportionate number of pesticide-related fatalities and serious neurological and developmental injuries occurs among children. Although chapter 1 gave data showing that pesticide use could be cut by half, without serious economic consequences, instead U.S. pesticide use has increased by more than 50 percent in the last three decades. In the United States, it now amounts annually to 8 pounds per person.[31] Consumers are clearly responsible for this pesticide-induced environmental injustice because pesticides save them money. Organic food averages about 50 percent more than inorganic. Yet these consumer cost-savings for pesticide-laden food come at the expense of children's (and farm workers') lives and health. Those who buy pesticide-laden food do not bear the full financial or health costs of the chemicals. Fairness suggests that consumers need to pay the full costs of foods they eat, not impose them on others, especially children.[32]

Similar environmental injustice likewise occurs because of the ways that developed-nation citizens save on their health and economic costs by imposing waste-incineration risks on others, especially on the children of the poor. A 2005 WHO study showed that current levels of air pollution, including that from waste incinerators, are implicated in much childhood disease and death; at least in the United States, waste incinerators, metal-processing facilities and other industries annually release over one million tons of lead, other heavy metals, and dioxins that are known to cause immune dysfunction, cancer, hormonal changes, and developmental abnormalities.[33] Annual U.S. waste-incinerator ash annually totals 17 million tons, of which 51,000 tons are lead.[34] In part because children absorb much more of this lead than do adults, chapter 1 showed that the U.S. Centers for Disease Control confirm that sources like incinerators and lead paint have caused 900,000 U.S. children under age five—4.4 percent of all U.S. children—to have blood-lead levels able to cause irreversible cognitive, behavioral, internal-organ, blood-forming, and developmental damage, as well as reduced IQ, delinquency, and criminality. Moreover, as chapter 1 emphasized, the children who are hurt by airborne lead from waste incinerators tend to be the children of poor people and minorities, because more incinerators are sited in their neighborhoods. In poorer areas like south-side Chicago, waste from states far away is trucked in, to be burned. Because most upper-middle-class and wealthy people do not bear the waste-incinerator risks from their own garbage, but impose them on others, especially children, they fail to pay the full health costs of their own waste-generation. Consequently, they are partly ethically responsible for the health harms imposed on the children of the poor.

Whenever certain neighborhoods in northwest Indiana, New Jersey, Houston, or elsewhere receive disproportionately higher pollution, it is likely because other people receive undeserved economic benefits or less pollution. They do not bear the full costs of their own products or activities, and their money allows them to impose these costs on others. Consider the many metal-fabrication plants in the "Cancer Alley" of northwest Indiana, discussed in chapter 1. They produce goods whose consumer prices likely would be higher if the manufacturers controlled more pollution. Thus the consumers of these goods receive unearned economic benefits—borne on the backs of residents of northwest Indiana. Largely minority, south-side Chicago has filthy air partly because it has a disproportionate number of waste incinerators. To the degree that wealthy garbage-creators do not bear the full risks and costs of their own waste, they receive unearned and disproportionate economic benefits from what they impose on the poor. Although the wealthy may neither know nor intend this transfer of burdens, they have duties to inform themselves and are at least partly causally responsible for it.[35]

Often people become causally and ethically responsible for health and human-rights threats because of where they shop and what they buy. Many people shop at Wal-Mart because it has lower prices. But critics charge that Wal-Mart has lower prices because it often pays and treats its own U.S. workers unfairly and because it purchases most of its goods from Chinese companies that use child laborers, slave laborers, or unfairly compensated workers, many of whom labor in environmental conditions harmful to their lives and health. If citizens either fail to try to inform themselves of these possible misdeeds or know about them but continue shopping at Wal-Mart, but without doing anything to help reform it, they are *prima facie* partly responsible for any harm done by Wal-Mart. Why? People have obvious negative duties not to uphold injustice. They have duties not to contribute to, profit from, or participate in, the unjust treatment of others. This is not to say, of course, that harm-causing institutions like Wal-Mart do no good. Virtually all organizations that contribute to life-threatening and rights-threatening environmental injustice also do great good. They may provide jobs to workers and cheaper goods to consumers. Yet such benefits do not completely excuse unjust behavior. A person would not be excused for committing murder merely because she also did much good in her life. Likewise, an institution is not fully exonerated from life-threatening environmental injustice, merely because it also generates significant benefits.[36]

Sweatshops are another example of why citizens have partial ethical responsibility for environmental injustice. Recall the chapter 1 examples of Central-American sweatshops. In developing nations, sweatshops sometimes may provide the best work available. In the United States, however, such excuses do not work because sweatshops are illegal. In the United States sweatshops are defined as providing wages violating the federal minimum and working conditions violating the U.S. Fair Labor Standards Act. United States sweatshops typically rely on child, slave, or immigrant labor, and nonenforcement of labor laws. Numerous studies have shown that, beginning in the early 1980s, sweatshops returned to the United States. Because some U.S. sweatshop laws are not enforced, female immigrants often work on apparel behind barbed wire, inside locked rooms, without legally required health and safety protections. They often work for $1.60 an hour, for as long as 17 hours each day. Concentrated in New York, California, and Texas, these sweatshops produce merchandise destined for stores like Macy's, Filene's, and J. C. Penney's. The U.S. Labor Department estimates that more than half the garment shops in these U.S. areas violate U.S. laws. Other social scientists say 75 percent of U.S. apparel workers labor in sweatshop conditions—conditions of environmental injustice. Yet partly because they fail to protect workers' health and human rights, environmentally unsafe sweatshops provide much cheaper textiles to U.S. consumers. Currently, the average U.S. household spends about 4 percent of its annual income on clothing, of which roughly half is thought to be produced under sweatshop conditions. Partly as a consequence of such sweatshop purchases, the percentage of U.S. household income, now spent on clothing, is less than half of what it was 50 years ago. Sweatshop-produced apparel is now estimated to cost U.S. consumers only about 58 percent of non-sweatshop-produced clothing. These figures suggest that, without the environmental injustice of sweatshops, the average U.S. household might have to spend about 5.5 (as opposed to 4) percent of its annual income to purchase the same clothing.[37] The average U.S. household thus saves about $650—1.5 percent of its annual income of $43,300—because of its (perhaps unintentional) participation in the oppression of apparel workers and its not paying the full costs of its clothing.

In comparing what U.S. consumers save because of sweatshops, note that the average U.S. household gives about $0.30 per day in government foreign aid, plus another $0.12 per day in private donations to the global poor. This means the annual foreign-aid total (government and private) contribution of the average U.S. household is about $153. Per person, this is about half of what the French and the English give, and about one-eighth of what the Norwegians give.[38] These figures suggest that the average U.S. household annually saves more than four times more money, just by buying sweatshop-produced apparel, than it spends on all its foreign-aid contributions, which are less than those in some other nations.

Because of environmental injustice, U.S. consumers also may fail to pay the true costs not only of sweatshop-produced clothing but of other goods, like authomobiles, pesticides, and incinerator wastes, all discussed earlier. Consider the environmental injustice to indigenous people that is often associated with the extraction and use of oil.

Shell, for instance, has taken roughly a million barrels of oil, every day, from Nigeria during the last 60 years. At 2006 prices, this means that for 60 years, Shell has extracted Nigerian oil now worth up to about $22 billion annually. During this time, it has paid only about $9,600 annually ($575,000 total) in compensation for oil-spill damages, despite the fact that 30,000 Ogoni tribespeople in Nigeria have been made homeless, and 2,000 Ogoni have been killed because of Shell operations. Shell has failed to clean up oil spills, destroyed farmland, and flared virtually all of its natural gas. The flaring has released many developmental and neurological toxins and carcinogens—such as unburned polycyclic aromatic hydrocarbons, particulate matter, aldehydes, ketones, and volatile organic compounds like benzene, toluene, and xylene. When local people, like the Ogoni, nonviolently protest oil-company destruction of their homelands, Shell and other companies sometimes put pressure on the military to kill or injure the protestors. Although they typically give oil-related royalties to military dictatorships abroad, the companies often destroy the land of local agricultural people, who receive no compensation for their losses. The nonviolent indigenous group, Nigeria's Movement for the Survival of the Ogoni People says Shell owes it $6 billion in royalties and $4 billion for environmental devastation of its homelands. Is its demand reasonable? For comparison, recall that U.S. regulatory analysis presupposes that an environmentally induced death is worth at least $5 million. If this U.S. standard were applied to the Ogoni demand, and if one ignored the 30,000 Ogoni made homeless by Shell, just the 2,000 Ogoni deaths could arguably deserve compensation of at least $10 billion (2,000 x $5 million). This $10 billion is double what the Ogoni seek for loss of their lands and people, and it is only a fraction of the annual value of the Ogoni oil that has been extracted for 60 years. Should Shell pay the Ogoni? According to the U.S. Department of Energy, in June 2000 a Nigerian court found Shell guilty of a large leak that contaminated Ogoni land in the 1970s. The court ordered Shell to pay $40 million in clean-up costs and damages. Instead Shell has filed appeals contesting the Nigerian court ruling and has claimed that the facts are not clear in the Ogoni case. Is such behavior justified? In 1995, most nations agreed that Shell encouraged the Nigerian government to hang 8 nonviolent Ogoni activists. As a result, virtually all developed nations protested Shell's behavior and withdrew their diplomats from Nigeria. Shell had to hire seven U.S. PR firms to try to clean up its image. A huge global coalition of nations, companies, and organizations has boycotted not only Shell but also ChevronTexaco and ExxonMobil.[39]

ExxonMobil and ChevronTexaco, the top two U.S. oil companies, extract about half of Nigerian oil, and Shell extracts the other half. ExxonMobil and ChevronTexaco are expected to double their extractions by 2010, and they appear to behave in ways similar to Shell. ChevronTexaco, for instance, has leased helicopters to the African military for the purpose of attacking demonstrators whose lands and homes are being destroyed. ChevronTexaco has provided dollars and infrastructure to the Nigerian military that kills nonviolent environmental activists.[40]

Apart from their benefits to consumers and to the economy, oil and gas explorations in the Amazon, Africa, Asia, and the Arctic also have devastated scores of indigenous people around the globe. They have caused native peoples to lose their lives and health, their territories, their economic stability, and their collective identities. In this century alone, one-third of all indigenous cultures existing in Brazil have gone extinct—roughly one per year. This is what occurred, for instance, with the Tetetes of Ecuador who disappeared after Texaco began oil extraction on their lands in the 1970s. In such situations, indigenous people are able to exercise no rights of self-determination and consent. Often oil and gas companies will offer them medical and educational services, but only in exchange for giving up all their rights regarding petroleum extraction. As a result of oil projects like those in Nigeria, indigenous populations all over the globe have experienced air, water, and soil contamination—and thus increased respiratory diseases, reproductive and neurological disorders, and cancer. Water samples in oil-extraction regions of countries like Nigeria and Ecuador reveal levels of toxic contamination many times what is allowed in Western nations. Projects like the 620-mile Chad-Cameroon pipeline, built by ExxonMobil, ChevronTexaco, and Petronas, appear typical. It has displaced people against their wills, polluted their homelands, strengthened the Chad dictator, funded his new arms purchases, and begun the pattern of death, displacement, extinction, disease, and prostitution that marks oil development. The Gwich'in of Alaska, the Achuar and Nahua of Peru, the U'wa of Colombia, the Khant-Mansy of Siberia, the Nukak and Mascho-Piro of the Amazon basin, and the Baka and Efe of the Congo basin all seek to end oil and gas projects imposed on them. Military dictatorships, relying on foreign dollars, often allow oil extractions to be done in ways that violate local people's rights to life, to consent, and to due process—as has occurred in places like Nigeria, Thailand, Ecuador, Colombia, and Myanmar. Trying to prevent such human-rights violations, the state of Massachusetts ruled that it would not provide government contracts to companies doing business with the military dictatorship in Myanmar. In response, oil companies like ChevronTexaco and the National Free Trade Council sued Massachusetts. In 1999, the U.S. Supreme Court ruled against the Massachusetts law, which was modeled on successful U.S. anti-apartheid laws of the 1990s. The ChevronTexaco behavior in Massachusetts suggests not only that oil companies sometimes participate in Third-World human-rights violations but also that they actively oppose those who seek to stop these violations. Interestingly, as CEO of Halliburton, U.S. vice-president Dick Cheney signed an *amicus* brief against the Massachusetts law about Myanmar.[41]

If the oil-company behavior outlined in the preceding paragraphs is typical, the 1997 Kyoto Oilwatch Declaration may be correct. It argues that "climate change is only one part of the ecological debt accumulated by the industrialized countries through their exploitation of resources in the South." It claims that "transnational corporations and state-owned energy companies have primary responsibility for the exploitation of fossil fuel reserves" and for "the destruction of . . . biological and cultural diversity." According to the declaration, instead of promoting economic prosperity through ethically defensible oil extraction, companies often have done what saves them the most money. "Corruption, cultural destruction, involuntary resettlement, and violence are too often the outcomes of fossil-fuel development." Why? "Taxpayer funds from Northern countries that are intended for poverty alleviation and sustainable development, which must be paid back by Southern taxpayers, are instead being used by multilateral and bilateral aid agencies for corporate welfare in the form of investments in fossil-fuel projects, which benefit mainly multinational corporations and local elites in the borrowing countries" because of the unethical ways these projects are designed and implemented. "Fossil fuels comprise the bulk of that energy lending."[42]

Are U.S. citizens partly responsible for the environmental injustice often accompanying flawed ways of engaging in fossil-fuel development? After all, U.S. citizens comprise 4 percent of the global population but use 25 percent of global oil, more than half of which is imported.

One reason U.S. consumers are partly responsible for oil-related environmental injustice is that they use the oil that often has been obtained in questionable ways. That is, consumers participate in oil-related economic and trade relationships that are sometimes unethical. A second reason for their partial responsibility is that U.S. consumers elect the leaders who have subsidized the oil industry and, as a result, have subsidized or allowed environmental injustice like that in Nigeria. Annually the U.S. government alone provides about $35.2 billion in subsidies to U.S. oil companies—or about $350 per U.S. household; independent economists claim that the U.S. oil subsidy is actually roughly $55 billion per year.[43] Of course, oil subsidies may not be cost effective, especially from an environmental perspective. Nevertheless, because subsidies and resulting environmental injustice may help current U.S. consumers pay less than the full price for gas, this is a third reason that they are partly responsible for the environmental injustice. All things being equal, consumers gain disproportionate and unethical economic advantages whenever oil companies treat indigenous people unjustly and destroy their lands. Oil companies' failure to pay the full costs of their oil extraction results in cheaper gas expenses for U.S. households.[44] Such costs include human-rights abuses, land and water degradation, the disappearance of native peoples and habitats, global warming, and so on. Because U.S. oil consumers receive the economic benefits of the failure to pay these full costs, they also are partly responsible for oil-related injustice. As citizens, they may not have worked to promote market fairness, to prevent subsidies that appear to allow environmental injustice, or to produce a system in which consumers bear the full costs of the products they use.

If the clothing, automobile, pesticides, waste-incinerator, and oil-industry examples are typical, they suggest that just in economic terms, U.S. consumers gain far more, from *prima facie* injustice abroad, than they offer in aid to the foreign poor. They also suggest that the average U.S. household may gain in many ways because it fails to pay the full, human-rights, environmental-injustice price of the goods it uses. Almost all Americans are thus partly complicit in human-rights abuses, even if they do not intend them, and even though there is no simple algorithm for determining each person's precise level of responsibility. Therefore, as the second premise of the responsibility argument maintains, they bear *ethical responsibility* for these abuses. This responsibility differs, depending on factors such as the level of harm caused, the benefits gained, whether beneficiaries intend the harm, whether they bear culpable ignorance for it, whether they try to prevent it, and so on. Each person's level of ethical responsibility needs to be assessed, case by case, situation by situation. Regardless of these individual differences, however, because sweatshop-analogue arguments hold for many environmental and institutional harms, consumers bear partial responsibility for them. Many harms arise from market failures to take account of externalities like dirty air. Others arise from various trade agreements, like those discussed in chapter 1. For example, some economists say that in 2004, the United States "collected $1.8 billion from tariffs—taxes—imposed on imported clothing and other goods from India, Indonesia, Sri Lanka, and Thailand, five times what it promised those tsunami-hit countries in emergency aid."[45] In various ways, wealthy members of developed nations participate in economic networks that save them money, often at the expense of the health and human rights of the poor. If so, they are complicit in this harm and bear partial ethical responsibility for it, as noted in premise 2. To varying degrees, they may contribute to what harms "innocent people for minor gains."[46]

How do pollution-related failures in *democratic* responsibility occur? Instead of electing leaders who substantially reduce life-threatening pollution and then distribute it equally, many citizens elect those who do the opposite. In other ways citizens also fail to do the work of democracy, such as lobbying leaders to enforce pollution laws, or helping educate fellow citizens about pollution. The APHA suggests that one prominent way in which citizens fail in democratic responsibility is by electing leaders who spend the U.S. budget inappropriately. The APHA condemns budget cuts for things like health and pollution enforcement, while leaders increase spending on militarism. In its resolution 8531, for instance, the APHA said the "escalating military budget" harms "preventive public health" and has "serious actual and potential negative effects on the health of people in the United States."[47]

It is not easy to distinguish different levels of democratic responsibility for the harms done by the government institutions of which people are a part. There is no simple algorithm, and instead responsibility must be determined, case by case, by means of a variety of ethical considerations. For instance, citizens have more democratic responsibility, all things being equal, to the degree that nation-caused harms are serious, citizens have personally benefited from them, and citizens have the ability to change things. To help distinguish different levels of democratic responsibility, consider the following six situations of responsibility, greatest to least. There is no space here to discuss levels of responsibility in detail. Nevertheless, all things being equal, polluters, government leaders, or other citizens bear less democratic responsibility (for life-threatening or rights-threatening environmental injustice) as one moves down the list. Citizens' democratic responsibility also varies, from most to least, insofar as they elect leaders (or do nothing to stop leaders) who err in the following ways.

1. *Legally requiring harm to others.* For instance, citizens do nothing when officials legally require polluters (who do not reduce pollution) either to buy pollution credits that create life-threatening "hot spots"

or not to release information about life-threatening pollution—
to which citizens have rights to know.

2. *Legally allowing harm to others.* For instance, citizens do nothing
   when leaders permit polluters either to buy pollution credits or not
   to release information about life-threatening pollution.

3. *Foreseeing but indirectly failing to prohibit or prevent harm to
   others when it could be prevented.* For instance, citizens do nothing
   when leaders fail to prevent polluters from withholding information
   about life-threatening pollution.

4. *Failing to enforce prohibitions against harms to others.* For instance,
   citizens do nothing when officials fail to enforce polluters' reporting
   their emissions through the Toxics Release Inventory to which
   citizens have rights to know.

5. *Failing to alleviate naturally induced harms.* For instance, citizens
   do nothing when leaders fail to alleviate pollution harms to those
   who were born genetically more susceptible to such harms.

6. *Failing to alleviate victim-induced harms.* For instance, citizens do
   nothing when leaders fail to alleviate additional harms to smokers
   that occur primarily because they smoke in an area of already high
   pollution.[48]

Besides these six illustrations, many other sets of circumstances affect levels
of democratic responsibility. For instance, consider citizens who work in a
nongovernmental organization (NGO) that tries to protect against environmental injustice. Obviously, they are less responsible for environmental injustice than those who never do such work.

Without going through all the factors affecting citizen's democratic
and ethical responsibility for environmental injustice and human-rights
violations—a discussion too lengthy to be presented here—the preceding discussion is sufficient to show three important points. First, a variety of factors
makes people more or less responsible for harms like environmental injustice.
Second, each case must be analyzed individually to determine someone's precise level of responsibility. Third, most people probably bear far more responsibility for environmental injustice than they realize.

Premise 3: Duties Based on Responsibility for Harm

Earlier sections and chapters defended premises 1 and 2 of the responsibility argument. They show that citizens (premise 3) must either defend the
prima facie unjust institutional order from which they unfairly benefit, or stop
participating in it, or compensate for this injustice by working for reform.

Why do citizens face this either-or situation? If some *prima-facie unjust*
institutional order exists (premise 1), citizens are responsible for this injustice

if they either unfairly profit from it, bear culpable ignorance about it, or elect those who cause the injustice (premise 2). As a result, premise 3 requires them either to forgo their institutional membership (often not a realistic option); to compensate for their unethically obtained benefits; or to show that the alleged injustice is, *ultima facie*, just. Why? Justice requires avoiding complicity in pollution-related serious harms, and therefore justice also requires compensating for this complicity. All criminal and civil law is built on this same fundamental presupposition of compensation. Not to rectify some injustice or compensate for it would destroy the very concept of justice itself. The best compensation for some injustice is working to stop it—to change the social order that allows it. One also might work to benefit those most victimized by that injustice. Recognizing that such compensation is required, the APHA "urges affected communities and populations, patients, caregivers, and all concerned persons, to work in coalition," to make "urgent efforts, through legislation . . . advocacy and litigation, to stem further" threats to public health. It even goes so far as to endorse public-interest law groups, saying they have "stimulated citizen participation in environmental decision-making, have brought suits on behalf of citizens seeking to stop pollution, have prevented the marketing of harmful drugs and pesticides . . . and . . . given support and backing to the actions of regulatory agencies involved in consumer and environmental protection."[49] In short, the APHA presupposes something like the responsibility argument and its third premise when it urges citizens to work for public health and environmental justice.

Premise 4: Excuses for Environmentally Unjust Institutions

For the responsibility argument to establish someone's partial and *ultima facie* accountability for a specific case of environmental injustice in an institution in which she participates, however, one also would need to show that none of the three "excusing" claims mentioned earlier (claims 4.1–4.3) is true. That is, one would need to show that the *prima facie* environmental injustice cannot be excused, *ultima facie*, on grounds that it involves no real injustice and has occurred naturally (or without human causation), has been compensated, or cannot be remedied. If any of these excuses holds, ultimately one bears no (or less) responsibility for alleged environmental injustice.

To assess each of these three excuses for alleged environmental injustice, one must investigate case-specific details. For now, however, consider how one might respond, in general, to those who use these excuses to deny the responsibility argument. Objectors might say the alleged environmental injustice arose naturally (without human causation) rather than through injustice, was compensated, and cannot be fixed by means of any alternatives. I call these, respectively, the nature-versus-injustice objection, the compensation objection, and the no-viable-alternatives objection to the responsibility argument.

The Nature-Versus-Injustice Objection: Tax Policies

Perhaps the most common response to some case of life-threatening and rights-threatening environmental injustice is that the pollution is "just business" or has occurred naturally (without human causation), not because of any injustice. This nature-versus-injustice response is *correct*, insofar as there are some natural factors that exacerbate most pollution effects. Weather patterns like air inversions, for instance, might keep polluted air in a valley. This response is *incorrect*, however, insofar as none of the pollution harms outlined in chapter 1 arose only because of some natural occurrences. Rather, at least some of the harms have been worsened because of specific historical injustices. In general, environmental injustice typically is not wholly natural, as the APHA recognizes, because it is partly the result of information suppression, coverup, environmental crime, misrepresentation of science, and so on, all of which threaten rights to know, to consent, to life, and to equal treatment, as was outlined in chapters 2–3. Most manufacturers and government officials probably are not guilty of "orchestrating ignorance" about pollution. Nevertheless, to the degree that people are unable to give or withhold genuine consent to pollution, their rights are violated. To the degree that many are guilty, life-threatening pollution is not merely a natural occurrence. Indeed, the same factors responsible for attempts to cover up many threats to life and health are responsible for them in the first place. Both previous chapters and The APHA have argued that many coverups and life-threatening environmental crimes have occurred, for instance, in the institutional orders associated with some major chemical companies and with energy or nuclear interests. Since virtually all citizens participate in these two institutional orders, by virtue of using their products or consuming their energy, virtually all bear partial ethical responsibility for the harm done by these orders.[50]

A second bit of evidence, suggesting that at least some pollution-induced harm is not wholly natural, is that it is not evenly distributed across the United States or across the world. Instead there are pockets of severe pollution, traceable to local contaminants imposed disproportionately (and therefore unfairly) on children, poor people, blue-collar workers, and minorities, often as a result of bearing others' burdens, like trucked-in garbage. The disparity of these burdens indicates that natural factors like poor genetics are not the main or sole cause of pollution-induced death and disease. Neither nature nor accidents has caused minorities and poor people to become the canaries in the coal mines of environmental injustice. In the case of minorities, as the APHA affirms (see chapter 1), environmental injustice in the United States is partly a legacy of slavery, civil-rights violations, and racism that continue to the present day. Given this history of racism, it will be difficult to excuse serious and disproportionate pollution threats to minorities.

In the case of poor people, environmental injustice also is not wholly natural. Instead, as the APHA—and earlier chapters and sections—have shown, it is partly the result of historically unjust U.S. tax and regulatory policies. At least since the mid-1970s, these policies have benefited the rich at the expense of the poorer 80 percent of the U.S. population. Although environmental injustice has occurred because pollution policies threaten people's rights to life, to know, to consent, and so on, tax policies have exacerbated these rights violations. Higher taxes have made poor people more vulnerable both to deadly pollution and to information-suppression about it because they have fewer socioeconomic resources, like medical care and good education, to deal with pollution-related threats. Because of their poverty and powerlessness, dealing with life-threatening pollution is not their first priority. First, they must work harder than others just to survive, feed their families, and hold down several jobs. For them, the urgent comes before the important, and environmental justice is not the most urgent problem of their lives.

How has this partly natural, partly unjust "poverty creation" exacerbated pollution threats to life and human rights? Partly it has been caused by tax policies that have helped increase U.S. economic inequality. In 1949, the wealthiest 1 percent of the population held 22 percent of U.S. wealth. In 1990, the wealthiest 1 percent held 35 percent of the wealth. In 2002, the wealthiest 1 percent held just under 50 percent of U.S. wealth. In only a half century, the holdings of the top 1 percent of U.S. citizens doubled. Likewise, in 1970, the ratio between U.S. CEO pay and U.S. worker pay was roughly 33 to 1, whereas in 2001 it was roughly 465 to 1.[51] By the year 2000, the United States

> was the most unequal society in the advanced democratic world.... The bottom 40 percent of Americans owned less than 1 percent of the nation's wealth. The bottom 60 percent...less than 5 percent of wealth....The typical African-American household had 54 cents of income...for every corresponding dollar in the typical white American household. Hispanics had 62 cents.[52]

The U.S. Congressional Budget Office says such wealth concentration has not occurred purely naturally but has arisen partly because the rich have been taxed less.[53] In constant dollars over the last 25 years, the 400 richest Americans increased their net worth by 500 percent, while the top 1 percent increased it by 150 percent. Yet the net worth of the middle 20 percent of all Americans decreased by 10 percent. Today, the U.S. upper-middle class is effectively in a higher tax bracket than multimillionaires. This is largely because of tax legislation with "special provisions"—like the 650 loopholes in the 1986 so-called U.S. Tax Reform Act and the 1990 "tax reform" overhaul. These "special provisions" put families earning $70,000–170,000 in the 33 percent tax bracket and those earning over $170,000 in the 28 percent tax bracket. Yet in 1948, the median U.S. family's effective tax rate was 5.3 percent, while that of the top 1 percent of families was 77 percent. By 1985, both the median and top 1 percent rates were roughly 24 percent. Over the last half century, the bottom 80 percent of Americans has borne a 500 percent increase in its share of federal tax burdens. This is partly because corporations and wealthy people have successfully lobbied to pay less. In 1950, corporations paid 27 percent of the federal tax burden, while workers' payroll taxes covered 7 percent. By 2000, corporations were paying only 10 percent of the federal tax burden, while payroll taxes covered 31 percent. Yet, in the last 20 years, U.S. corporate profits have increased by 80 percent, while hourly compensation in private industry has increased by only 2 percent.[54]

Even without illegal activities, such lobby-based and campaign-contribution-based economic and tax policies have created a tilted playing field that contributes to environmental injustice. This tilted field makes it more difficult for ordinary citizens to have the time and money to get adequate information about, and to prevent, environmental-health threats. And such difficulties are continuing. The Washington-based Citizens for Tax Justice showed that 1980s tax cuts for the richest million Americans added $1 trillion to the national debt—to be paid by future generations. The 2002 and 2003 U.S. tax cuts will have similar effects. Yet in 2000, with almost no public awareness, 12 of the largest U.S. corporations, including Goodyear, Texaco, Colgate-Palmolive, MCI, and Kmart, paid no corporate-income taxes whatsoever. They earned tax credits during the Clinton years of 1996–98, despite earning profits of tens of billions of dollars. During 1996–98 alone, U.S. corporate profits rose 23.5 percent, while corporate tax revenues rose only 7.7 percent. The data presented here, along with that in earlier chapters, is enough to make a *prima facie* case that special interests have influenced tax-related legislative outcomes, helped cause increasing economic inequality, and consequently threatened the ability of many poor and middle-class people to fulfill their rights to life, to know, and to consent to pollution-related risks.[55]

United States citizens have become less able to protect their environmental health, all things being equal, because after adjusting for inflation, most Americans have lost economic and therefore political ground over the last 5 decades. In constant dollars over the last half-century, U.S. workers' taxes, debts, and hours have all increased. U.S. workers also have been laboring longer but earning less than many of their western European counterparts. Using market-exchange rates, Germany, Denmark, Netherlands, Norway, Sweden, and Switzerland now pay their average manufacturing-production workers, respectively, 51, 22, 11, 28, 19, and 31 percent higher hourly compensation than does the United States. Yet U.S. workers now have longer hours than they did in 1950 and longer hours than the Europeans.[56] Compared to Europeans, U.S. workers likewise have weaker pension coverage, health coverage, vacation time, and maternity leaves. Yet they have one of the highest rates of hypertension. As a consequence, virtually all social indicators show that U.S. quality of life, for the bottom 80 percent of the population, after adjusting for inflation, has been declining at least since the 1970s. Based on measures such as wages, unemployment, health care, child poverty, dropout rates, drug use, violent crime, elderly poverty, and infant morality, the indices show that the current U.S. quality of life is about 66 percent of what it was 25 years ago. Since the middle 1970s, the poverty rate also has been increasing, from about 11.5 percent in 1976, to about 12.7 percent (37 million people) in 2004. Such census data suggest that specific historical, socioeconomic policies of the government have contributed to poverty and racism, and thus to environmental injustice. Because this injustice has not occurred wholly naturally, citizens bear some responsibility for it—for what their government has done.[57]

The Compensation Objection

To the preceding economic and tax statistics, however, objectors might make at least two responses. As a *general* response, proponents of the compensation objection may claim that these tax policies and environmental injustices have improved everyone's welfare. Without these government policies, they say, everyone would be poorer. As a *specific* response, objectors may say that particular sets of circumstances have compensated victims of environmental injustice.

Consider first the general objection. It is true that Americans today have a far greater array of consumer goods than they did three decades ago. Nevertheless, this increase in available goods and consumer gadgets hardly excuses or compensates for environmental injustice. Why not? Because the preceding census data show that for the last 30 years, the poverty rate in the United States has increased, and the bottom 80 percent of Americans has become worse off; both in terms of economic welfare and of quality-of-life indicators, this 80 percent has little access to increased goods. Consequently, those who deserve the most compensation for environmental-injustice are probably those who have received the least—because the poorest people are typically environmental-injustice victims, yet the United States has become more economically unequal, as the previous data show. Over these last three decades, the share of U.S. wealth held by the top 1 percent of people increased from 20 percent to 50 percent. Even during the stock-market gains between 1989 and 1997, the wealthiest 10 percent of Americans took 86 percent of the gains, and the bottom 90 percent took only 14 percent, mostly through their corporate-invested retirement funds. There was virtually no "trickle-down" to 90 percent of Americans. This increased economic inequality might be ethically justified, however, if it made everyone better off—if it increased overall welfare. But because earlier census data show that increased economic inequality and decreased quality of life have undercut the supposed benefits of economic expansion, there is no apparent "increased welfare" to compensate for environmental injustice, for the declining economic welfare of 80 percent of Americans, and for the increased percentage of people living in poverty.[58]

More recent Internal Revenue Service data likewise illustrate that there has been little trickle-down in U.S. economic growth and therefore little compensation for environmental injustice. Between 2002 and 2004, the overall share of increased wealth going to 99 percent of Americans decreased.

Roughly 40 percent of the increased wealth went to the top 1 percent of wealthiest Americans, and 80 percent went to the top 10 percent of wealthiest Americans. Only about 20 percent of wealth went to the bottom 80 percent of Americans. Whose overall share of income increased during this period? Only the top one-tenth of 1 percent of Americans increased in wealth. At the same time, the effective-income-tax rates paid by this top one-tenth of 1 percent of wealthiest Americans declined at more than 10 times the rate reduction for middle-class taxpayers. Thus for 99 percent of all U.S. taxpayers, their incomes during this 2002–2004 period did not keep pace with inflation. Their overall economic welfare declined, as economic inequality increased. Yet their relative taxes increased. Only the incomes of the top 1 percent wealthiest Americans kept pace with or exceeded the rate of inflation. The top one-tenth of 1 percent had more income in 2003 than did the bottom third of the U.S. population. This is a sharp change from 1979, in which the poorest third of Americans had incomes that, together, tripled the incomes of the top one-tenth of 1 percent. Yet the reasons for this failed trickle-down are not purely natural. They are not only the intelligence or hard work of investors. Instead, economists studying the IRS and census data say, changed federal tax rules, large increases in CEO pay, and failures in worker pay to keep up with inflation have all caused 99 percent of Americans to receive no trickle-down—no increased economic benefits or increased quality of life—in exchange for increased economic inequality.[59]

But perhaps proponents of the compensation argument believe victims of environmental injustice are somehow compensated noneconomically? Victims do not appear to have more democratic or human-rights opportunities, especially since earlier statistics show that U.S. quality of life is about 66 percent of what it was 25 years ago. All but the top 20 percent of wealthiest Americans are economically relatively worse off, in the early twenty-first century, than they were a quarter century ago. Consequently, as earlier chapters and sections showed, this increasing economic inequality has made it harder for most citizens to fulfill their human rights, equal opportunity, and democratic participation in government. The *urgent*, economic survival, has provided them with less time for the *important*, democratic citizenship.

Nor can proponents of the compensation argument easily show that victims of environmental injustice are compensated through better health or health care. If anything, those most deserving environmental-injustice compensation today are those least likely to have good health care, simply because the poorest people (without health care) are typically environmental-injustice victims. As chapter 1 noted, although the United States is the richest nation in the world, the average health of its citizens is poor, relative to that in other Western democracies. For instance, U.S. infant mortality is higher than in 41 other countries.[60]

- Of all industrialized nations, U.S. rates of income inequality, poverty, and child poverty are the worst.[61]

- The U.S. premature-death rate is higher, and life expectancy is lower, than that in nearly all other industrialized nations.[62]

- Women in the United States are 70 percent more likely to die in childbirth than in Europe. The U.S. CDC say U.S. black women die in childbirth at nearly four times the rate of white women.[63]

- Harvard statistics show that mortality is strongly related to income *inequality* but not to median or per capita income.[64]

The upshot? Proponents of the compensation argument err if they say quality-of-life, economic, democratic, or health-related opportunities somehow compensate victims of environmental injustice. In the last three decades in the United States, instead, these four opportunities appear to have decreased, as environmental injustice has increased.[65]

Perhaps the same factors, responsible for environmental injustice, also are responsible for blocking its compensation and for increasing quality-of-life, economic, democratic, and health-related inequality. As Thomas Jefferson realized, whenever special interests have excessive concentrations of wealth, they can control life, information, and even democratic government.[66] The economic successes of the tobacco industry show how wealth can often trump democracy. Courts showed that this industry engaged in fraud, claimed its "light" brands were less hazardous, and deliberately made cigarettes addictive. Yet tobacco has weathered 50 years of legal challenges, including the federal government's continuing attempts to claim $280 billion in a racketeering case. Phillip Morris, which has half the market, has been a defendant in 454 U.S. tobacco cases and 151 cases in other countries. Just between 2002 and 2004, Phillip Morris spent $933 million in legal costs. Still, tobacco stock remains high—a lucrative investment. The reason? Wall Street investment analysts say the cigarette industry can pay lawyers $850, often $1,000, per hour and beat its challengers in court. "With such legal [and economic] power, the tobacco companies have enjoyed a reasonable measure of success in court." Since the large 1998 tobacco settlement, Phillip Morris has enjoyed 27 verdicts in its favor, while plaintiffs have had only 16. As Wall Street analysts put it, "if tobacco companies lose in one court, they [have the money to] simply move to the next [court]. . . . In general the litigation environment has gotten better for them, and their stock prices reflect it." Plaintiffs seeking damages from cigarettes, pollutants, or dangerous products, however, often do not have the money to keep appealing decisions. Nor can they afford to pay their attorneys $1,000 per hour. What is the democratic result of pollution victims' more limited economic resources? They bear higher evidentiary and informational burdens whenever they try to challenge those who harm them, withhold information, or threaten their human rights. At some point—a point already reached in tobacco and other cases—economic inequality thus tips the scales against democracy, human rights, and even life. For the *general* version of the compensation objection to succeed, however, proponents would have to show that, despite the increased quality-of-life, economic, democratic, and health inequalities of the last three decades, victims have been compensated for environmental injustice. The preceding arguments do not suggest that proponents can easily do so.[67]

Suppose proponents make a more *specific* compensation objection? Suppose they argue, as many libertarians do, that those who live in areas having dirty air or water are compensated in many specific ways? Libertarians claim these citizens pay less for housing and taxes, live closer to their jobs, and thus save in transportation costs. Are such compensation claims correct?[68]

On the positive side, in principle, compensation for environmental injustice makes sense. It is better to compensate innocent people for injustice than merely to impose uncompensated harms on them. In addition, compensation often provides a practical way of siting needed but polluting facilities, so-called LULUs—locally unacceptable land uses. For instance, the 1982 Wisconsin provisions for landfill negotiation specify compensation provisions that have made siting successful. *On the negative side,* several reasons suggest that supposed housing, tax, or transportation benefits rarely compensate pollution victims. For one thing, pollution victims rarely consent to living in dirty air, in exchange for compensation. What poor person, worrying that her children were at risk, would willingly choose to live in dirty air, merely because housing prices were cheaper there? Rather, social-scientific data show that people often live in dangerous places, against their wills, because they have no other options. While they may be partially compensated through lower housing prices or better pay, they do not agree that this compensation is either adequate or worth the health of their children. Instead, they often say they are unaware of the health threats, that threats were not disclosed, or that they were exploited. Perhaps they "agreed" to cheap housing and dirty air involuntarily, merely because they had no other options. If these are the responses of pollution victims, then they have not consented to pollution risks. Whenever they have not genuinely consented, the compensation objection fails. Besides, if the supposed compensation were genuine, other people would willingly move into dirty areas, just to receive the supposed housing or tax "breaks." But people, who are not forced to do so, typically do not choose to move into dirty areas. Therefore, benefits like cheaper housing probably do not adequately compensate for environmental injustice.[69]

A third ethical problem with this more specific compensation objection is that while lower housing or tax costs theoretically might help compensate adults for their pollution burdens, children could never be compensated in this way. They are most damaged by pollution, least able to choose it, and largely innocent victims. For this objection to succeed, there can be no innocent third parties, seriously harmed by pollution, despite compensation. Yet as chapter 1 reveals, there are many innocent victims of pollution.

Even if pollution victims were somehow compensated, it is not obviously ethical to impose life-threatening pollutants on them. In cases of medical ethics, experimenters are not allowed to expose people to serious known harms, in exchange for compensation, because this would amount to treating persons like commodities, to be bought and sold. Another classical, medical-ethics requirement is not to target vulnerable groups and thus exploit them. If nonvulnerable people do not agree to participate in some experiment, medical ethicists take this as *prima facie* evidence that the experiment is ethically suspect, and that vulnerable people are somehow being targeted and exploited. Both examples suggest that, because medical-risk victims have protections against being targeted or deliberately harmed in exchange for money, victims of environmental risk arguably also ought to have the same protections. Because they do not, the compensation argument is ethically suspect.[70]

Apart from ethics, for the compensation objection to succeed, proponents must show that pollution victims actually receive housing or tax breaks because they breathe dirtier air. Yet much economic literature says the opposite. Especially among the poorest people with the least socioeconomic power, supposed compensation is limited or nonexistent. In poor neighborhoods, landlords often are able to get away with almost anything, including high rents and substandard housing. Why? Their clients are poor and thus less powerful. Typically, even grocery stores in low-income neighborhoods are overpriced, and their food is beyond the package-expiration dates. Typically, even the risky jobs of the poor have no hazard pay. Many studies show that only college-educated, unionized, male, skilled, non-minority, or non-low-wage workers enjoy a compensating wage differential or hazard pay, while all others do not.[71] Indeed, many economists say that for nonunionized and nonskilled workers, there is a *negative* compensating wage differential; they say that wages get lower as environmental-health threats increase.[72] This negative compensating wage differential likely occurs because, in many hazardous jobs, workers do not know the environmental-health threats they face, and they do not have other employment options, so they must work for whatever pay they can get. In other words, the same socioeconomic factors, that are responsible for environmental injustice, also limit compensation for that injustice. Consequently, both factual and ethical reasons suggest that the compensation objection fails.[73]

The No-Viable-Alternatives Objection

Citizens might be absolved from their *prima facie* responsibility for pollution-induced health and human-rights threats, however, if there were no alternatives to such threats. On the *positive* side, proponents of the no-viable-alternatives objection are partly correct. A bloody loaf of bread is better than no bread at all. Besides, people are morally obliged to do only what is possible. If it is not possible to reduce life- and rights-threatening pollution, people have no duty to try to reduce it. After all, ethicists agree that "ought implies can." Consequently, "cannot implies the absence of an ought." On the *negative* side, the objection errs in that it begs the question. To assume there are no alternatives to some environmental injustice, rather than to do a detailed empirical investigation in a specific case, merely creates a self-fulfilling prophecy. Besides, showing that there are "no alternatives" to some deadly pollution seems unlikely, because of advancing technology and the impossibility of proving negatives. For pesticidal chemicals, for instance, alternatives exist. As chapter 1 noted, at least half of pesticides are not necessary, and can be replaced with economically viable, biological forms of pest control.[74]

Instead, those who make the no-viable-alternatives objection may be claiming that "it is too costly" to remedy pollution-induced human-rights violations. But this begs a second question: "Costly for whom?" For the victims of pollution or for those who profit from pollution? Obviously objectors are wrong if they assume that some people have rights to jeopardize others' lives and health simply because their own profits are at stake. This assumption relies on free-market environmentalism and the cost-benefit state criticized in earlier chapters. Even when polluters bear high pollution-abatement costs, two reasons suggest these costs alone do not always outweigh pollution victims' claims to equal human rights, to equal protection from deadly pollution. The *first* reason is that, historically, the only ethically legitimate argument, considered sufficient for allowing some inequity to persist, is that it would lead to greater overall equality or fairness in the long run. This means that, at best, the no-viable-alternatives objection is incomplete. In addition to demonstrating empirically that there are no viable alternatives to some situation of environmental injustice, objectors also would have to show that the pollution and associated harms would lead to greater overall equality in the long run. Yet this would be something notoriously difficult to do, because economic expansion, as such, does not decrease inequality—as the just-discussed U.S. economic and tax history illustrates. The *second* reason (that high pollution-abatement costs do not outweigh claims to equal human rights) is that victims of life-threatening pollution typically are not requesting charity. They want an end to injustice from which other people have profited. Given polluters' profits, their imposition of injustice, and deadly threats to life, it is not reasonable for polluters to say that because pollution control is not cost effective for them, therefore it need not be pursued. Why not? An analogous argument would not work in the case of murder. People are not allowed to murder others, merely because doing so is more cost effective than not murdering them. Consequently proponents of the no-alternatives objection face overwhelming ethical and factual obstacles.[75]

The No-Will-to-Reform Objection

Perhaps those who object to the responsibility argument are making a different point. Regardless of what is technically or economically possible, perhaps they mean to claim that citizens *do not have the will* to accomplish significant reductions in environmental injustice or in life-threatening pollution. On the one hand, this objection might be right. Given the lobbying and advertising schemes outlined in earlier chapters, polluters seem to be persuading some people not to reduce pollution. Yet manipulated consumer preferences may not indicate genuine consumer opinion. On the other hand, several factors suggest that people either have, or can develop, the will to reduce harmful pollution. For one thing, as chapter 1 showed, Europeans and Japanese often enjoy greater longevity and have better pollution-control than Americans. Even if there is no causal connection between pollution-control and longevity, European and Japanese successes suggest that Americans also could be convinced to reduce pollution. They suggest that developed countries can have a strong sense of community, corporate ethical obligation, and commitment to the norm that individual polluters ought not gain at the expense of the entire community.[76]

Earlier chapters' accounts of polluter information-suppression also suggest that once people have more accurate information, they may have the will to control pollution. If most people were surprised by the public-health statistics outlined in chapter 1, this fact alone suggests that these data have not played a role in their thinking about pollution. Perhaps such data will do so in the future. After all, there could hardly be a more powerful motivator than people's desire to avoid bodily harm to themselves and their children. Asking whether or not people have the moral will to help reduce life-threatening pollution is like asking people on a runaway train whether they want to stop it. As epidemiologist Devra Davis emphasized, we already have a scientific blueprint for what must be done, and we should waste no more time in getting started.[77]

People also might have the will to control pollution if they recognized, as chapter 1 notes, that polluters often appeal to economics when it does not support their position. Economics rarely justifies some pollutant's massive death toll and other externalities or social costs. Earlier chapters' arguments against free-market environmentalism and the cost-benefit state show why not. So do the earlier examples of heavily subsidized nuclear energy, criticized by *The Economist*. The nuclear industry, like many other polluters, claims to make an economic argument for atomic energy. In reality, however, it is making a purely self-interested argument, one dependent more on subsidies than on actual market performance. Yet history shows that, once people recognize egoistic or self-interested arguments, they are not sympathetic to them and instead can be mobilized to support what is right. Moral force helped mobilize the nineteenth-century abolitionist movement, forcing the British government to suppress the slave trade. Moral force also was mobilized to end apartheid in South Africa. It was behind the 1964 U.S. Civil Rights Act. Similar moral force might be mobilized to reduce life- and rights-threatening pollution.[78]

Contemporary decision theorists, examining the prisoner's dilemma, help explain why moral force often helps mobilize people. They have shown empirically that often it is rational to be moral, that life is not a zero-sum game, and that all parties can gain when everyone cooperates. After all, failing to help those in need, failing to pay one's debts, failing to forgive, being envious, killing people with pollution, or allowing environmental injustice do not make people happy. They make people miserable. Many people cannot even be happy when they travel to a Second-World or Third-World resort for vacation. After seeing the poverty and injustice around them, they find it difficult to relax. Plato, Aristotle, Aquinas, and others explained why. They argued that humans are inherently social and other-directed. As a consequence, they said human happiness depends on living in a social and other-directed way—caring for others. But because only good people genuinely care for others, only good people fulfill their deepest natures and are thus authentically happy, that is, joyful and peaceful. Only good people lead a social, other-directed life of purpose and meaning—rather than a life focused largely on their own money, power, or pleasure. Zen Buddhists and other Asian thinkers also located the source of happiness in being good or virtuous, not in things like money, power, or pleasure. Their insights suggest that people can be motivated to recognize the *prima facie* duty to reduce life-threatening environmental-injustice because accepting this duty fulfills their essentially social, other-directed nature. As a consequence, it also will make them authentically happy. Accepting this argument also may promote one's own survival, not just that of environmental-injustice victims. Speaking of his experiences in a Nazi concentration camp, Viennese Jewish psychologist Viktor Frankl claimed that the only inmates who were able to survive the horrific conditions were those who looked out for others, who remained idealistic, or who found meaning in something beyond themselves. Those who did not turn outward, he said, succumbed to torture, despair, infection, or injury. They eventually died. Frankl even quotes the German philosopher Nietzsche: "He who has a why to live for can bear almost any how."[79]

Princeton philosopher Peter Singer makes a related point. People who have spent their lives working to reduce injustice to others will know that they have not lived and died for nothing. Harvard University child psychiatrist Robert Coles said something similar. He won a Pulitzer Prize for telling the stories of people who found rich and full lives by giving themselves to others. They lived lives of service and idealism. University of California sociologist Robert Bellah has documented the same thing. Humans share a deep sense of justice and community. These give them the will and the ability to help undo environmental threats to life and to human rights.[80]

Conclusion

This chapter argues that the three "excuses" fail, and thus that the responsibility argument has at least a *prima facie* plausibility. How should people respond to this argument? What should they do? Chapter 6 begins to address both these questions in more detail. For now, it is important to remember that what this argument requires is the efforts of ordinary people. The museum of Yad Vashem, established in Jerusalem to commemorate victims of the Holocaust, is a dramatic reminder of what ordinary people can accomplish. Leading toward Yad Vashem is a long, tree-lined avenue, the Alée des Justes, on which every tree commemorates a non-Jewish person who risked her life to save a Jew during the Nazi era. Each helper's case is carefully evaluated by a committee before a tree is planted. In many cases, these ordinary people who helped Jews were helping complete strangers. Only those who helped without hope of any reward have a tree planted for them. There are now more than 6,000 trees, spilling over onto a hillside, but the trees needed may number 500,000. Most of those who helped Jews were not famous—like businessman Oskar Schindler, who rescued those who were being taken to concentration camps by arguing that their special skills were needed for his factory. The Yad Vashem stories instead are mainly those of ordinary citizens who helped Jews. One was a Dutch mother of eight who, during 1944, went hungry herself and rationed food for her own children so that she could feed her hidden Jewish guests.[81]

The power of ordinary people also was evident in the American Revolution. Commenting on the era, some historians claim that only about 17 percent of the colonial population supported breaking away from the British. The merchant and industry class did not because it was bad for business.[82] The task of fighting for justice was left to others, just as it is today. What would happen today if 17 percent of people became aware of environmental-health threats and their responsibility for them? What would happen if they were convinced by the health data, inspired by ethics, and committed to do something about them? This book argues for another revolution, an ethical transformation directed at full citizen participation and institutional reform, to "make democracy work." The preceding arguments show that this is not a revolution recommended merely by charity, but one demanded by justice. It also is not a revolution that relies on accepting some new ethics. Instead it asks only that people rededicate themselves to same goal that inspired our ancestors more than two centuries ago—universal human rights.

5

Obstacles to Responsibility

Reverend Adolph Coleman is pastor of the West Pullman Church of God. In Chicago's south side, it is in Robbins, Illinois—incorporated in 1917 as the North's first all–African-American town. Robbins had been the first in the North to be wholly governed by blacks, and it was home to the nation's first airport managed by African-Americans. Yet today, with its small old clapboard houses, its narrow front yards and cracked sidewalks, it is among the poorest towns in America. Its per-capita income is about $7,000. The town's annual budget is roughly $1.6 million, but local property taxes produce only about $250,000 each year. Robbins has no gas station, no laundromat, and no fast-food franchises. Its 34 churches outnumber its 26 tax-paying businesses. By the late 1980s, Robbins was $6 million in debt. Reverend Coleman and other community leaders knew they had to do something.

In the early 1990s, a Philadelphia company proposed trucking in garbage from the East and building a local waste incinerator. Many of the 7,000 residents of Robbins viewed the proposed electricity-generating garbage burner as an economic boon. Pointing to nearly a million dollars in annual royalties, lease fees, and taxes, the mayor said the incinerator would bring jobs and economic recovery to Robbins.[1] Coleman disagreed. He knew that other towns had already rejected the incinerator as unsafe. Organizing community opposition, he argued that it would harm public health in his already highly polluted community. Even the U.S. Environmental Protection Agency (EPA) had declared Chicago "a severe non-attainment area" for air pollution. And Robbins was the dirtiest neighborhood in Chicago.[2]

With his sisters and his supporters, Reverend Coleman called or visited virtually every Robbins household to rally opposition to the facility. As they did so, the mayor and Robbins officials had him arrested and jailed. They claimed he had no right to leaflet against the proposed incinerator. But Coleman argued that because electric power in Robbins was cheaper than what the waste burner could produce, people were supporting the incinerator mainly because of the tax subsidies it promised. He explained that the Pennsylvania Energy Company was eager to build the plant because it would receive $300 million in no-interest loans and more than $400 million in tax incentives. Yet over 10 years, the incinerator would cost Chicago residents an additional $42 million in lost revenues.[3] Although Coleman showed that the Pennsylvania company would give Robbins several payments in the hundreds of thousands of dollars, for the next 23 years the Robbins tax base would slowly decline. Why? The agreement froze the incinerator's taxes.[4] As a result, schools and public services in Robbins would not benefit from the higher property-tax revenues that traditionally occur when the value of improved land increases. Moraine Valley Community College, for example, calculated that over 20 years, it would lose $21 million in tax revenues because of incinerator tax breaks.[5] Coleman also warned that a housing project, a senior-citizen home, and a medical center were within a few blocks of the proposed facility.

Accusing Coleman of acting against the best interests of his own African-American community, every school and church in Robbins refused to give him a meeting place to discuss the proposed incinerator. Coleman was forced to meet in a Pentecostal church in Blue Island—a working-class, racially mixed town near Robbins. There he joined forces with Reverend David Scott, an African-American Church of God pastor. Scott had already helped defeat three proposed incinerators for Blue Island. Nearby, citizens had stopped other waste burners proposed for south Chicago in Stickney, Harvey, Crestwood, Dolton, Ford Heights, and East Chicago Heights. What disturbed Coleman, however, was that few other African-American clergy in Robbins were willing to speak out against the incinerator. "Leadership gets bought out," he said. Preaching to his community, Coleman showed that the incinerator would compete with recycling efforts and the many jobs brought by recycling much of the trash, instead of burning it. He explained that the plant would threaten the health of anyone within a 30-mile radius because it would belch out high volumes of heavy metals. Each year the incinerator would put an additional 1,000 pounds of lead and 4,400 pounds of mercury into Robbins air, apart from its cadmium, dioxin, and furan emissions. Coleman showed that Robbins children, six times more likely to suffer from dangerous effects of air pollution than adults, already faced almost unbreathable air. Even the American Public Health Association (APHA) had said no one should build more incinerators in south-side Chicago because it already was so heavily polluted. One African-American radio announcer called the proposed Robbins incinerator another cause of the economic and environmental "apartheid" on the south side of Chicago.[6]

Lessons from the Chicago Case

Without even requiring cost studies of incinerator alternatives like recycling, in 1994 the Illinois EPA issued the permit for the Robbins plant. Coleman and others appealed this apparent regulatory capture, but the Illinois Supreme

Court sided with the EPA. It ruled that it was not unfair to site the incinerator in this already heavily polluted, poor, minority neighborhood.[7] The EPA and the court ignored the fact that incinerators have major capital costs and provide almost no jobs, whereas recycling has few costs and provides many jobs. Soon other south Chicago towns passed resolutions or filed suits against the incinerator. They claimed decisionmakers violated the law by failing to inform them about the proposed plant and its health threats. But it was too late. Too few had joined Reverend Coleman's community coalitions, and the incinerator opened in 1997.[8] Five new waste incinerators, all slated to burn trucked-in waste from wealthier areas, have been proposed for poor minority communities in south-side Chicago.[9]

If Adolph Coleman's case is typical, protecting public health may not be easy. Even community leaders like Coleman may be treated like the doctor in Henrik Ibsen's play *An Enemy of the People*. The doctor told citizens what they did not want to hear, even though hearing it was necessary to save them. Just as people turned against the doctor, they turned against Coleman. Another lesson of the Robbins case is that, compared to other citizens, community leaders like Coleman have greater responsibilities to try to protect public health precisely because they have greater abilities to do so. They have enjoyed greater privileges of education, professional leadership, and community trust. *Noblesse oblige*. Perhaps most important, the Robbins case illustrates the ethical and political necessity of carefully considering and answering the objections of those who support some polluting facility or action. Robbins officials believed that the short-term economic benefits of the proposed incinerator were an important way to promote community welfare. Coleman, however, tried to evaluate their objections through all the means of democratic deliberation available to him. Although he did not succeed in stopping the incinerator, he invigorated the process of community-building, public education, and citizen interaction. He made it more likely that future citizens would be able to protect public health.

Chapter Overview

Coleman's behavior is a model of how to behave ethically and reasonably in attempting to reduce pollution threats. He carefully considered and answered the objections of fellow citizens who disagreed with him. He worked interactively and democratically with them, trying to forge a community consensus. To clarify these duties of civic virtue, ethical analysis, and democratic deliberation, this chapter surveys some of the main objections that might be brought against the responsibility argument. Chapters 1, 3, and 4 already considered eight of these objections. This chapter evaluates eight additional concerns. I call them the unfairness objection, the burden objection, the neutrality objection, the uncertainty objection, the conflicting-duties objection, the economics objection, the collective-responsibility objection, and the failure objection.

Eight Earlier Objections

Chapter 1 responded to the *longevity* objection, the claim that pollution is not a serious public-health threat because people are getting healthier and living longer. Chapter 1 also responded to the *health-successes* objection, the claim that because public health is improving in a variety of ways, one ought not be concerned about pollution-induced threats to life and human rights. Chapters 3 and 4 evaluated the *natural-occurrences* objection, the argument that although pollution sometimes causes *prima facie* environmental injustice, citizens bear no responsibility for it because this harm is trivial compared to natural (non-human-caused) harms, to which citizens ought to direct their efforts. Also considered in chapter 4, the *rising-tide* objection is that those most victimized by environmental injustice are often helped by the economic prosperity that lenient pollution rules allow.

Chapter 4 considered four main attacks on the responsibility argument. The first, the *nature-versus-injustice* objection, is that citizens are not responsible for alleged environmental injustice because it arises naturally, not because of injustice. Second, the chapter responded to the *compensation* objection, the claim that alleged environmental injustice need not be corrected because its victims enjoy counterbalancing benefits, such as cheaper housing prices. Third, the chapter answered the *no-viable-alternatives* objection, the allegation that situations of environmental injustice cannot be improved. Finally, the chapter responded to the *no-will-to-reform* objection, the claim that, while environmental injustice could be prevented, people do not have the will to do so. Earlier chapters have shown that all of these objections rely on questionable ethical and factual premises. What remaining worries might someone have about the responsibility argument?

Special Responsibilities and the Unfairness Objection

One common objection is based on the fact that many people fail to be active in civic life and are "free riders." As a result, this objector argues that it seems unfair for the most conscientious people—like Reverend Coleman—to bear the heaviest burdens of helping reform societal institutions. In part, this objection is correct. All things being equal, people may have fewer civic responsibilities when others fail to do their fair share. Yet others' failures do not completely remove all responsibility for public health. After all, a high murder rate would not remove citizens' duties not to commit murder. Why not? Failure to accept either the responsibility argument or the murder prohibition could cause or allow great harms. If the statistics in chapter 1 are correct, the severity of the harm trumps even legitimate worries about fairness and free riders. Worrying about the unfairness imposed by assuming partial responsibility for life-threatening pollution needs to be put in perspective. It is like being in choppy seas on a crowded lifeboat and worrying that some passengers are rowing harder than others. Obviously, the free riders and lazy rowers are wrong. Yet those who overemphasize their own burdens, amid serious threats to life, often do so at their own peril. They would do better to emphasize the severity of life-threatening pollution. Doing so might both protect them and induce others to do more to protect themselves. As Reverend Coleman realized, unfairness and severe pollution have similar solutions—citizen education and citizen advocacy for prevention. Besides, no distribution of burdens in life is ever completely fair, because there are always people who do less than they should. One solution to such unavoidable unfairness is to recall the end of the previous chapter, and the connection between being virtuous and being happy.

Focusing on the unfairness of civic burdens, however, some ethicists deny that conscientious people like Adolph Coleman have greater duties to correct societal harms, just because they have greater abilities to "make a difference." They claim one should "distinguish between causing evil, on the one hand, and preventing evil or promoting good, on the other." They say people are responsible primarily to avoid causing evil.[10]

While there can be a distinction between causing evil and promoting good, this objection is not relevant to the responsibility argument. Why not? This argument is based on the premise that people have contributed to evil through the institutions in which they participate and from which they benefit. Thus the responsibility argument is about compensation for harm that one does, not about doing good. It is about justice, not merely charity. Moreover, apart from whether they are partly responsible for harm, virtuous people would try to protect others if they were easily able to do so. They would not forgo being benevolent, compassionate, or courageous merely because others did not help. Instead, they would recognize shared needs, shared conceptions of the good life, and membership in the same species. They might also recognize that sometimes accepting even unfair burdens is the right thing to do. Virtuous people also might recognize that all moral duties, including justice, presuppose beneficence. As a consequence, they might say everyone has *prima facie* responsibilities to be beneficent or to help prevent harm, especially whenever the sacrifice involved is trivial.[11]

The most important problem with the unfairness objection, however, is what it ignores. It ignores the fact that people with greater rights and opportunities often voluntarily accept these privileges. Consequently, they arguably have greater responsibilities. One reason that Reverend Coleman had greater duties to help prevent life-threatening pollution is that he had more education, leadership opportunities, and community trust than others. His chosen profession brought him these advantages. When people receive special rights and benefits because of professional, parental, or spousal roles, their doing so likewise imposes greater responsibilities on them. Even when people accept benefits (like buying cheaper clothing made in sweatshops) because of their roles as consumers, they thereby accept partial responsibility for the harm caused by those benefits. Otherwise the price of some people's benefits would be the blood of others. This is one reason that boycotting unethical or illegal activities is often morally required, a matter of justice and not charity. Fairness thus dictates that people bear greater moral responsibility for harm either when they have greater abilities to prevent it or when they themselves benefit from it.[12]

Following this "greater abilities" argument, ethics requires professionals, in particular, to meet a higher standard than that of nonprofessionals. Professionals have greater responsibilities to prevent societal harm than nonprofessionals not only because of their greater professional privileges and rights, but also because of the community trust they enjoy; their greater abilities, opportunities, and education; their being licensed and regulated by the community; and so on. No professionals are wholly self-made. Virtually no professional students, even in private schools, ever pay the full costs of their education. Because taxes and donations always supplement it, professionals owe society something more than others owe.[13] The intellectual capital or expertise of professionals is thus partly a "public resource," just as medical research is. Because it is often supported by the public, medical research is not merely a commodity to be bought and sold but something to be distributed partly according to public need.[14] For similar reasons, professionals' abilities, work, and privileges are not merely their own, to use as they wish. They also are something to which the public can lay rightful, if only partial, claim. As Hans Jonas expresses it: "the scope and kind of power determine the scope and kind of responsibility."[15]

Accepting this special responsibility because of their special power, scientists representing the Ecological Society of America routinely issue policy recommendations, as when they warned the public about lax federal regulations for biotechnology.[16] The APHA, in particular, has accepted its special responsibility for public welfare, and each year it issues about 20 policy recommendations. For instance, in 1981 the APHA responded to the Nestlé violations of international codes on marketing infant formula. As mentioned in earlier chapters, it warned of health threats from flawed Third-World marketing, and it called for a Nestlé boycott until those marketing strategies were changed. Because the APHA took this stance, it was easier for health advocates to gain support from other groups, like three major British pop bands—Pulp, Dodgy, and Ian Brown. Supporting the Nestlé boycott, the bands refused to take part in the V2001 music festival because it was sponsored by Nestlé. They charged that because Nestlé induces poor mothers to abandon cheaper, healthier breast-feeding, many babies die. Their parents are unable to keep buying formula and to provide sterile bottles. As Ian Brown's manager put it, we have the ability to give this cause "some street cred." As fathers, we know that "only by raising public awareness" can we "pressure companies to act in a socially responsible manner."[17]

As such examples suggest, if those with special talents or opportunities did not accept special responsibilities to prevent harm, the results could be catastrophic Even the courts have said as much. In cases involving client privilege and privacy, courts say professionals' first duty is to protect public health and safety. Thus a pharmacist, for example, may be liable for negligence in filling a prescription, exactly as written by an erring physician. In

Riff v. Morgan Pharmacy, the court found that every professional has "a duty to be, to a limited extent, his brother's keeper."[18]

Contrary to the unfairness objection, most codes of professional ethics also presuppose that greater abilities generate greater responsibilities. For scientists and engineers, their codes specify public health and safety as their highest priority. The National Society of Professional Engineers, for instance, says: "he [the engineer] will regard his duty to the public welfare as paramount. He shall seek opportunities to be of constructive service in civic affairs and work for the advancement of the safety, health, and well-being of his community." The American Association for the Advancement of Science emphasizes the "added responsibility of members of the scientific community, individually and through their formal organizations, to speak out," whenever public health or safety requires their doing so.[19] *The U.S. Code of Ethics for Government Service* says something similar: "public service is a public trust, requiring employees to place loyalty to the Constitution, the laws, and ethical principles above private gain." If professionals' primary and special responsibilities are to the public, obviously they ought to try to prevent harms to public health.[20]

A central reason that professionals have special duties under the responsibility argument is their near-monopoly over specific information and services. Neither the competitive marketplace nor public awareness can effectively police this near-monopoly and its potential harms. Consequently, professionals have greater responsibility to do so. As the leaders of the Scientific Research Society, Sigma Xi, said:

> Because the pathways that we pursue as research scientists are infinite and unfrequented, we cannot police them as we protect our streets and personal property. We depend on those other travelers—other research scientists whose work happens to take them along such lonely byways of knowledge—to assist in ensuring that the research environment is a safe one.[21]

Professionals also have special duties, under the responsibility argument, because of citizens' rights to free informed consent. To help ensure that citizens can exercise these rights and are not misled by information manipulation, professionals have duties to speak out. They must provide the public with whatever special information is necessary to prevent harm. Otherwise, as chapters 2 and 3 show, special interests may "get away with" disinformation.[22]

Television and the Burden Objection

As the unfairness objection suggests, however, it is not always easy to specify the limits on the duties imposed by the responsibility argument. Thus someone might make the burden objection: "I have duties to my own family and children. I have no extra time for anything. I should be free of the burden to help reform social institutions, even if they cause harm."

Obviously, this objection is partly reasonable. People are morally required to "prevent great harm" only when it is possible to do so and only when the personal costs are not excessive. Yet even small costs sometimes can be too great a burden. Some people may have other serious responsibilities. And even small costs, applied to many situations of harm, could be enormous. If people have only a modest number of occasions to help others or to reform harm-causing institutions of which they are a part, says political scientist Joel Fishkin, the burden is not great. But as moral philosopher Brad Hooker notes, such "minimal altruism" might have the *cumulative* effect of "overload." It might impose great burdens and severely restrict people's choices. If people were required *always* to make small sacrifices, their aggregate sacrifice could be overwhelming.[23] As a result, there must be an upper bound to obligations presupposed by the responsibility argument.

Contrary to Hooker's language, however, the issue here is not one of altruism. The argument of this book is not the altruistic argument of philosopher Peter Unger. He says we have obligations to make great sacrifices to aid the needy, for example, to give away most of an already-small salary. Instead the duties imposed by the responsibility argument are duties to help reform harm-causing institutions in which we participate. We have these duties precisely because our participation contributes to harm, and our benefits from participation make us partly responsible for this harm. These duties are a matter of justice, not charity. Nevertheless, we have rights to pursue our own commitments, apart from our duties to help reform institutions from which we derive benefits. We also have duties to do only as much as we are able, without jeopardizing our cheerfulness, sanity, or important relationships. The point is that we have *prima facie* duties to reform harm-causing institutions in which we participate. How those duties are specified, *ultima facie*, depends on analyzing each individual case.

What observations might help clarify the individual-case burdens imposed by the responsibility argument? In a context of charity, rather than justice, social philosopher Joel Feinberg recognizes that there are many needy people and pressing causes. Because people cannot do everything, he says they have some rights to choose among the eligible recipients of their aid.[24] Obviously, however, people have fewer rights to make such choices when they have helped to cause harm that requires compensation. People's rights to choose (where and how to compensate for harm) *decrease* because of many factors. These include a clear and immediate emergency, the necessity to prevent a great tragedy, one's level of responsibility for harm, or the ease of addressing the harm. However, people's rights to choose obviously *increase* because of many factors. These include one's innocence of harm, assistance that is mere charity, or the absence of professional duties of assistance. Because of such rights to choose, ethics does not require everyone in every situation to help reform harm-causing institutions for which one is partly responsible. Nevertheless, because the risk or cost of much help is minimal, most people probably can do far more than they are doing. For example, suppose some U.S. trade and aid policies toward Tanzania have been exploitative, yet citizens have done nothing to correct them. As a result, U.S. citizens are partly responsible for poor health in Tanzania. But suppose U.S. citizens also are partly responsible for poor health in 100 other nations, because of harms caused by the institutional orders from which they benefit. Would it be impossible to compensate for health harms in many of these nations? Perhaps not. Per capita medical spending in Tanzania is about $1.37 per year. About 26 percent of the people live on less than $1 per day. A majority of children under age 5 have vomiting, fever, convulsions, cough, diarrhea, or difficulty breathing, eating, or drinking. If only a few dollars a day would help alleviate such problems, there are good reasons to provide them, and for more than just one nation. Using criteria like those just mentioned (the immediacy of the threat and so on), one might have to choose recipients among the 100 nations. Nevertheless, many people can afford compensation, even widespread compensation.[25]

Precisely because the burdens of much compensation would be minor, if everyone contributed, philosophers like Peter Singer, Peter Unger, and W. D. Ross argue that people ought not forgo making small sacrifices in order to do great good for others. But again the argument here is even more modest than theirs. This argument is that because people owe duties of compensation, by virtue of their membership in harm-causing institutions, they ought not forgo minor sacrifices in order to prevent harm. But when is a sacrifice minor? Two characteristics come to mind. The sacrifices do not jeopardize important relationships or other duties. And they do not put sacrificers at a disadvantage relative to free riders who have sacrificed less.

While the precise level of sacrifice is not always clear, most people probably can sacrifice more time and money than they do. Consider that 54 percent of Americans over age 18 drink coffee daily, averaging more than three cups per day. Another 25 percent of people drink coffee occasionally. Consider also that one-third of these 54 percent, who are daily drinkers, drink expensive specialty coffees. Americans annually spend about $9 billion buying coffee retail, and another $9 billion purchasing it already brewed. Following the responsibility argument, what would happen if people donated the money for several Starbucks lattes each week? It might make a significant difference to organizations working to prevent environmental injustice. Something similar holds for donating time. Consider that the average U.S. adult watches more than 4 hours of TV each day. The average U.S. home has the TV set going daily for more than 8 hours. The average U.S. child spends nearly 4 hours daily watching television. Among 8- to 13-year-olds, that average is 4.5 hours. Sleeping and going to work are the only activities on which average U.S. adults spend more time than watching TV. A higher proportion of students in most U.S. states watches TV far more than do students in all other 18 countries reporting TV-watching data to the U.S. Department of Education. In 12 of these 18 countries, less than 80 percent of students watch 2 or more hours of television daily. Yet in 47 U.S. states, more than 80 percent of students watch more than 2 hours daily. One result of such TV habits? Homogenized, advertised, heavily edited, corporate values often replace personal interaction, learning, and community work. As chapters 2 and 3 warned, they also contribute to the way advertising, PR, and front groups can dominate public-health information. Other results? In 1999, U.S. 17-year-olds were far less likely either to read for pleasure or to spend 1–2 hours daily on homework than were their 1984 counterparts. Only about half of U.S. adults, aged 25 and older, read regularly—defined as reading a newspaper once a week or a book in the last 6 months. Such statistics suggest that it need not be burdensome for many Americans to contribute some time to public-interest groups working to prevent public-health harms. If many people contributed some of the roughly 30 hours weekly they spend on TV, they could easily fulfill the responsibility argument, promote social interaction and deliberative democracy, and address some of the social, political, and scientific problems surveyed in chapters 2 and 3.[26]

A third consideration also helps reduce the burdens of the responsibility argument. This is Henry Shue's distinction between the *scope* and *magnitude* of justice. Regarding *scope*, everyone on the planet has rights and duties grounded in human interdependencies and interactions. Yet, as already mentioned, the *magnitude* of the duties—their burden—is not the same for all because of the limits set by other duties and by what it is possible to do. What is a good test for whether duties are too burdensome? Would people with healthy self-interest, who are able to make a difference, *freely* and *noncoercively* accept them? If not, the burdens may be too great. Neither the responsibility argument nor any other moral argument can require people to "pay any price." Even benefits like public health are not worth the price of harmed personal relationships, reduced mental health, injustice, bloody revolution, or totalitarian enforcement. Whenever "an unbloody half loaf is better than a bloody loaf," duties under the responsibility argument are limited. People cannot always and everywhere make amends for the harms that their institutions cause. They can, however, as Henry Shue puts it, protect "a few at a time until it becomes too heavy a burden."[27]

Ethical Objectivity and the Neutrality Objection

But suppose people believe that while they ought to compensate for the harms done by institutions in which they participate, they ought to remain neutral and objective? They may object that their compensation ought to take the form of medical or social assistance, not political reform. Confronted with the problems outlined in earlier chapters, such objectors might say people ought to assist those harmed by faulty chemical regulations. Yet they might deny obligations to help reform the political system that produces such faulty regulations.

While this objection represents a noble effort to avoid subjectivity and bias, it errs in misunderstanding objectivity. And although there is not enough space here to go into the details of the extensive scientific debate over objectivity and value judgments, it is clear that objectivity is not neutrality or passivity, in the sense of avoiding all value judgments. Why not? It is *impossible* for someone to avoid all value judgments. To see why, consider value judgments of three types—bias, contextual, and methodological. *Bias* values occur whenever people deliberately misinterpret or omit something so as to serve their own purposes. These values can always be avoided. *Contextual* values include personal, social, cultural, or philosophical influences, such as where and how people grew up, or how much money they have. Contextual values play a role even in science, as when Korenbrot showed the influence of the value of limiting population growth. This contextual value caused many medical researchers to overemphasize the benefits of oral contraceptives and underestimate the risks. Because all knowing takes place in some context and is done by knowers who always have some context, contextual values often cannot be eliminated. As a result, the best strategy is to be aware of them and to ensure they do not lead to bias. *Methodological* values are even less possible to avoid. They are the judgments that people make in choosing one decision rule, scientific method, or data set, rather than another. Scientists collecting data, for instance, must make value judgments about what data to gather or ignore, how to interpret observations, and how to avoid erroneous ones. These methodological value judgments are unavoidable because they are essential to all knowing. Why? Human perception does not provide people with pure facts, but with observations that can be understood only through people's beliefs, values, theories, or categories of interpretation. Trackers do not "see" a certain animal's prints in the dirt. Instead, their methodological value judgments enable them to recognize the marks as made by one animal rather than another. Likewise, high-energy physicists do not count all the marks on their cloud-chamber photographs as observations of pions. Rather, they count only those streaks that their beliefs, training, and experience—their methodological values—indicate are pions. One reason contextual and methodological values play such a large role in life is that all belief is hampered by incomplete information. Facing unavoidable data gaps, people must either use contextual or methodological value judgments to bridge the gap or stop work. Because everyone, even scientists, must sometimes rely on incomplete information and theories, not all value judgments can be avoided. If not, it makes sense to use the best contextual and methodological value judgments possible.[28]

But if objectivity does not require neutrality, but making the best contextual and methodological value judgments, how does one do so? The first step is realizing that although all values are partially subjective, in the sense that none can be empirically confirmed, not all are subjective *in a reprehensible way*. Rather, some can be objective in the sense of being *unbiased* and evenhanded. Others can be objective in the sense that there are *good reasons* for them, like their consistency with other facts. Much science is objective in this sense. There were good reasons, like consistency, for accepting the unseen neutrino, a century ago, even though it had not been seen.

Likewise, there often are good logical and conceptual reasons for accepting one value judgment over another. The second step in moving toward objective value judgments is to criticize those that are obviously biased—subjective in a reprehensible way. This is what chapters 2 and 3 attempted to do. Thus one might criticize methodological value judgments to use small sample sizes or only short-term studies to assess effects of pollutants.[29]

A third step in moving toward objective value judgments—to reliably guide institutional reform and protect public health—is realizing that they have two main characteristics. First, objective value judgments are tied to fair and evenhanded representation of situations, as just discussed. They avoid bias values, like conflicts of interest. As Mary Midgley recognized, what constitutes bias is not the acceptance of one's own scheme of values but the refusal to look at anyone else's.[30] Second, objective value judgments are recognized by testing them. As just discussed, do they survive relevant criticism by the community of people who understand the situation? The results of such testing/criticism illustrate why, as chapters 2 and 3 suggest, people can be *blamed* for their failure to be objective in making value judgments like those about small samples. But if people can be blamed, it must be possible to be more or less objective. It must be possible to be more or less evenhanded in judgments, more or less responsive to criticisms of those judgments.

But what makes criticisms of value judgments and social institutions more or less objective? At least four factors come to mind: empirical factors like data, conceptual factors like consistency, ethical factors like conflicts of interest, and explanatory factors like predictive power. Regarding *empirical* factors, chapter 2 showed that *The Economist* used economic data to criticize the 2005 Bush administration decision to subsidize risky commercial nuclear technology. *Conceptual* factors, like consistency, also can anchor objectivity. Chapter 2 showed that it is inconsistent for the nuclear industry to make the value judgment that its plants are safe, yet to demand from the federal government a liability limit that protects it from 98 percent of nuclear damages. *Ethical* factors likewise can help anchor objectivity. As chapter 2 showed, the value judgments of chemical companies like Dow and Monsanto were not objective when they violated ethics and suppressed information about the hazards of dioxin. Finally, *explanatory* factors can anchor the objectivity of value judgments. As chapter 3 showed, it is more objective to make the value judgment that scientists on federal regulatory-advisory committees ought not be consultants for the regulated industries than to allow it. Why? Allowing such consulting has been shown to explain repeated instances of obvious committee bias. The upshot? While the preceding empirical, conceptual, ethical, and explanatory factors provide no algorithm for making objective value judgments, they do explain what reasonable people call "objective." Reasonable people—even scientists—make value judgments every day. They accumulate observations and inferences until the probability of their judgments is so great that they do not doubt them. They call their judgments "objective" when the balance of empirical, conceptual, ethical, and explanatory evidence supports them. They believe that objectivity requires neither infallibility nor perfect judgments nor neutrality. It requires only evenhanded, well-supported judgments that are able to survive repeated testing and criticism. In other words, scientists, lawyers, and ordinary people typically rely on value judgments that are *prima facie* true (reasonably probable, or because of a presumption in favor). People can never show something is infallibly true. They can establish that an action is *prima facie* ethical, never perfect. Because they can not, only *prima facie* truth or *prima facie* ethical behavior often is necessary in order to behave ethically. If people need only prima facie knowledge that their attempts to reform harm-causing institutions are reasonable and unbiased, their attempts easily can be said to be objective.[31]

What would happen if people tried to follow the neutrality objection against the responsibility argument? The consequences would be disastrous. People would have to avoid all criticism, even criticisms of unjust ethical positions, faulty science, heinous crimes, or irrational inferences. But obviously they ought not be avoided, just as seeking to reform harm-causing institutions ought not be avoided. In fact, non-neutral but objective criticism may be the only way to avoid biases like those surveyed in chapters 2 and 3. Consider the case of John Graham, former director of Harvard University's Center for Risk Analysis. He later became director of U.S. president Bush's Office of Information and Regulatory Affairs at the Office of Management and Budget. Graham's Harvard center was completely funded by the worst corporate polluters, such as tobacco and chemical companies. Perhaps as a result, it produced research that consistently took anti-regulatory stances. Graham's studies denied risks of secondhand smoke; they downplayed risks to children from pesticides; they repeatedly contradicted U.S. National Academy of Science and U.S. Environmental Protection Agency findings. What would happen if citizens remained neutral and failed to criticize Graham's "hire education" or cases like those in chapters 2 and 3? These omissions would only increase flawed science and self-interested politics. They would merely endorse whatever values were dominant. Proponents of the neutrality objection thus tacitly endorse dominant values, even flawed values. They are *inconsistent* in implicitly *sanctioning* dominant or status quo values yet explicitly *condemn*ing making value judgments. Thus the most objective thing to do, in the presence of questionable value judgments, is not to remain neutral but to engage in unbiased and evenhanded criticism.[32]

Why do so many people confuse objectivity and neutrality and, perhaps as a result, avoid all political activity? Perhaps people confuse three different questions, and thus what objectivity requires. (1) Are there *general principles* (e.g., postulate environmental risk probabilities that are consistent with observed accident frequencies) that promote objective knowledge? (2) Are there *particular methodological procedures* (e.g., observe accident frequencies for a period of at least 5 years before concluding they are consistent with postulated probabilities) that promote objective judgments? (3) Does a specific knowledge-claim or action, *in fact*, always illustrate either the general principles or the particular procedures? Some people erroneously assume

that whenever one answers questions (2) and (3) in the negative, the answer
to question (1) is negative. This is false. Debate about question (2) does not
jeopardize objectivity, so long as people agree on question (1). In fact, debate
over question (2) must presuppose objectivity in the sense of question (1).
Otherwise the discussion would be futile. Therefore, whenever people can
answer question (1), even if they cannot answer questions (2) and (3), they
can have objective knowledge.[33]

A second reason people may confuse objectivity and neutrality is their
forgetting that both ethics and knowing generally exhibit a hierarchy of rules
and value judgments. Different degrees of certainty and objectivity are appropriate at different levels of ethical or epistemological generality. Whenever
people demand certainty that is inappropriate for some level, they may believe objectivity is impossible. In ethics, for instance, the *most general* rules
are the *most certain*. For example: "Postulate risk probabilities consistent
with observed accident frequencies." "Do good and avoid evil." The *least
general* rules or value judgments are the *least certain*. For example, "person X
errs in killing person Y under circumstances Z." In order to apply rules from
the most general level, people must make a number of value judgments at the
least-general, lower levels. The objectivity of these lower-level value judgments may be anchored in the four ways discussed above. For instance, some
value judgments are better than others because they are better *means* to the
end of explaining behavior.[34] By thus understanding objectivity in terms of
different levels of certainty and *prima facie* truth, one relies on the insights of
Karl Popper, John Wisdom, and Ludwig Wittgenstein. These philosophers
identify objectivity with actions, as well as with explanatory and predictive
power. They do not define objectivity only in terms of some simple algorithm
or an impossible notion of justification. Instead, they also tie objectivity to
actions—the criticisms made by the relevant knowledge communities. According to this scheme, when is a value judgment about the safety of some
food additive objective? When it is able to survive and answer the criticisms of
those informed about, and potentially affected by, the additive. Although there
is not enough space here for this social and critical account of knowing
to address more detailed debates over objectivity and neutrality, in general
this account presupposes that objectivity, in its final or least-general stages,
requires people to appeal to particular cases, just as legal justification requires. This account does not presuppose an appeal to *specific rules* of knowing and acting, applicable to all situations. Nevertheless, *general rules*—such
as surviving evaluation by means of consistency, fairness, and consequences
likely to occur—always are used by the critical community of knowers. Using
techniques illustrated in chapters 1 and 3, community members can employ
democratic deliberation to discover which judgments are more objective.[35]

But this point about the community of knowers emphasizes a third reason
that people often confuse ethical objectivity with ethical neutrality. Knowing
is social. It takes place within a varied community of knowers, each having
a multiplicity of different values and insights. These different perspectives—
exhibited in public debate, open exchange, criticism, and amendment of

one's views—all help secure objectivity. Seen from the vantage point of a community of knowers, objectivity does not require neutrality. Instead, it requires only the existence of a diverse and critical community within which bias can be detected, criticized, and laid to rest. For those who use a purely individual model of knowing, however, there is no obvious way to correct error. This is why, despite their differences, Phillip Kitcher and Helen Longino say even an unbiased individual knower is an inadequate focus for objective understanding and action. Why must objectivity also rely on the criticisms and amendments of community members? Because any single observation is "always selective," the best way to be objective is to multiply standpoints, to "increase experience," to adopt a critical attitude, to be ready to modify views on the basis of criticism and interaction. Alternative standpoints, including those of women, minorities, heavily impacted environmental stakeholders, or oppressed people, are particularly important in ethics. Otherwise, people could fall victim to the dogmatism of their own selective standpoint. As philosopher John Stuart Mill recognized, the surest way of getting to the truth on any question is to examine all the important objections that can be brought against candidate opinions. As Philip Kitcher put it, knowing requires a "division of cognitive labor," a community whose richness and diversity suggests the inadequacy of privileging any particular observer or agent as alone "objective."[36]

If the preceding arguments are correct (even though they have not gone into the technical details of the debate), proponents of the neutrality objection are wrong to reject attempts at institutional reform as always biased. They erroneously tie objectivity to neutrality, to freedom from all value judgments, and to privileged observers like scientists. Instead, objectivity should be tied to a social account of knowing, to the very community interactions that underlie democratic deliberation, as defined in chapter 1. Psychologists Daniel Kahneman and Amos Tversky suggest there are good reasons for supporting this account of objectivity. They have shown that once experts move beyond pure data, their value judgments often are no more reliable than those of laypeople. Philosopher Anthony Kenny said something similar. The opinions of scientists about facts are reliable only within their own science and only to the degree that they make no questionable value judgments. If science cannot avoid at least some value judgments, and if even science can fall victim to the sorts of flawed value judgments illustrated in chapter 3, there is an antidote—the social account of knowing just defended. Even committees of the United States National Academy of Sciences have argued for such an account. They argue that experts and laypeople should have equal roles in human-health risk assessment because assessment is as value laden as it is scientific. This means that *what* a pluralistic community ought to *believe* about objectivity is bootstrapped, in part, onto *how* that community ought to *act*. It ought to act with procedural fairness. It ought to evenhandedly evaluate and predictively test all relevant perspectives, including those of stakeholders, scientists, women, children, minorities, environmentalists, industrialists, and so on. It ought to provide a marketplace of ideas for analyzing, defending, and criticizing alternative beliefs, actions, and positions—so as to secure objective beliefs. As Israel Scheffler points out, "objectivity requires simply the possibility of intelligible debate over the merits of rival paradigms." Similarly, objective social reforms, in response to the responsibility argument, require not neutrality but objectivity in the sense of democratic deliberation, tested by the community.[37]

Precaution and the Uncertainty Objection

Frequently, however, people are not sure about what is objective in a particular situation. Often there is no community consensus on criticisms of social institutions that might cause harm to public health or human rights. After all, for much of the twentieth century, there was no obvious community consensus on the harms caused by cigarette smoking. Proponents of the uncertainty objection thus might complain that, in individual cases, people often disagree. They even disagree over the three conditions, outlined in chapter 4, that could undercut the responsibility argument. As a result, proponents of the uncertainty objection claim that attempts to reform institutions, or to compensate for alleged threats to health, are premature, if not wrong, because of various uncertainties. Is this objection a sound one?

First of all, as chapter 1 reveals, many health data are known. These data reveal an amazing consistency about many serious problems, despite some uncertainties about other health concerns. Besides, many uncertainties are not as great as they seem. As chapters 2–3 showed, sometimes they are manufactured by hire education and front groups, like those funded by the tobacco industry.

A third way to address uncertainty is to rely on the insights and arguments of philosophers such as Peter Singer and Peter Unger. They illustrate how detailed factual analysis of some uncertainty can help illuminate a particular case. Unger, for instance, asks whether donating to UNICEF is a reasonably certain way to help prevent Third-World childhood deaths. Reasoning about case specifics, he shows that donation does make sense. Why? The per-child cost of UNICEF vaccinations for tuberculosis, measles, whooping cough, diptheria, tetanus, and polio is only about $17. Besides, Unger shows that UNICEF vaccination programs have already been highly successful. They have cut Third-World childhood deaths from some diseases by 33 percent, and the majority of vulnerable children in the world live in countries where UNICEF is able to operate productively. Case-specific, factual analysis thus can reduce many uncertainties.[38]

The social account of knowing just defended also provides a way to reduce many uncertainties. According to this account, one ought to respond to uncertainty by immersing oneself in the community of knowers, by interacting and debating various aspects of this uncertainty in order to arrive at the best way of reducing it. Although there is no algorithm for reducing uncertainty, one requirement for doing so is the open interaction and critical exchange of deliberative democracy.

A fifth response to those who are worried about human-health uncertainties is that they can learn. After all, one could hardly respond, after taking on the responsibilities of parenthood, that one is absolved from being a good parent because one does not know enough. Why not? People are at least partially responsible for their ignorance and for the characters they have developed. In book III of the *Nicomachean Ethics*, Aristotle says ignorance does not always excuse people from ethical responsibility or from acting. They may be ignorant in part through their own fault and, as a consequence, may become unjust. This is why Aristotle argues that wickedness is in part voluntary, in the sense that wicked people often could have made other choices or could have become informed. For Aristotle, only unavoidable ignorance of a situation causes failure to be partially responsible for it.[39]

A sixth response to human-health uncertainties has already been provided by the APHA. As a default principle for dealing with uncertainty, the APHA recommends adopting the "precautionary principle." The APHA formulates the principle as the claim that situations characterized by potentially life-threatening uncertainty should be assumed harmful until proved safe. According to this principle, one should try to prevent potentially serious public-health harms even before all the details are known about them. What is the APHA rationale for this principle? Whenever one waits for potentially serious harms to become obvious or widespread before doing anything about them, it often is too late to stop the harms. As a result, AHPA recommends treating all chemicals as dangerous until they are proved otherwise. Following this principle not only protects human health against potentially serious threats but also provides an incentive for reducing future uncertainty. If polluters know that, in the absence of reliable data about their pollutants and products, government will follow the precautionary principle, they will be less likely to prolong uncertainty or to discourage doing the requisite scientific studies. When used as a default rule, the precautionary principle is a useful antidote to the informational problems like those discussed in chapters 2 and 3.

Some people, however, might reject the APHA recommendation to adopt the precautionary principle. Instead, they might say that in situations of uncertainty, citizens should follow what both law and science prescribe. The law requires people to be treated as innocent until proved guilty. In situations of uncertainty, pure science requires researchers to avoid false positives, false assertions of harm, rather than false negatives, false assertions of no harm. Proponents of the uncertainty objection believe that public-health protection requires following these same legal and pure-science rules. But does it?

Adopting these legal and pure-science default rules in areas of public health, contrary to the precautionary principle, is problematic on both factual and ethical grounds. Because I have given these arguments elsewhere, they will not be repeated here. In brief, however, they show that the analogy between either law or pure science and public health is fundamentally misguided. It is misguided for at least six reasons, as follows.

1. Legal presumptions of defendants' innocence are not always appropriate for polluters precisely because polluters, by definition, already are known to have released materials likely to be harmful. Moreover, the presumption of polluter innocence does not guarantee polluters the right to continue their activities, until some verdict is reached. Why not? The presumption of a serial-murderer defendant's innocence allows him no right to remain at large, out on bail, until his trial. While both defendants should be presumed innocent, community protection may require restricting their activities. Denying bail to high-risk defendants is like denying polluters the right to pollute until some verdict resolves the matter. Neither denial jeopardizes the presumption of legal innocence.

2. In civil cases, juries are required to determine guilt or innocence based on the preponderance of evidence. That evidence may be only 51 percent in favor of a particular verdict and 49 percent against it. Given the evidence presented in chapters 1–3, there already is a preponderance of evidence suggesting that some polluters cause harms to both life and human rights. Because of this evidence, although polluters must be assumed innocent, in general they ought not be allowed to continue polluting until their activities have been assessed.

3. Why did the founding fathers and mothers of the United States establish the legal default rule of "innocent until proved guilty"? One reason is that individual citizens typically were the defendants, and they often were more vulnerable than plaintiffs—who frequently were wealthy government or manufacturing interests. In cases of American public-health threats, however, corporations and not individual citizens are the typical defendants. Because corporations usually are not the more vulnerable party, the plaintiffs may have at least equal need for the presumption of innocence.

4. Why do pure scientists employ the default rule of avoiding false positives, false assertions of some effect? They typically do so for two reasons. One is that they would rather make no assertion than make a false one. The other reason is that their assertions, in any pure-science case, have no consequences for human welfare or human rights. In situations involving pollutant threats, however, most ethicists believe that one instead should follow the default rule of avoiding false negatives, false assertions of no harm. The reason? False assertions of no harm from pollution could have disastrous consequences for human welfare and rights. Consequently, pollution cases are radically disanalogous to the pure-science cases and ought not employ the same default rule.

5. In addition, as chapters 2 and 3 showed, phenomena such as regulatory capture, information suppression, and flawed private-interest science suggest that polluters sometimes have financial interests in covering up their harm and guilt. Thus, it may be naïve to assume that because polluters are presumed innocent, they should be allowed to pollute until some verdict resolves the matter.

6. Because polluters receive economic benefits from failing to control their releases, it likewise is unfair for their potential victims to bear the entire

burden of proof for harm. Those who receive the greater benefits from pollution should bear the greater costs, including many of the costs associated with the burden of proof.

If these six arguments, developed fully elsewhere, are correct, what follows? In the face of life-threatening uncertainty, ethics dictates following the APHA precautionary principle.[40]

Metaphysical Guilt and the Conflicting-Duties Objection

Suppose, however, people make a very practical, conflicting-duties objection to the responsibility argument. Suppose people say, with philosopher Fred Feldman, that they are not morally reprehensible just because they choose to try to make the world better in ways *other than* reforming institutions that promote environmental injustice. Perhaps instead they work for economic development or compose music.

The most basic problem with this objection, like the main problem with the burden objection, is its failure to recognize that the issue is not one of choosing among several options for *charity*. Rather, if the previous chapters are correct, the issue here is one of *justice*, compensating for harm caused by institutions from which one benefits. In addition, compensating for harms to which one contributes is more important than doing good in other ways, such as composing music. With philosopher Peter Unger, one also might question the conflicting-duties objection and argue that some obligations are not optional, not merely part of "nice charity thinking."[41] In situations of severe need, Unger says, people are not completely free in deciding when and how to practice charity, much less justice. Why not? A trivial sacrifice from donors might produce massive benefits for those in need. What follows if Unger is right that great needs create duties that are not merely part of charity? It follows that Feldman's objection begs the question. He assumes that alleviating even grave needs is purely optional. Suppose a parent took good care of only two of her three young children. The parent ought not object that her conflicting duties to those two justified her failure to care for the third child. The obvious problem with such a parental response is that it begs the question of whether the duties to the third child are as important as those to the first two. Like Feldman, she could be faulted for presupposing that care of all three of her children was merely a matter of choice. Presumably she gave up this choice when she assumed responsibility by virtue of her parenthood. Likewise, citizens' responsibility for institutional harms might be something they accept by virtue of citizenship or membership. After all, would it have made sense for citizens in Nazi Germany to claim they were not responsible for Nazi atrocities because they were attending to other good things, like composing music? If not, the conflicting-duties objection does not undercut the responsibility argument of the previous chapter.

Trying to explain why Nazism triumphed, French and German philosophers Jean-Paul Sartre and Karl Jaspers provide many insights into the conflicting-duties objection. What would be their likely response to people who say "other duties" prevent them from giving attention to pollution-induced deaths? Sartre and Jaspers ask why there are not more heroes when the times demand them. Their response is partly that people are morally guilty for their failures to act. Their more important point, however, is that people are guilty for the kinds of persons and institutions they allow themselves and their groups to become. They often allow themselves to become passive and weak people. As a result, they are unable to help stop major threats, like Nazism. "Metaphysical guilt" is the name Jaspers gave to people's responsibility for who they are and who they become. While not everyone bears moral guilt for Nazism, Jaspers says all people bear metaphysical guilt. They are morally responsible for not becoming the sorts of people who would have been able to help prevent harms like Nazi atrocities. Jaspers wrote:

> There exists a solidarity among men as human beings that makes each co-responsible for every wrong and every injustice in the world, especially for crimes committed in his presence or with his knowledge. If I fail to do whatever I can to prevent them, I too am guilty. If I was present at the murder of others without risking my life to prevent it, I feel guilty in a way not adequately conceivable either legally, politically or morally.[42]

Jean-Paul Sartre voiced a similar theme:

> If someone gives me this world with its injustices, it is not so that I may coolly contemplate them but so that I may animate them by my indignation, expose them and show their nature as injustices, that is, as abuses to be suppressed.[43]

No matter how restricted are people's options, no matter how many other duties they have, Sartre and Jaspers believe they always have some ability to confront injustice. At least they have some ability to avoid metaphysical guilt by becoming capable of responding to injustice. Sartre and Jaspers believe people can choose to be "authentic," can choose to accept responsibility for themselves and for the world they are helping create. With Aristotle, they believe people choose their character, through their repeated attitudes and actions. As a result, they also choose the subsequent behavior of which they are capable.[44]

Jaspers's account of metaphysical guilt suggests why, in the face of grave social harms like pollution-induced deaths, people cannot easily absolve themselves of responsibility by appealing to the conflicting-duties objection. People may have other duties, and this may excuse them from acting. Yet if people have failed to become the sort of individuals who are genuinely capable of confronting grave social harms, they are guilty nonetheless. If people have no "will to reform" harm-causing institutions and instead complain that the burden is too great or that other duties conflict, they may bear metaphysical guilt.

One way to correct this character flaw—that militates against civic responsibility and often appeals to "other duties"—is to begin to exercise control over our character. Among other things, this involves being sensitive to how our attitudes, actions, and omissions affect others. Because we sometimes can change bad behaviors, the ways we respond to others, we know we can change the behavior that ultimately shapes our character. We know that we are not mere victims of instinct or inclination. Education, psychotherapy, self-examination, and reflection all reveal that we are often able to improve and become more sensitive. We can overcome the tendency to associate only with certain kinds of individuals, to read only particular types of literature, or to remain passive participants in social institutions. Because we are able to improve, we can perform the moral duties necessary to accept the responsibility argument. These duties begin with self-improvement, with using means such as self-reflection to become more virtuous and more sensitive, with becoming more attentive to community needs, with reforming our attitudes and habits. As Aristotle notes: "While no one blames those who are ugly by nature, we blame those who are so owing to want of exercise and care."[45] While no one blames those who by nature cannot accept the responsibility argument, we blame those who are so owing to want of exercise and care.

Why do many people not take this first step of assuming responsibility for their own character? They might deny that they can change, that they are complicit in harm, or that change is needed. Or they might say, as in the current objection, that they have other duties with greater priority in their lives. Such responses may be legitimate, or they may indicate bad faith—moral blindness or lying to oneself about oneself. When Hannah Arendt covered the trial of Nazi war criminal Adolph Eichmann, she suggested why he was in bad faith. Why did he fail to take responsibility for his actions and those of the Nazis? Eichmann displayed an uncanny ability not to think about what he was doing, said Arendt. Extending this insight, Arendt coined the phrase "the banality of evil" to refer to the way apparently normal people, acting in groups, fail to think about what they are doing. As a result, they allow great harms. Arendt thus suggests that those who use the burden objection or the conflicting-duties objection must do at least two things. One is to avoid begging the question and instead to evaluate whether their other burdens and duties genuinely preclude following the responsibility argument. The other is to ensure that they are not in bad faith and not metaphysically guilty. Have they prevented themselves from becoming the sorts of people who, in principle, could take on the duties imposed by this argument?[46]

Equity and the Economics Objection

Suppose people reject the responsibility argument because they are not convinced that pollution reduction is a desirable way to prevent harm. Following the economics objection, suppose they claim that following this argument would threaten economic development, which is thought to benefit everyone overall. They also might say that reducing harm from pollution is contrary to promoting economic welfare—which benefits everyone equally.

Does economic development benefit everyone equally? Not if income is distributed unequally. Economists admit that economic growth does not change existing income distributions, but only exacerbates them. Hence economic growth is beneficial to all only if existing income distributions are beneficial to all. Moreover, recall earlier chapters' statistics about increasing inequalities in U.S. income distribution and about decreasing quality of life. Census data in earlier chapters suggest it is wrong to believe that economic growth is genuinely beneficial to all. A third problem with this objection is that reducing public-health threats and reforming institutions that threaten health need not jeopardize economic growth. Indeed, these actions promote the economic growth of the pollution-control, alternative-energy, alternative-manufacturing, and organic-foods sectors. The objection also errs in presupposing generally that economic growth ought to trump human life and human rights. After all, society does not let murderers go free just because it is not economically efficient to incarcerate them when it is unlikely that they will kill again. Instead, as already argued in earlier chapters, society recognizes that considerations like fairness, justice, and protecting human life typically take precedence over economic objections. Otherwise, as chapters 3 and 4 already argued, ethics would be irrelevant. Otherwise, innocent people would have their lives put at risk for the economic gains of others. Society could ignore equity and fairness and instead could impose social risks when it was profitable to do so. People would have no rights to consent to profitable risks imposed on them by polluters. Social decisionmaking would be reduced to economics. People would have to be "willing to pay" to protect their lives from profitable pollution. There would be no requirements for environmental justice or human rights, except in cases where it was profitable to recognize them. Obviously, none of these consequences makes sense.[47]

What about proponents of the economics objection who say that reducing pollutant-caused harm is contrary to economic welfare? Attorney Cass Sunstein makes this objection when he claims that because industries cannot spend regulatory-compliance monies on economic expansion and hiring, therefore regulatory compliance causes poverty. The fundamental problem with this claim is that it relies on several highly questionable presuppositions. One is that monies not spent on regulatory compliance would be spent on expansion rather than on CEO salaries or profits. Another assumption is that monies spent on regulatory compliance benefit no one. While these monies may not benefit polluters and their economic expansion, as already mentioned, they do benefit industries engaged in pollution control. These monies also encourage technological innovation to avoid or reduce pollution. They are not merely a drain on the economy but an addition to it. Such expenditures also benefit victims of pollution—who currently lose at least $25 billion per year because of health costs and lost workdays from pollution-induced sickness. Hence the assumption, that monies not spent on expansion of pollution-intensive industries are monies lost to the GNP, is clearly false.

Numerous ecotourist businesses demonstrate that sustainable development and environmental preservation can be profitable. Thus even economic considerations often favor preservation and pollution reduction.[48] Besides, as a 2004 U.S. National Academy of Sciences analysis has demonstrated, once one considers the full economic costs of ecosystem services damaged by pollution, not polluting is often cheaper in the long run. (As discussed earlier, ecosystem services include processes such as natural water filtration in undeveloped lands, nutrient cycling, and production of medically useful plants.)[49]

But suppose society prefers economic development to pollution control? Should these preferences affect citizens' duties under the responsibility argument? While no proponents of democracy can ignore *preferences,* the real issue is whether some preferences for pollution serve authentic welfare and respect human rights. To accept any preferences as a basis for social policy, including preferences for pollution over public-health protection, one would have to show that they did not unjustly harm other citizens. Otherwise, one would have to follow racist and murderous preferences. But in the case of preferring life-threatening pollution, it would be difficult to show these preferences harmed no one unjustly. One also would have to show that *future* people, assuming their welfare ought to be considered, would be likely to favor *present* pollution. If reasonable future people did not have this preference, it would not serve the greatest good for the greatest number of people, present and future. Therefore, the pollution could not be justified, even on utilitarian grounds.[50] This means a reasonable *prima facie* presupposition is that controlling life-threatening pollution may be a better way to protect the societal interests of everyone. Thus, because of the responsibility argument, citizens have *prima facie* duties to reform institutions that allow life-threatening pollution.

Ways of Life and the Collective-Responsibility Objection

One difficulty with affirming duties to prevent harm to public health, however, is that often they are collective. Ultimate moral responsibility for public-health protection rarely belongs to a single person. Because individuals typically cannot prevent threats to public welfare, people must act collectively. One objection to such collective action is that it is impossible to determine each individual's "share" of collective responsibility for the public good.

Rudyard Kipling's response is that "the sin they do by two and two they must pay for one by one." His notion of collective responsibility seems to place praise and blame on everyone for all acts, something that might make no one responsible, that might make the concept of responsibility vacuous.[51] People like H. D. Lewis go in the opposite direction. They think responsibility is like a pie. The more pie-eaters there are, the less responsibility there is. His physicalistic view is analogous to the position that, the more people one loves, the less love there is to go around. Larry May, Michael Zimmerman, and others agree more with Kipling. They argue that responsibility is not like a pie. It is not reduced by sharing, but decreases only as a result of things like duress, incapacity to accomplish some end, or the honest belief that particular actions will do no good. How does Larry May say individuals in some group can evaluate their level of responsibility for harm? His answer: by examining the group structures and solidarity through which members are related to one another. Do the relational structures among members of a group help cause the intentions, omissions, and actions of the members, such as failing to act to correct a public-health threat? Whenever they do, May says that one can attribute collective responsibility to the group.[52]

May's arguments provide grounds for believing the collective-responsibility objection is flawed. Why? People typically are able to influence the institutions of which they are members. As a result, people are responsible for institutional behavior, even if it is not always possible to pinpoint their precise levels of responsibility. Nevertheless, that responsibility is proportional to the degree of influence an individual has or could have on the group, if she developed her character in the ways she ought. Emphasizing that social groups enable individuals to do more harm or good than they otherwise could do, May explains that the *benefits* of community membership are possible only because of increased *responsibility* on the part of members. This responsibility is heightened because groups often are able to transform individual values, and individuals often are able to transform group values, as in the case of racism. Psychological studies show, for example, that racism is in part the result of groups' influencing individuals, and individuals' influencing groups. Thus, individuals bear some responsibility for group actions and omissions. As Joel Feinberg warns:

> No individual person can be blamed for not being a hero or a saint... but a whole people can be blamed for not producing a hero when the times require it, especially when the failure can be charged to some discernible element in the group's "way of life" that militates against heroism.[53]

The issue here, of course, is not heroism but compensating for the harm done by institutions in which one participates. For example, to the degree that people help produce a "way of life," a climate of social insensitivity, they are collectively responsible for harms like the murder of Kitty Genovese. Although 58 residents of a New York apartment building heard Genovese's screams for help, during an attack lasting 55 minutes, they did nothing. She was beaten, stabbed, and eventually killed. This "Genovese syndrome" again occurred when Breann Voth was brutally murdered in 2003 in Vancouver, British Columbia. At least three nearby residents heard Breann's screams. They continued for 10 minutes. Again residents did nothing. After her daughter's death, Mrs. Voth returned to the scene of the crime and posted several lines of the famous anti-Nazi poem of Pastor Martin Niemoller. "When they came to get the slaves, I did nothing. When they came to get the Jews, I did nothing. When they came to get me, what did you do? I did nothing."[54]

German philosopher Hannah Arendt probably would say that those who heard Kitty Genovese's and Breann Voth's screams, but did nothing, are not the only ones responsible for their deaths. Arendt does not believe members' direct causal responsibility for harm is necessary for making them responsible for institutional harm. Her starting point is that all people are members of communities that they influence. Because they share their lives and influence, she says, "this taking upon ourselves the consequences for things we are entirely innocent of, is the price we pay for the fact that we live our lives not by ourselves but...[within] a human community." Her rationale for collective responsibility is that the world is one we have all created, that "we all share, wrong-doer, wrong-sufferer and spectator." She also believes that people must be collectively responsible, for practical reasons. The world itself "is at stake". Gandhi echoed a similar theme: community interconnectedness creates responsibility for other members of the community. "Whenever I live in a situation where others are in need...whether or not I am responsible for it, I have become a thief."[55]

Why and how are people collectively responsible for harm because they "all share" the same world or the same community? One reason is that they have influenced, for good or for ill, a climate of social insensitivity. That climate is partly responsible for tragedies like the Genovese death or pollution deaths. At least some of this social insensitivity should be blamed on professionals, like university ethicists. Contemporary academic ethics does not emphasize personal responsibility for group welfare, in part because of controversies over each person's "share" of collective responsibility. And many virtue ethicists, like Alasdair MacIntyre, are skeptical of humans' ability even to know what is good and to agree on it. As a result, they are reluctant to argue for duties of collective responsibility, even when they preach the importance of community.[56] Except for discussions of the Holocaust, collective responsibility likewise is not an important theme in contemporary postmodern ethics, which tends to be nihilistic. Nor is it an important theme in contemporary analytic philosophy, which tends to be quietest.[57] Yet if academic ethics shapes current attitudes, and if current attitudes condone moral insensitivity and ignore collective responsibility, then academics themselves bear some responsibility for current threats to life.

The point here is not that proponents of the collective-responsibility objection are wrong when they say it is difficult to specify precise shares of personal responsibility for group harm. Of course such specifications are difficult. The point is that, faced with serious threats to life and human rights, one does not need precise specifications to know either that these threats have occurred or that they ought to be stopped. A second point is that the difficulty of such collective-responsibility specifications does not absolve one of moral responsibility for collective harm. Why not? The difficulty of specifying a parent's precise level of responsibility for her child's self-esteem does not mean no such responsibility exists. Instead, in both cases, one is at least responsible for failing to do many obvious things that one ought to do. There are obvious ways to help prevent collective harm, like allowing life-threatening pollution. One can instead speak out. There are obvious ways to help prevent harm to a child's self-esteem. One can avoid destructive criticism. A third point regarding this objection is that it is beside the point. Squabbling over "precise shares" of responsibility, given current pollution threats, is like rearranging deck chairs on the *Titanic*. It is like fighting over who is rowing hardest when everyone must row as hard as possible just to keep the lifeboat from capsizing. Once some of the worst threats to life and human rights are reduced, there will be time to argue for what everyone's precise share of collective responsibility ought to be. The previous chapters suggested that whatever those shares, most people in developed nations could do more than they presently do. David Copp, Robert Goodin, John Harris, Virginia Held, Larry May, O'Nora O'Neill, Tom Pogge, James Rachels, Peter Singer, Peter Unger, and others argue that people have responsibilities to prevent harm wherever they can. Those duties exist, regardless of whether people can precisely specify all of them in detail and regardless of whether they err through commission or omission, directly or indirectly, actively or passively.[58]

But what collective responsibilities do people have, if they cannot always specify them precisely? Ethicist Robert Goodin says that, regardless of their specific duties, many people probably err in collective responsibility because they fail to join with others in ways that might make a difference. Joining with others, to make a difference, is precisely what the APHA recommends when it calls for "advocacy and litigation" to protect public health; it asks citizens "to work in coalition" to achieve public-health goals, and it specifically promotes action through public-interest law groups. To help prevent life-threatening pollution, people could work with some non-governmental organization (NGO)—like Physicians for Social Responsibility. Yet often people do not. Often they assume such work is purely optional. Yet if people ought to follow the responsibility argument, and if the only realistic way of achieving effective institutional reform is through such NGOs, then people have duties to work within these NGOs. As Goodin puts it, "in the real world, it is these failures to organize [so as to coordinate individual action] to which collective responsibility most often attaches."[59] People are thus collectively responsible for harms like pollutant-induced deaths, whenever they fail to work with a group capable of preventing them, and whenever such groups are the only realistic ways of preventing harms. They are especially responsible whenever there is an embarrassing wealth of appropriate collectives—Human Rights Watch, Public Citizen, and so on.[60]

NGOs, Small Wins, and the Failure Objection

Perhaps the most worrisome objection to the responsibility argument is that attempting to reform harm-causing institutions will fail. This failure objection is that people are powerless to effect meaningful social change. In fact the very severity of the problems outlined in chapters 1–3 might encourage such an objection. The more widespread and serious the problem, the more likely are people to feel powerless and frustrated in their efforts to solve it. Whenever one's efforts are likely to fail, then better to devote one's energies to solvable problems. Hans Jonas recognizes this point. "There is no moral obligation to sacrifice one's life in the sure knowledge that nothing will have been gained."[61]

What can be said in response to the failure objection? The first and most obvious point is that people acting alone are likely to fail in reforming harm-causing institutions. In addition, collective actions through NGOs often are necessary. Gwen Pearson founded IRATE. Karen Silkwood worked with her union. Reason Warehime began NARS. Adam Finkel worked with PEER. Once one examines such efforts, it is obvious that the failure objection is wrong—at least with respect to NGOs. Migrant-worker advocate Cesar Chavez worked with the United Farmworkers and won many benefits for them. Ralph Nader and his two NGOs, Public Citizen and the Public Interest Research Group (PIRG), accomplished extraordinary things. They fired the opening guns of campaigns that brought improved regulation of the U.S. automobile, chemical, gas, meat, nuclear, and textile industries. The work of these two NGOs, almost single-handedly, led to dozens of laws. These include the 1966 Freedom of Information Act, the 1966 National Traffic and Motor Vehicle Safety Act, and the 1972 Consumer Product Safety Act. They helped create the EPA and the Occupational Safety and Health Adminis-tration, prototype agencies of their kind. They campaigned for mandatory air bags in cars, and they soon became standard equipment.[62] Such successes reveal that people working together can accomplish what otherwise would be impossible for someone working alone.

Besides citing health-protective successes and the importance of NGOs, understanding the personal and political nature of civic reforms is another way to avoid failure. Psychologists say people often feel powerless, despite the obvious power of effective and organized collective action, when they define social problems in ways that overwhelm their ability to do anything about them.[63] Sometimes they define the needed protections of life and hu-man rights in purely external ways. They forget that the point of the re-sponsibility argument is not merely to reduce threats to life and public health. The point also is to be changed oneself. When people become the change they seek, they will be personally transformed in ways that help sustain com-munities that respect life and human rights. Recall this chapter's discussion of Aristotle, Hans Jonas, and Jean-Paul Sartre. Why did they argue that people are collectively responsible for threats to life and to human rights? One reason is that people are first responsible for the kind of individuals they become, for their levels of moral sensitivity. Becoming responsible in this earlier sense helps fulfill the responsibility argument and is enhanced by it. The transformation required by the responsibility argument thus must be personal as well as political. Otherwise, the resulting political action runs the risk of being unethical, self-serving, or despairing. There is never an in-oculation against despair, never a perfect answer to the failure objection. Nevertheless, to the degree that one begins and continues both organized collective action and a personal ethical transformation, frustration and feelings of powerlessness are likely to diminish. Don Quixote understood this point. He did not justify his knight-errantry mainly because he thought it would be effective or successful. He also celebrated, and wanted others to celebrate, the pleasures of a life pursuing what is noble and good. No one fails who takes pleasure in pursuing what is good—even if the pursuit leads to less good than one wishes.

A third response to the failure objection is the small-wins strategy, described by social psychologist Karl Weick. This strategy consists of redefining massive problems as a series of smaller, less frustrating, more controllable difficulties. These offer more opportunities for success, for immediate and "visible results." On a more mundane level, this might be called the strategy of divide and conquer. Breaking an overpowering problem into a series of smaller difficulties makes it easier to resolve, step by step. Suppose one is faced with counting thousands of sheets of paper while being continuously interrupted. To reduce recounting time and ensure the ability to complete the counting task, it can be divided into "small wins"—100-count piles. The "small wins" strategy is premised in part on psychologists' Yerkes-Dodson Law. According to this law, concern about a problem initially increases efficiency of action to address it, but as energy and frustration about it increases, they impair the performance efficiency needed to resolve the problem. This empirically substantiated law documents an inverse relationship between concern about some problem and one's effectiveness in addressing it. Why? Social psychologists have confirmed the fact that as levels of problem arousal increase, three damaging things occur. People miss crucial informational cues about the problem and are less able to concentrate and to devise novel strategies. As a result, they make more primitive responses—perhaps reverting to earlier learned behavior, even when it is not appropriate to the situation. Social psychologists also have documented the fact that high arousal caused by realizing the severity of some situation can improve performance only when it occurs after a person has decided what to do about a problem and overlearned how to do it. To keep problem arousal at modest levels but responses at high levels, they say people need to work for small wins. For instance, when activist Saul Alinsky found a massive social problem, such as a demoralized, low-income, high-crime neighborhood, he persuaded the residents to picket for reinstating government-provided infant medical care at the local clinic. He knew this "small win" would be easy and immediate. Most important, he knew it would energize people who had given up. He knew this small win would empower them to move toward other "small wins."[64]

There are many cases demonstrating the wisdom and success of using the "small wins" strategy. For instance, sports analysts showed that the Pittsburgh Steelers did not become a great football team because of "the big win." Instead, they consistently beat many weaker teams. How did they attain their typical four-to-one ratio of games won to games lost? They won only about half their games against teams whose wins exceeded their losses. Yet they won

98 percent of their games against teams whose losses exceeded their wins. Likewise, 35 years ago, facing massive prejudice against gays, the Task Force on Gay Liberation knew that an immediate big victory was impossible. Instead, the task force pursued a small-wins strategy. One small win occurred in 1972 when the task force succeeded in changing the Library of Congress classification for gay books. Instead of being listed in the category for abnormal sexual relations, sexual crimes, and sexual perversions, gay books now have a classification described merely as "varieties of sexual life." Similar small-win strategies are behind the "One day at a time" philosophy of Alcoholics Anonymous. They also are behind feminist attention to seemingly trivial linguistic details. One example is the gender bias in calling a married couple "man and wife." Nearly four decades ago, William Ruckelshaus, as the first administrator of the EPA, also followed a small-wins strategy. He achieved quick, opportunistic, tangible first steps toward pollution control. He did not attack the worst problem—air pollution—first. Instead, Ruckelshaus did his homework, discovered that many cities were violating federal water-pollution laws, sued those cities, and gained quick wins. He thus established a beachhead for later, greater environmental work.[65]

The small-wins strategy is successful for both theoretical and practical reasons. On the theoretical side, different people employ different notions of rationality to address massive social problems like pollution. Consequently, they often disagree on how to solve them. Some people may prefer the bounded rationality of neoclassical economics—solving pollution problems by means of citizens' willingness to pay for cleaner air. Others may prefer the political rationality of direct action—believing that virtually no powerful people ever willingly give up power, including the power to pollute. Still others may prefer the conventional rationality of legal rights—attempting to establish rights to a livable environment based on the enforceable right to life. None of these three groups might agree on an overall strategy for reducing pollution. However, they are more likely to agree on a series of small steps toward reducing it. They might agree, for example, on ensuring adequate information about levels of pollutants actually released, on recognizing citizens' rights to know about these levels, and on taking steps to enforce accurate reporting of them.[66] By circumventing theoretical disagreements over different rationalities, the small-wins strategy instead focuses on subproblems on which virtually everyone can agree. It then uses subproblem agreement as a basis for further wins. In short, the small-wins strategy sidesteps problems of bounded and opposed rationality. Instead it defines as problems those very limited, very clear situations for which complete remedies are easily achievable. On the practical side, this strategy is successful because psychometric evidence has established that most people prefer small changes to larger changes. Most people are able to change their opinions when alternative positions are advocated within the rationality limits they personally accept. They learn best through a gradual progression. These three findings are explained in part because big wins typically evoke big countermeasures or opposition. Big wins also alter the expectations of the winners and the public. Such expectations can make future wins difficult. One illustration is the early acclaim given promising novelists' first books or the adulation and attention accorded Nobel Prize winners. As a result of this acclaim, they may become less able to work, because expectations have been raised so high. Pursuing a small-wins strategy, however, provides information that facilities learning and adaptation. It offers stable and uncontroversial building blocks for future change. It empowers and energizes those who need to effect change. It initiates a pattern that can attract allies, deter opponents, lower resistance to subsequent proposals, and give hope for the future. As such, the small-wins strategy follows Alinsky's three criteria for activist goals: they should be highly specific or concrete; realizable or confidence building; and immediate. Why does pursuing small wins, when following the responsibility argument, reduce frustration and despair? These small wins are more achievable, and people's existing skills are seen as more obviously adequate to the task.[67]

A small-wins strategy also enables citizens seeking social change to be "hardy." According to social psychologist S. C. Kobasa, hardy people have at least three characteristics: commitment, control, and challenge. They have commitment, or a sense of purpose that enables them to impose meaning on things. They have control, or the tendency to act as if they can influence situations. They also accept challenge—the belief that change is an incentive to grow rather than a threat to their security. Small wins promote hardiness because they promote commitment and the vision of an orderly series of steps to an ultimate goal. They reinforce control through achievable successes that provide incentives to realize bigger and bigger wins. Especially in a policy world with few clear solutions, small wins make political sense because they make achieving consensus easier. Of course, more radical social reformers may accuse small-wins strategists of being naïve or optimistic, especially about the necessity to play political hardball. This supposed naïveté, however, might better be described as openness and optimism. Both traits are necessary, over the long haul, for addressing serious social problems, such as environmental threats to life and public health. Suppose some small win seems too easy, ineffective, or naïve? Psychologically resilient reformers—who can tolerate high levels of problem-concern and stress—should go for bigger wins. But for those facing frustration, powerlessness, and possible failure, it makes sense to work for small wins.[68]

A particularly striking example of the effectiveness of the small-wins strategy occurred in the late 1970s in Poland, when the people lived under the totalitarian rule of General Wojcíech Jaruzelski. Nuclear weapons and 200 divisions of the Russian army were behind him. Instead of succumbing to the failure objection, workers organized themselves into the Polish Workers Defense Committee. Through this organization, they rejected the belief that all their resistance was doomed to fail. They searched for very narrow windows of opportunity, within which together they could organize actions that would promote life and health. After large meetings were outlawed, members sponsored small meetings, 10 workers each, to hear uncensored lectures on Polish history. They banded together to publish a newsletter in which factory-workplace conditions were accurately described. They evaluated their situation and soon saw the massive needs of different members of their group for medical, legal, and financial assistance. As a result, they pooled their resources, evaluated individual workers' needs, and arranged to provide assistance, as a group, whenever they could.

Together the Polish workes effectively set up an alternative set of educational, informational, financial, medical, and legal institutions that was able to meet many of the needs of individual workers. The totalitarian government met virtually none of these needs. The Polish Workers Defense Committee, however, enabled workers to build community among themselves, to "restore social bonds outside official institutions." It enabled them to avoid trying to seize power, in the hope that they could use it to do good. Instead, they largely ignored state power and themselves devised ways to do good, through their own collective action. Pursuing their own personal transformation, they did not expect to be able to overthrow their oppressors directly. They realized that, by transforming themselves, they could blunt the force of their oppression. How did the Polish Workers Defense Committee encourage this personal transformation? It allowed members great autonomy, the ability to act freely. It imposed no detailed lists of what members could and could not do. Instead, it encouraged people to do whatever they could to help workers, provided it was not contrary to the few principles on which they had all agreed. By encouraging workers to behave autonomously, when government recognized no rights to autonomy, the Polish Workers Defense Committee encouraged community and personal transformation. This community began as individuals' forming different small groups organized around particular issues that were of concern to them, like pollution or working conditions. These practices of autonomy, community, and mutual trust, in turn, created empowered, hopeful workers. They were committed to small local actions on behalf of "militant decency," rather than waiting for large-scale political change to help accomplish good. The Polish Workers Defense Committee encouraged a strategy of personal transformation through which each worker was encouraged to "start doing the things you think should be done—start being what you think society should become." The organization's assisting in the personal transformation of thousands of workers thus resulted in a visible, day-to-day community of free people. They were filled with "angerless wisdom." They did not wait for either their own violence or the government to change things. Instead, they ignored their oppressors and became the change themselves. The depth of this personal transformation—especially the humility and lack of vanity of the organization's members—became apparent after Solidarity was formed. Once the union, Solidarity, was organized and successful, the Polish Workers Defense Committee voted to abolish itself because it was no longer needed.

At the heart of these steps leading to the workers' organized action was the small-wins strategy, using the successes of many small victories—like publishing newsletters and helping other members with medical needs. These small victories helped to build community, to energize and empower members, and to provide alternative, freeing institutions in the face of totalitarian ones. They proved that evolution is a powerful form of revolution. They created an alternative society within which workers behaved as if Poland were already free. Why was this organized action ethical and successful? It created community instead of strangers, responsibility instead of despair, agreements instead of disagreements, personal virtue instead of wasted anger, enthusiasm instead of hopelessness, autonomy instead of rigid rules, and persistent acts of decency instead of naïve hopes for an impossible "big win."

Conclusion

This chapter argues that many objections to the responsibility argument can be answered. If citizens use the small-wins strategy, work through NGOs, and carefully evaluate their own abilities and opportunities, they can help accomplish both political change and personal transformation. They can compensate for the harms caused by institutions of which they are members, and they themselves can become the change they seek. Most Americans have not fully recognized either of these duties. They have forgotten Plato's warning, that all people are essentially social or political animals. By their nature, people must be concerned with the affairs of the "polis" or state. They also have forgotten Thucydides' warning to the Athenians: if people believe "someone else" will carry their political responsibilities for them, the common cause will imperceptibly decay.[69]

Where We Go from Here

Ella Baker, an organizer in the civil-rights movement, spoke bluntly about what is necessary for oppressed people to reclaim their rights. They have to learn one thing: "in the long run they themselves are the only protection they have."[1] Juana Gutierrez, a grandmother who lives in East Los Angeles, learned that Baker is right. There has been no one but herself and her neighbors to protect local residents as more and more noxious facilities move into East LA and spew out increasing amounts of pollutants. Every year they discharge more than 33 million pounds of chemical wastes into East LA air and water. Local children are often sick. Many have asthma. Still pollutants increase, partly because the companies know that East LA is home to poor people, and the poor have little power to demand cleaner air. The median annual income is about $7,500, and unemployment hovers around 33 percent.[2]

Juana Gutierrez

The daughter of a Mexican farmer, Gutierrez came to the United States when she was 15. Although her father told her not to "get involved," she says she did so anyway because "I was worried about my kids."[3] In 1985, when California governor George Deukmejian proposed building a sixth prison in already troubled East LA, Gutierrez and the predominantly Hispanic population were outraged. The additional prison symbolized everything that was already wrong with their neighborhood. They were angry that Deukmejian could find tens of millions of dollars to incarcerate those who had not become productive adults but could not find the thousands of dollars needed to fund their community schools and the war on drugs.[4]

Gutierrez decided to fight the proposed prison. In 1986, she joined Aurora Castillo to cofound Mothers of East Los Angeles (MELA). Their parish priest, Father John Moretta, suggested the name. To inform the Hispanic community about the planned prison, Gutierrez used her most available network, people streaming out of Sunday Mass. Every Monday, through church leafleting, MELA organized protest marches against the prison. Pushing baby strollers and wearing white kerchiefs to symbolize nonviolence, for months and months MELA marched. Eventually they enlisted the help of the men, who carried signs calling themselves the "chauffeurs" of the mothers. Finally state officials dropped the prison plan. Energized by the small win against the prison, MELA began to fight other threats to the community. An above-ground oil pipeline, a hazardous-waste storage site, and a toxic-waste incinerator were all proposed for East LA. The toxic incinerator was slated to burn 125,000 pounds of hazardous materials per day, including used motor oil and industrial sludge. From their church, again and again MELA protestors walked more than a mile to the gates of the $20-million incinerator project. As they marched, they chanted: "El pueblo parara el incinerador!" (The people will stop the incinerator!) "Pueblo que lucha triunfa." (People who fight win.) The facility owners and operators had sited it in East LA because they said residents would not fight. Yet Gutierrez and MELA fought through 6 years of agitation, 4 lawsuits, 16 hearings, and 6 mile-long protests. Finally, in June 1991, the Mothers passed around cookies to their 400 members to celebrate cancellation of the incinerator. Soon after, MELA began other public-health projects, like a lead-poisoning-education campaign that now employs 10 youths. The group also organized a water-conservation program that offers free low-flush toilets and recycles old ones. Defying "a system that penalizes low-income communities," Gutierrez and MELA have dispelled the myth that poor people do not care about public health and the environment.[5]

Juana Gutierrez began MELA because no one else was doing enough to help local children and because she saw, firsthand, health problems in her own Latino community. Wealthier people often are far removed from such problems. As a result, they often fail to see the damage that environmental injustice can do. Their garbage, trucked to places like east LA or south Chicago to be burned, increases air pollution in the neighborhoods of the poor. Their expensive consumer goods often come from unsafe blue-collar workplaces, and they are none the wiser. People like Juana Gutierrez and MELA often take up the work of public-health protection because they experience threats to their own lives. Earlier chapters showed that Gwen Pearson and IRATE members personally experienced these threats. So did Reason Warehime and NARS members. People also experience these threats vicariously, through learning health statistics like those in chapter 1 and through understanding their socioeconomic and institutional causes, as presented in chapters 2–4. What happens when people do not experience these threats directly? Before they act, they often must experience harms to others as their own. As Indian pacifist Gandhi realized, the ultimate motivation is that people themselves must identify with the dreams and the sufferings of those whose lives are at risk.

Chapter Overview

Earlier chapters showed how Karen Silkwood identified with the dreams and sufferings of fellow radiation workers. Adam Finkel identified with the dreams and sufferings of government safety inspectors who were at risk from beryllium. Adolph Coleman identified with the dreams and sufferings of African-Americans who were breathing south Chicago pollution. Not everyone may identify as they did, and not everyone may agree with the positions they took. Yet everyone probably can agree that citizens should try to prevent harm, as best they can, and they should use the tools of democracy to do so. The purpose of this chapter is to suggest several ways in which citizens might live out the responsibility argument and thus help to protect life and human rights.[6]

Chapter 1 revealed the massiveness of environmental threats to life. Chapters 2 and 3 showed why people often fail to recognize these threats. Advertisers, front groups, and PR machines spend billions of dollars annually in ways that often mislead people about health and jeopardize their rights to know and to consent. Building on the problems outlined in chapters 1–3, chapter 4 used the responsibility argument to show that all citizens have *prima facie* duties to respond to these problems in one of two ways. Either they must stop their participation in any institutional order that threatens life and human rights or, if they remain in these institutional orders, they must compensate for doing so and work for their reform. Chapter 5 answered a number of objections to this responsibility argument. This chapter suggests several ways citizens might begin to implement the duties demanded by this argument.

Divided into three parts, the chapter first surveys a brief, four-step strategy for practicing duties to help stop harms to life and to human rights. Recalling the last chapter's arguments for the small-wins strategy, the chapter next argues that these four steps are best accomplished through piecemeal reform rather than revolution. The third part of the chapter provides a number of specific reforms for which citizens might work to reduce harms to life and to rights to know and to consent.

Public Involvement, Private Fulfillment

How should citizens begin to prevent life-threatening harms caused in part by institutions in which they participate and from which they receive benefits? If Glaucon in Plato's *Republic* is right, many people might not do so. Glaucon tells the story of the ring of Gyges to explain why. The ring was able to make its wearers invisible, so that they could do evil without being caught. Glaucon argues that people do good only because they fear punishment, retaliation, or what others will think of them. If no one ever found out what evildoers did, Glaucon says most people would behave unethically. They would serve their own private gain at the expense of others. In response, Socrates argues that wrongdoing only *seems* to be profitable. Why? Only those who live virtuously are genuinely happy, because only they live in ways that are genuinely social. If people are essentially social, as Socrates believed, their purely egoistic or unethical behavior destroys the very psychological and biological foundations needed for their own happiness. "No man is an island." Thus, if the Greeks, the Asians, and the game theorists mentioned in chapter 4 are right, citizens who follow the responsibility argument are behaving not only ethically but also socially and rationally. Confronting threats to life and to human rights, they are not part of a system in which altruists need be hurt. They are not part of a zero-sum game, like poker, in which if anyone wins, others must lose the same amount. Instead, as chapter 4 argued, and as Princeton University ethicist Peter Singer puts it, ethics and self-interest often point in the same direction.[7]

If ethics and authentic self interest often point in the same direction, and if all parties gain from cooperation and altruism, then ethical duties like those dictated by the responsibility argument also have a psychological and practical foundation. Public involvement can bring private fulfillment. Without public involvement, without people's trying to correct harms caused by institutions from which they benefit, people are likely to experience the paradox of hedonism. That is, the more they deliberately seek pleasure, the less likely they are to find it. Analogously, if humans are by nature social, the more people seek meaning only privately and individually, the less likely they are to find it.[8] Why? Once people's basic material needs are met, nonegoistic and nonmaterial sources of fulfillment probably play the dominant role in their happiness. As chapter 4 notes, sociologists like Robert Bellah say much the same thing. They question the tendency of many people to turn only inward in search of meaning. Looking at the lives of ordinary people, Bellah discovered that those who were turned outward in public service, directed at some self-transcending cause, rarely experienced any crisis of meaning.[9]

Practical Strategies: Four Steps for Public Citizens

The point here is not that making our lives meaningful should be our main goal. Rather, if we follow the ethical mandates of the responsibility argument and try to prevent threats to life and human rights, one side effect is likely to be a full and meaningful life. How might we begin to serve others and to implement the responsibility argument? Earlier chapters suggested general strategies such as deliberative democracy, small wins, and work with health-protecting nongovernmental organizations or NGOs. In using these three general strategies, citizens might pursue four steps—getting information, cooperating with others, evaluating alternatives, and pursuing organized action. While these four steps are not mutually exclusive and are recursive rather than sequential, nevertheless they offer some initial ethical suggestions. More detailed steps are better left to practical, case-by-case analyses.

The first step, getting *information* about public-health threats, is both the easiest and the hardest of the four. It is the easiest because it may require nothing beyond reading and thinking, something people can do daily. It is the hardest because, as chapters 2 and 3 revealed, special interests sometimes distort available information. In addition, many citizens receive their information only from limited and perhaps biased sources. Often people fail to get opinions and evidence from the greatest variety of people and groups possible. Many citizens likewise have not made the lifestyle commitments necessary to remain informed about public health. Instead, they may spend too much time on activities like television. As a result, citizens may have a false complacency that allows unscrupulous groups to "whitewash" or "greenwash" their behavior. Whitewash, of course, can arise from any agenda-driven groups—environmental organizations, churches, labor unions, corporations, and even government agencies. The greater the group's economic or social power, the greater their potential threat to legitimate information—as the recent coverup of sexual predators in the Roman Catholic Church reveals. As earlier chapters suggested, because corporate groups donate about 80 percent of U.S. campaign contributions and spend about 100 times more dollars on scientific research than do environmental groups, their greater power and potential for abuse suggests that their behavior ought to receive proportionate scrutiny from those seeking reliable information.

Cooperating with others is the second step in using deliberative democracy to pursue the responsibility argument. Cooperation is difficult because people frequently recognize its necessity only when they see some threat before them. Yet often no threat is obvious until after people have already cooperated and thus gained public-health information. As already mentioned, perhaps the most crucial vehicle of such cooperation is working with NGOs such as civil-rights groups, church groups, and professional societies. One health-related NGO is Bread for the World. Promoting food assistance and child immunization in developing nations, it offers "action kits" that show citizens how to support its food and public-health programs.[10] It is a valuable source of both health information and cooperation. As this example suggests, however, cooperatively working with such an NGO is not merely a matter of paying annual dues or reading a book. It involves keeping informed, helping to educate others, and supporting ongoing group activities and meetings. It involves commitments of both time and money—organizing, leafleting, educating, canvassing, and other activities characteristic of deliberative democracy. Without cooperation through a variety of focused groups, like Bread for the World, it is difficult for citizens to obtain accurate information, to evaluate conflicting viewpoints, to succeed in alleviating societal problems, or to sustain and motivate their own efforts to do good. The reason? If the social model of gaining knowledge—defended in chapter 5—is correct, cooperation and a cognitive division of labor are necessary to make much information readily available. The U.S. founding fathers and mothers recognized this point and organized New England town meetings. Benjamin Barber speaks of neighborhood meetings. James Fishkin urges deliberative opinion polls. Such cooperative ideals identify deliberative democracy not with structures or institutions but instead with processes of wide communication among various people and social sectors. These processes are necessary both to build democratic consensus and to debate and amend conflicting social proposals.[11]

A third step in using deliberative democracy to implement the responsibility argument is *evaluating* health threats and alternative solutions to them. This likewise is something best achieved through open interaction with a variety of other people and points of view. Yet most citizens associate only with certain groups of people and typically hear only a few points of view. As a result, their evaluations of social problems often are incomplete. To understand public-health threats, people need to hear a diversity of opinions about them. They also need emotive, narrative, and scientific or factual understanding, as well as ongoing evaluation—vigilance and criticism. Otherwise, there is little hope of recognizing and countering the massive informational problems outlined in chapters 2–3.[12] One way of exercising such vigilance, at least in scientific evaluation, is to look for the characteristic errors of private-interest science, some of which were surveyed in chapter 3. Another way is to avoid acting on the basis of unevaluated opinions that have not survived the testing and analysis described in chapter 5. This means that people cannot follow the responsibility argument merely by having good intentions and then following preexisting opinions. Instead, they need to aim at evaluation that is open, transparent, empirical, accessible to all, and democratic. They need to follow a method like that of John Stuart Mill. He argued for examining and trying to answer all relevant opinions and objections. He urged not being limited only to several sources of information.

Evaluation is particularly necessary if citizens who hope to reform life-threatening social institutions find themselves at odds with at least some members of those institutions. If they are eventually forced either into whistle-blowing, as Karen Silkwood and Adam Finkel were, or into civil disobedience, as Adolph Coleman was, their actions will require special evaluation. Although there is no time to discuss civil disobedience in detail, the classic ethical conditions for engaging in civil disobedience also provide useful tools for evaluating citizen behavior under the responsibility argument. Civil disobedience is generally defined as a public, nonviolent, conscientious violation of some law or policy. Through it violators aim both to change an unethical law or policy and to accept the legal consequences of their disobedience. The rationale behind civil disobedience is fidelity to conscience and to a higher morality that may require citizens to disobey what is merely a civil law. If civil laws fail to protect victims of environmental injustice, as they did in Reverend Coleman's neighborhood, civil disobedients can hold civil authorities to a higher standard—that of human rights. In his famous "Letter from Birmingham Jail," civil-rights leader Martin Luther King appeals to this higher standard. He reminds his readers that everything Adolph Hitler did was legal, but everything the Hungarian freedom fighters did was illegal. He also quotes St. Augustine, that an unjust law is no law at all. Warning that the United States would never have arisen without civil disobedience, King warns civil-rights advocates that privileged groups rarely forgo their privileges voluntarily. Because they do not, he says citizens must disobey in order to obtain change.

As generally understood, there are at least seven conditions, all of which must be satisfied for ethically legitimate civil disobedience.

- Certain limits of injustice are exceeded in a serious and life-threatening way.
- Conditions for free cooperation among people, to resolve the injustice, do not exist.
- Disobedience is necessary to support basic ethical or democratic principles, such as civil rights.
- Dissidents agree to "pay the price" of their disobedience by accepting the penalties for it.
- Dissidents evaluate their proposed action, its likely consequences, and their own intentions.
- Dissidents behave nonviolently.
- Dissidents accept the existing political system, but not a particular law that is unjust.[13]

One form of civil disobedience, whistleblowing, is directed at an organization, including government. As such, it must satisfy all the preceding conditions for civil disobedience. Karen Silkwood's organizational disobedience or whistleblowing, discussed earlier, was directed at Kerr-McGee, and it appears to have satisfied these conditions. According to the standard paradigm, an act of whistleblowing must have five characteristics.

- The act disobeys an organizational policy.
- An employee (citizen) of the organization (nation) in question performs the act.
- The goal of the act is to rescind an organizational policy.
- The act tries to appeal to a higher moral standard to challenge the questionable policy.
- The employee or citizen acts under the belief that the policy seriously threatens public or organizational interests and acts to protect that interest.

Most ethicists believe that whistleblowing is justified only if four conditions, analogous to those for civil disobedience, are met. (1) The policy seriously threatens the public. (2) It cannot be overturned within a reasonable period of time through normal, internal channels. (3) Whistleblowing is likely to be effective in overturning the policy. (4) The whistleblowing will not violate any higher ethical obligations. Failure to meet any of these conditions typically makes whistleblowing unethical. Often this means it is unfair to the accused or endangers the whistleblower.[14]

Organized action, the fourth step in using deliberative democracy to implement the responsibility argument, is a natural response to the three previous steps. As earlier chapters emphasized, because individuals acting alone often can do little to help correct public-health problems, concerted and well-organized collective action usually is necessary. That is why the 50,000-member American Public Health Association (APHA) encourages "work in coalition," including "advocacy and litigation." Through organizations like "public-interest law groups," APHA says citizens can help exercise their "maximum responsibility" for public health. Explaining its activities on its website, the APHA says it "has been influencing policies and setting priorities in public health for over 125 years." It claims to serve the public not only "through its scientific and practice programs" but also through its "advocacy efforts." Showing how such advocacy and organized action can help overcome citizens' feelings of frustration and powerlessness, the previous chapter used the example of the Polish Workers Defense Committee. If these earlier arguments are correct, organized action must build on small wins and on personal transformation—working to become virtuous oneself, to become the change one seeks. Because it is so easy for advocates and any special interests to fall into bias, however, it is important to evaluate all collective actions from alternative points of view. This includes evaluating different proposed beliefs and actions, including doing nothing. In fact, organized and enlightened responses to the responsibility argument require ongoing and iterative evaluation of alternative perspectives and actions. This continuing evaluation is important to help make organized action less self-serving and more affirming of those who have been disenfranchised. As philosophers Hilary Putnam and John Dewey recognized, evaluation also is necessary to keep collective policies and actions inclusive, participative, and objective.[15]

The Case for Piecemeal Reform

Using deliberative democracy to implement the responsibility argument, through the preceding four steps, citizens might respond in two incorrect ways: uncritical activism or passivity. Uncritical public-health activists can fall into the same ethical traps as other special interests criticized in chapters 2 and 3. They typically assume that their own ends justify any means, even unethical means. Those who remain passive also err. This is not only because they ignore duties to help prevent harm done by institutions in which they participate and from which they gain benefits. They also err because they beg the question of whether enlightened public citizenship, as outlined so far, can make a difference. If earlier examples are right, it often can make a difference. As the beginning of each chapter shows, ordinary people, working with others, sometimes can do extraordinary things.

As the small-wins strategy and ethical conditions for acts like civil disobedience and whistleblowing make clear, citizens implementing the responsibility argument virtually always must pursue incremental change. Why? Change accomplished in more radical ways is likely to be either undemocratic, to neglect some citizens' rights, or to fall victim to some of the biases discussed in chapters 2 and 3. Directed at preventing harm, this incremental change is what Kai Nielsen calls "intelligent piecemeal social engineering." It can occur through the rich associational life of governmental, professional, and NGO groups, such as neighborhood volunteer organizations or the APHA.[16]

How should one try to carry out this piecemeal social change? Karl Popper offers several insights. Mirroring the small-wins philosophy, he condemns *ideology* and *utopianism*, yet praises *reformism*.

> Work for the elimination of concrete evils rather than for the realization of abstract goods. Do not aim at establishing happiness by political means. Rather aim at the elimination of concrete miseries.... Choose what you consider the most urgent evil of the society in which you live, and try patiently to convince people that we can get rid of it.[17]

Popper's words suggest that those who follow the responsibility argument should work to eliminate obvious and serious problems such as environmentally induced death, hunger, and exploitation of native peoples, not some particular good. The reason? The responsibility argument requires preventing life-threatening harm for which people are partly culpable because of the institutions in which they participate. Their *stopping harm* has a higher priority than *doing good*. Why? Justice always requires trying to correct a serious wrong, for which one is partly responsible, whereas justice does not always require doing some particular good. Another reason, mentioned earlier, regarding the small-wins strategy, is that people tend to agree more about what is bad, like environmental racism. They agree less about what is good—like particular religions. For example, in the United States, New Zealand, the United Kingdom, the Netherlands, and Belgium, there is overwhelming evidence that, independent of income, racial discrimination results in segregation that, in turn, results in minorities' breathing dirtier air and drinking dirtier water. In all these nations, this inequality is recognized as a "bad." [18] A third reason for the priority of stopping harm, before promoting particular goods, is that promoting these goods often involves different rationalities, as the last chapter mentioned. Yet people rarely change their forms of rationality. Stopping harms, however, need not involve different rationalities and hence is often easier to accomplish. It requires only minimal cooperation and agreement that something is bad—for whatever reason. As such, the broad cooperation necessary for incremental social change obviously requires avoiding specific commitments both to any particular ideologies and to doctrinaire left-versus-right approaches. Such avoidance also helps keep people open, inclusive, reflectively self-critical, able to compromise, and capable of democratic deliberation. But attempting to accommodate the diverse democratic needs and interests of all citizens means most social problems also must be addressed piecemeal, directly, and nonviolently. Even Marxist Rosa Luxemburg said a revolutionary should not oppose piecemeal reform.[19]

Pursuing incremental change and small wins requires those following the responsibility argument to remain public and democratic in their efforts. This is accomplished in part by employing ethical standards (like those already mentioned) for information gathering, cooperation, evaluation, and action that are transparent, empirical, and accessible to everyone. Because scientific knowledge is typically the most accessible and empirically available, public citizens ought both to rely on it yet remain vigilant about its misuse, illustrated in chapter 3. As the second step of democratic deliberation (cooperation) suggests, citizens pursuing incremental change likewise should be willing to see other points of view, including scientific ones. They should avoid strident, polemical, ideological, and impractical actions that discourage cooperation or sustained incremental change.[20]

Although earlier discussions have outlined both conditions for ethical action (like those for whistleblowing) and iterative steps to follow (getting information, cooperating with others, evaluating alternatives, and pursuing organized action), there is no simple recipe for how to fulfill the responsibility argument. This is partly because, as already emphasized, following this argument requires a *personal*, as well as a *political*, transformation. This personal transformation must be dictated, in part, by each person's unique abilities, experiences, and relationships—as illustrated by one well-to-do retiree, a former corporate executive and friend of the author. Critical of increased government funding for health, education, and welfare, he spent a year as a part-time volunteer in a public grammar school in Florida. He went into this service work as a person deeply committed to private enterprise and to the corporate model that had made him a multimillionaire. After seeing the inadequately funded schools, the overcrowded classes, the poor equipment, the poorly paid teachers, and many children whose basic needs were not met, he had a conversion experience. Slowly he became an outspoken proponent of improved public education, smaller class sizes, higher teacher pay, and increased health, education, and welfare funding. His own firsthand experience—like that of Gwen Pearson, Kate Burns, Reason Warehime, and others in this book—changed him. His service work personally transformed him in ways that years of study or reading, alone, probably could never do. As a result, he learned what he needed to do, as a citizen, and who he needed to become. The same is probably true for most people. Earlier chapters have tried to supply part of the ethical *why* for this personal and political transformation. The service itself and the hearts of the servers themselves will teach people much of the *how*.

What specific policies and actions might citizens pursue, as part of the political transformation urged by the responsibility argument? The rest of this chapter has some suggestions, many taken from recommendations of the APHA. These suggestions follow the small-wins strategy of chapter 5 and are divided into those protecting rights to life, to know, and to consent. Ideally, citizens' political work should help to address the same sorts of harms from which they benefit or for which they themselves are most responsible. If people live in a town that ships its waste out of state to be burned in poor neighborhoods, they might work first to redistribute and reduce these waste-related burdens. If people buy consumer goods that likely are made in sweatshops, they might work with NGOs addressing sweatshop abuses, and so on.

Proposals for Fulfilling Rights to Life

How might citizens help correct many threats to life, to some of which their own governments have contributed? The largest association of public-health professionals in the world, the APHA, has hundreds of such suggestions, not all of which can be mentioned here. These include both general policy recommendations as well as specific practical proposals for implementing them. On the policy side, for instance, the APHA calls on the United States "to assume a leadership role" internationally in adopting "a deliberate...energy strategy" built on conservation, more stringent "fuel-economy standards," "renewable fuel sources...strengthened controls for greenhouse-gas emissions and hazardous air pollutants, and the expedited institution of safe and renewable energy sources." On the more practical level, examples of APHA recommendations include those "to cease man-made mercury emissions from all sources," especially coal plants; to require more stringent diesel-exhaust standards by "using a health-based Permissible Exposure Limit"; to tighten the blood-lead "level of concern" standard; to tighten benzene-exposure limits, partly by ratifying the 1971 International Labor Organization mandate on benzene; and to reduce toxic pollutants in human breast milk by having the United States ratify the Stockholm Convention on Persistent Organic Pollutants and fund the CDC to develop a national human-milk monitoring program. In many ways, APHA has repeatedly called for pollution prevention through toxics reduction, especially reduction of "synthetic organic chemicals and heavy metals [which are]...one factor contributing to critical public-health threats such as cancer, neurological problems, reproductive effects, and asthma." Consistent with the stances defended earlier in the book, the APHA also has taken positions on various proposals likely to affect health. For example, the APHA recommends that Congress "declare the Yucca Mountain site unsuitable for development of a nuclear repository"; "reject any proposed legislation for high-level-nuclear waste storage which mandates weakening the existing radiation standards"; and support "alternative methods to safeguard...nuclear waste and minimize the risks to public health for all generations." [21]

Apart from such APHA-recommended improvements in health standards, pollution prevention, and energy policy, a crucial part of protecting rights to life is promoting full enforcement of existing health, safety, and environmental laws, in part by working with NGOs to prevent regulatory capture. As earlier chapters showed, especially since the year 2000, U.S. health-enforcement monies have been cut massively. For instance, FDA inspections declined from 8 percent of total imports in 1991 to less than 2 percent 10 years later. Full enforcement also is needed, as the APHA points out, because current trade agreements often are misused to allow other nations to ship into the United States products that are made under conditions that violate U.S. human-rights, environmental, or public-health laws. Since 2003, the president has had the right, under NAFTA (the North American Free Trade Agreement) Fast Track and without any congressional approval, to approve trade deals that can circumvent these health and safety laws. One possible result, according to the U.S. Centers for Disease Control (CDC), is that 9,000 Americans die each year from food-related illnesses, and another 6 million annually become seriously ill. According to government investigators, food identified as pesticide contaminated—half of all imported food—has been marketed without either penalties to the producers or warnings to consumers. Many U.S. fruits and vegetables come from Mexico, for instance, yet over 15 percent of beans and 12 percent of peppers imported from Mexico violate FDA (U.S. Food and Drug Administration) pesticide-residue standards. Half of imported green coffee beans contain measurable levels of banned pesticides. The U.S. government oversight agency, the GAO (Government Accountability Office) estimates that 14 percent of all U.S. meat is now contaminated with illegal residues.[22]

According to the GAO, enforcement in the Department of Agriculture (USDA) food-monitoring program also is inadequate for at least three reasons. (1) It does not adjust its testing of imported meat in response to known problems with heavy-metal residues. (2) It does not take account of animal-drug and pesticide compounds banned in the United States but used by exporting nations. (As mentioned earlier, one-third of all pesticides manufactured in the United States are banned or not registered in the United States, are shipped abroad for use there, but often returned on imported food.)[23] (3) Because manufacturers introduce thousands of new chemical compounds annually, there is never complete information on what residues might be present. As a result, the USDA must rely on limited sampling and testing at the end of the food-production process. Government enforcers do not require manufacturers even to provide reference standards and test methods for unregistered pesticides, shipped abroad, that return to the United States via food imports.[24]

Another part of improving health enforcement would be using the small-wins strategy to help ensure that all dangerous pollutants are included on the Toxics Release Inventory. It now covers only 1 percent of all chemicals. Another needed reform, recommended by the APHA, is ensuring that all industries and agencies, including the Department of Defense and the Department of Energy, report their Toxics Release Inventory data. Still other enforcement improvements could be achieved by avoiding current policies of "jail for crime in the streets, but bail for crime in the suites." Reformers could demand that penalties for white-collar environmental crime be proportional to the harm done.[25]

As argued in earlier chapters, there also are at least three legal incentives that could help prevent white-collar, environmental crime. One is returning to the pre-2000 Corporate Responsibility Rule, prohibiting persistent and serious corporate criminals from receiving government contracts. Another incentive would be to remove current liability limits that protect polluters at taxpayer expense. As already mentioned, the U.S. Price-Anderson Act is a good example of a law that should be repealed, as recommended by the APHA. It gives nuclear polluters freedom from up to 98 percent of liability claims, even for intentional safety violations.[26] Still another incentive for protecting pollution victims would be to use the small-wins strategy to work for statutory reform of toxic-tort law, as the APHA also suggests. The earlier example of Reason Warehime and other atomic veterans illustrates that because pollution victims often bear too high an evidentiary burden, their legitimate claims fail. Recent tobacco-industry settlements also show that well-financed industry attorneys can often prevail, simply because they are the less economically vulnerable party. The U.S. judicial system, however, began with the premise that it ought to protect the more vulnerable party. In eighteenth-century America, this was usually the defendant. In twenty-first-century toxic torts, however, the more vulnerable party often is the plaintiff, the person injured by pollution but economically unable to untangle the complicated causal chain of harm. As a result, even in worker–compensation claims, pollution victims almost always lose. The antidote is to work for reform of toxic-tort law.[27]

Citizens also could help protect life by forcing government to follow the recommendations of the APHA to phase out of most uses of chlorine. As already mentioned, special-interest polluters instead joined with committees in the U.S. House of Representatives to prevent tighter chlorine regulation. Likewise, the APHA specifically recommended following the precautionary principle—the better-safe-than-sorry view that "every chemical should be considered potentially dangerous until the extent of toxicity is sufficiently known." Yet the U.S. government continues to follow the opposite default rule. It has not tested 98 percent of chemicals that are in use but instead assumes they are harmless until shown otherwise. Citizens could work with groups to improve this default rule.[28]

They also could work for better safety regulations, illustrated through a variety of repeated APHA recommendations. One such recommendation is for disaggregation of all health and safety standards. This recommendation entails re-examining all standards, to ensure they provide adequately protective exposure limits for different groups, such as women and children. Complaining that pollutant regulations are not adequately attentive to vulnerable populations, the APHA recently called for such a reexamination. It urged agencies responsible for setting pollution standards to "evaluate the effects on more sensitive populations not previously considered in [regulatory] standard development." The APHA also gave three arguments for doing so. It noted that many regulations were set up to "40 years ago." Many were "set near the maximum acutely tolerable level, with little regard for the risks of long-term serious or irreversible damage for men, women, and children [or for]...effects on growth and development, and toxic illnesses." Even worse, the APHA noted, many of the regulatory standards were not set by disinterested parties. Instead they were set by "employees of various multinational chemical companies" whose role "was not balanced by those representing" health interests.[29]

As chapter 1 revealed, disaggregated drinking-water standards are particularly needed for infants because of their (relative to body weight) higher water, therefore higher pollutant, intake. Disaggregated standards also would better protect the one-third of Americans who have been estimated to be especially sensitive to toxic chemicals because of prior high exposures.[30] Such standards likewise would help ensure that polluters could not merely defend their polluting actions by claiming their overall benefits exceeded losses. In addition, they also would be forced to address pollution effects on the most vulnerable groups. As argued in earlier chapters, overall societal benefit is never allowed as legitimate justification for putting a medical subject at serious risk to life. If not, overall benefits ought not be said to allow (at least not without adequate compensation and legitimate consent) serious pollution risks, especially to vulnerable groups. Part of what was so heinous about Nazi experimentation was that it made the lives of particular individuals expendable, supposedly in the name of group benefit. Yet as already mentioned, all ethical systems condemn such expedient, tyranny-of-the-majority thinking. If so, citizens need to publicize this condemnation and ensure that it is enforced regarding pollution.[31]

Protecting rights to life also requires citizens to use the small-wins strategy to seek reforms in contemporary legislative interpretations of property rights. As mentioned in chapters 2 and 3, front groups use hire education and private-interest science to promote "the cost-benefit state" and "free-market environmentalism." As a result, many citizens have been misled. In particular, they have been misled into thinking that polluters have property rights to despoil the commons of air and water; that citizens must be "willing to pay" polluters to stop this destruction; and that "pollution rights" are tradable market commodities. Yet, as argued earlier, no particular individuals like polluters can legitimately claim sole rights to the commons. If not, they cannot simply demand that others pay them not to pollute. Besides, if tradable pollution rights allow victims to be killed slowly by pollution, they are no more legitimate property rights than "murder rights" would be. Protecting rights to life thus requires citizens to accept the recommendations of the APHA regarding use of property and to promote a return to the classic account of property rights articulated by thinkers like British moral philosopher John Locke. One traditional Lockean constraint is that people not use their property rights in ways that seriously harm others (as pollution can do). Another constraint is that people have no property rights to resources (like clean air and water) to which others do not also have equal access.[32]

Protecting citizens from life-threatening environmental injustice likewise requires that citizens work for reforms in medical education and medical research. Physicians and scientists must be trained to be aware of environmentally and occupationally induced disease and death. In part this will require that medical scientists follow the recommendations of the APHA for greater emphasis on prevention of disease, not merely on cures or treatment, and on racism as a cause of ill health. It also will require that physicians not rely mainly on drug-industry representatives to obtain most of their continuing pharmaceutical education.[33]

Enlightened medical education and protection of life also require citizens to demand more regulatory and medical emphasis on using the precautionary principle as a default rule under uncertainty about serious threats to life. As already mentioned, the APHA recommends adopting this principle. By pushing government to follow this recommendation, citizens could ensure that pollution threats did not become catastrophic or widespread before government did anything about them.[34] The principle also would promote greater testing of industrial pollutants as well as swifter development of green technology and products.[35]

Organizing themselves as consumers, through NGOs that use the small-wins strategy, ordinary people can be especially powerful in preventing threats to life and to human rights. They can use consumer boycotts to make it more costly for firms *not* to use, than to use, worker-safe and environmentally safe technologies. By boycotting lettuce from nonunion farmworkers and boycotting Nestlé because of its infant-formula practices, as APHA has recommended, well-organized Western consumers have sent corporations a powerful message via their pocketbooks. The message? If companies jeopardize life and human rights, in the long run citizens will force them to reform or to go out of business.[36] Many university students have kept their institutions from buying goods made in sweatshop conditions of unsafe, slave, child, or underpaid labor.[37] Likewise people can force governments and manufacturers to recognize human rights. They can lobby to stop all forms of assistance to governments and to companies that do not recognize rights to life, to bodily security, to organize labor groups and to enjoy equal environmental protection.[38] One example of such needed lobbying is forcing abolition or reform of the U.S. Overseas Private Investment Corporation (OPIC). Designed to promote economic growth at home and abroad, OPIC gives American firms taxpayer funds for up to 75 percent of financing, plus investment insurance for overseas projects costing hundreds of millions of dollars. In reality, however, OPIC often helps firms locate abroad so they can avoid U.S. public-health, environmental-, and occupational-safety regulations. Once abroad, the firms impose serious health risks on those in poor nations who are unable to protect themselves. For example, although such plants are outlawed in the United States, OPIC has used taxpayer dollars to help U.S. companies build dangerous, asbestos plants in India and substandard smelting complexes in Africa.[39]

Other practical strategies for preventing threats to life and to human rights include encouraging the United States to endorse the International Criminal Tribunal.[40] People also could work with NGOs like Human Rights Watch,[41] for instance, to ensure reform of USAID (the U.S. Agency for International Development). USAID currently administers billions of U.S. aid dollars in over 100 countries. As chapter 1 showed, however, the agency mainly gives subsidies for U.S. businesses, rather than aid to the needy. The same is true for

OPIC.[42] Projects of USAID have included paying for the move of Decaturville Sportswear to El Salvador. Taxpayer money funded the loss of 650 jobs in Decaturville, Tennessee. It moved them to El Salvador sweatshops but lined the pockets of the company owners. As chapter 1 noted, reforms of USAID have never been carried out, largely because special interests have fought them.[43] The alternative? Citizens could lobby government so that USAID would support human rights, workplace safety, sustainable development, and natural-resource protection. Citizens could help promote foreign aid that provides medical care and food to the needy, not merely welfare for U.S. corporations. They could lobby groups such as CARE, the World Bank, and the Church World Service to use assistance guidelines that promote only projects that protect public health, democracy, and sustainable development.[44]

Proposals for Fulfilling Rights to Know

Citizens, however, cannot work with government to reduce threats to life unless they know what those threats are. This means that public-health duties must include using the small-wins strategy to help ensure fulfillment of citizens' rights to know about environmental contaminants. As the APHA put it, in one of its policy statements promoting rights to know, "respect for . . . individual autonomy and individual rights . . . requires that those who are at risk have the right to know . . . and the right to decide whether to undergo such risks." [45] One of the most important ways to help fulfill these rights is to demand, with the APHA, that Congress pass the 2002 National Health Tracking Act, already discussed in earlier chapters. Still another important way is to expand requirements for food labeling, also recommended by the APHA. Consider how weak labeling is, even for genetically engineered foods. Even before the first such foods came to market, the U.S. Food and Drug Administration (FDA) claimed they were "substantially equivalent" to traditional foods. As a result, FDA said they needed no special regulations or labels. Indeed, unless there is a known change in nutrient composition, or the engineered food is already known to contain some protein that induces allergic reactions, transgenic foods are "not subject to any pre-market approval process, public notification, or labelling." Even if transgenetic foods were completely safe and had caused no deaths—and they have caused deaths—it would make sense to label them. Why? Most of them are heavily loaded with pesticides. Indeed, 80 percent of transgenic foods are engineered for resistance to otherwise-lethal doses of herbicides, so that farmers can reduce labor costs by using more chemicals. Those who eat the resulting food, however, are not resistant to the higher levels of chemicals. Without the labeling as APHA recommended, people will be aware neither that their food is transgenic nor that, as a result, it likely has higher levels of chemicals.[46]

To prevent threats to children's rights to know, citizens could use the small-wins strategy to help implement the APHA recommendations to designate

schools as "advertising-free zones," to limit child-directed advertising on
television, to develop school-based initiatives on "consumer media literacy,"
to limit alcohol and tobacco advertising and product placement in films, and to
limit advertising that stimulates unnecessary use of legal drugs.[47] More generally, citizens could promote fuller citizen knowledge of public-health risks
by working with non-governmental organizations (NGOs) like Fairness in
Advertising and in Reporting (FAIR) to outlaw advertiser censorship of media, to limit the degree to which media ownership can be concentrated in the
hands of only a few people, and to monitor ways in which media-controlling
polluters may bias news coverage. Still other reforms include limiting tax
deductions for media advertising and using the proceeds to support public
broadcasting. Citizens also could work with NGOs like Public Employees for
Environmental Responsibility (PEER) to strengthen whistleblower laws. This
would help protect reporters (who may need to disclose advertiser or media-
owner conflicts of interest), university or private scientists (who may need to
disclose harmful effects of drugs or pollutants), and federal employees (who
may need to disclose details of regulatory capture). At present, even though
federal-scientist whistleblowers are better protected than those in private industry, the case of Adam Finkel shows they often face severe retaliation.
Frequently they must fight costly battles to protect both scientific information
and public health.[48]

Citizens also could enhance fulfillment of their rights to know by promoting campaign finance reform and public funding of elections. As earlier
chapters suggested, this would help prevent the legalized bribery through
which polluters are often able to capture regulatory agencies and politicians
and thereby suppress important health information. Lack of effective campaign finance reform could be a key reason that the Congress has not passed
the National Health Tracking Act.

Ultimately, however, fulfilling citizens' rights to know about health threats
requires better science, more science, and policing the manipulation of science. For instance, APHA notes that special interests have influenced the
White House Office of Management and Budget. Under the guise of "paperwork reduction," this office has "blocked information collections" and public-
health studies by government health and regulatory agencies. As a remedy, the
APHA recommends policing the Office of Management and Budget so that
it refrains "from interfering with scientific studies of occupational, environmental, and other health problems." "Special interests [also] have exploited the nature of science, specifically scientific uncertainty, to delay legal
protection and/or regulatory action" against dangerous pollutants, says the
APHA. "Under the guise of a call for 'sound science,'" these special interests
have rejected "established scientific methods as 'junk science.'" To balance
this influence of flawed, private-interest science, the APHA likewise recommends increasing public funding of science and the public-health work
force.[49] Yet if chapter 3 is right, public funding for both scientific research and
university education has decreased massively in recent years. Between 2001
and 2005, the average in-state tuition at public, four-year institutions in-

creased 36 percent; enrollment increased 12 percent; consumer prices increased 11 percent; while total state-taxpayer appropriations for their universities have remained flat, at about $68 billion per year. In real dollars, taxpayer support has declined, and the percentages of state budgets going to higher education have declined. Private-interest funding is often a substitute. The results? As earlier chapters suggested, the effects are less public control of information, less access to education, less knowledge of pollution risks, and less fulfillment of rights to know.[50]

Another way to promote better public information, science, and disclosure would be to follow the APHA recommendations to have independent clinical trials for new drugs, germicides, and products like pesticides. This would provide more checks and balances than the current system, in which testing is done and reported (typically without any real oversight) by the same companies that stand to profit from the results. Special interests might still do their own studies, but at least there would be more reliable, independent research to act as a check on errors or fraud. Better fulfillment of rights to know also would be achieved by requiring federal regulatory agencies to perform or fund alternative benefit-cost analyses and quantitative risk assessments. While the 1969 National Environmental Policy Act mandates agencies to evaluate alternatives, almost none do. As a result, benefit-cost analyses and quantitative risk assessments often reflect the biases and conflicts of interest of the polluters who conduct them. This bias often occurs, as the APHA warns, because of "administrative policies that attempt to define the characteristics of valid public health science, or dictate prescriptive scientific methodologies" instead of using "the best available science to protect the public health." One solution would be to conduct different analyses, relying on different factual and ethical assumptions reflecting different stakeholder interests. The different conclusions of these alternative assessments could then be assessed through some form of quasi-judicial "adversary assessment," like that used in U.S. congressional-committee hearings. If the pollution victims of Hammond, Indiana, had been able to perform their own quantitative risk assessments, they might have been protected from the flawed private-interest science that threatened both their children and their rights to know.[51]

Citizens likewise would be better able to fulfill their rights to know if there were fuller disclosure of conflicts of interest on all U.S. federal advisory committees. Using the small-wins strategy, citizens could urge government to require that all committee members reveal, to the public, their sources of income and stock, above some threshold, such as $5,000. As already argued, current U.S. law does not require this full disclosure on all committees. Even in cases where some internal disclosure is required, there is never disclosure to the public, and often government regulators grant waivers (of conflict-of-interest rules) based on the assertion that some individuals' talents are needed by a committee. Unjustified waivers would be less likely in the face of full public disclosure and a more transparent governmental health-advisory process. Citizens could go even further and promote the recommendation of the APHA that all federal committee members be "free of direct financial conflicts of interest" and that government employ universal criteria for avoiding such conflicts of interest and achieving committee balance. At present, the APHA notes that, because

> there are currently no government-wide uniform criteria for determining and managing conflicts of interest or achieving balance on federal scientific and public health advisory committees, or for determining the scientific or expert qualifications of candidates ... committees are heavily weighted toward business and industry interests.

Business and industry representation on federal scientific committees tends to be between three and four times that of citizen or nonprofit groups. Achieving more balance would help protect rights to know.[52]

Proposals for Fulfilling Rights to Consent

To help fulfill the public's right to consent to various pollution-related risks, citizens also could urge government to implement two important recommendations. In 1996 a U.S. National Academy of Sciences report, *Understanding Risk in a Democracy,* recommended that risk assessors give equal weight to stakeholder deliberation, as well as expert views. The 1997 APHA recommendations on chemical exposures said something similar. As already noted, the APHA called for reevaluating chemical-exposure regulations because they were set largely by chemical-company experts whose presence on the committees "was not balanced by those representing workers' [or public] interests." No health professionals or stakeholders were involved. Consequently, the APHA has said, many of the regulations are too lenient, partly because they were arrived at in ways that were "not balanced." Yet both government and other scientists have largely ignored these academy and APHA recommendations. A possible explanation is that balanced committees do not serve special interests. As chapter 3 suggested, it is far easier for special interests to control experts, whom they can pay as consultants, than to control citizens who are trying to protect their health. As a result, many government advisory committees are dominated by scientific employees of polluters and by university scientists having consulting relationships with the polluters. Of the roughly 15 members of typical government risk-assessment committees, usually pollution victims and their stakeholders are represented by only one or two people. They also often are not paid for their time, as the industry or academic members are. Instead, the victim- or stakeholder-members of the committee often must take off from their work and serve at their own expense. Often they find themselves outnumbered by well-financed special interests. If campaign finance reform requires public financing of elections, something similar seems necessary for government science advice. As it is, the current system of supposed "representative consent," through expert- and industry-dominated government advisory committees, puts stakeholders at a disadvantage. These disadvantages are so great that, because genuine citizen consent is questionable, citizens must use the small-wins strategy to help implement recommendations like those of the APHA.[53]

As mentioned earlier, another way to help citizens fulfill their rights to consent is to accord pollution victims the same protections as subjects of medical experiments. It makes sense, morally speaking, to disallow medical experimentation on especially vulnerable groups whose consent may be questionable. If so, allowing widespread pollutant experimentation on especially vulnerable groups, who have failed to consent at all, also is questionable. Individual medical subjects typically have the protection of written consent forms. Pollution victims, who are far greater in number, whose exposures are tracked far less carefully, who are less easily identifiable, and who receive few if any benefits from their exposure, however, have no written consent forms. Indeed, the relevant risks are rarely fully disclosed to them. What appears to have happened is that society has regulated the "easy case," medical risk. Perhaps it has done so because fewer special interests gain from medical, as opposed to pollution, experimentation. Whatever the reason, there is no obvious justification for not protecting pollution victims as well as medical subjects. Achieving this protection will be more difficult, since some pollution is unavoidable, and many pollutants are ubiquitous. One of the first steps to achieving fuller citizen consent to various pollutants would be improving techniques for full risk disclosure. In the case of worker pollution exposures, the APHA has recommended that all health-related guidelines, including those in the hazardous workplaces, be "linguistically and culturally appropriate" and not merely written in English. The APHA also has recommended institutional review boards for all private research conducted on workers, typically to study workplace pollutants or health effects. For members of the public, the APHA has promoted fuller consent by recommending increased funding for community-based participatory public-health research, for participatory processes to evaluate public-health protections and environmental-health programs, and for full citizen involvement and consent "that builds from the bottom up and that places maximum responsibility on the community: citizens." The APHA also has recommended that government publish and distribute informed-consent policies, so that all citizens will be aware of them, and that it increase funding for groups like the Consumer Product Safety Commission.[54]

Citizen Exemplars

Despite the many APHA policy recommendations and its assistance with community education, evaluation, cooperation, and advocacy,[55] it is not easy to help stop threats to health and human rights. As earlier chapters noted, one reason is that it often is not easy to identify pollution victims. They may be merely "statistical casualties." Or perhaps no reliable health studies have been done. As a consequence, those who do know about some pollution victims, or suspect some pollution problems, bear special responsibilities to tell their stories and to take action. Perhaps this is why most of the work of protecting pollution victims is done locally. Millions of unnoticed people throughout the world, people like Gwen Pearson, Juana Gutierrez, and Adolph Coleman, work to protect their own neighborhoods.

What might motivate more citizens to take on such duties of the responsibility argument? One way is to build on the information and arguments presented here, like the many APHA recommendations. Another way is to help people learn from, and become part of, existing traditions of public service and volunteerism, especially in the United States. Just among people aged 55 and older, 24 million Americans volunteer in some cause. Often they do so through their churches, schools, and neighborhoods. The federal Foster Grandparents Program, for instance, links older men and women with disabled or disadvantaged children. The National Service Corps' Program places volunteers in 1,300 programs nationwide. In centers like Samaritan House in San Francisco, it enables retired dentists and doctors provide free care to uninsured, homeless, and poor people. It is easy to think of ways to build on this already-existing generosity and use it to help prevent pollution-related threats.[56]

Pulitzer Prize–winning Harvard psychiatrist Robert Coles, in his book *The Call of Service*, recounts some of this generosity. He tells of dozens of ordinary people—of all ages—doing extraordinary things to help protect the lives and human rights of others. Many of them were transformed by crucial early experiences. Often the transformation was through programs that bring American youth to impoverished urban ghettos, to Appalachia, or to foreign lands. Coles says young people "especially disapprove" of dictatorships in Latin America. Yet they continue to serve there, trying to better the conditions of the people. Two government programs he mentions repeatedly are the Peace Corps and Volunteers in Service to America (VISTA). Coles quotes one young Peace Corps volunteer who spoke for the experiences of many. He said the best part of his service was not what he did for others, but how those in Latin America educated him, both as a moral person and as a citizen. VISTA Volunteers said much the same thing—that their transformation was personal, as well as political. As one volunteer in West Virginia said,

> I've learned how rotten the county system of government is, how corrupt. Here government is the major industry, along with coal—and government is tied up with the coal industry, lock, stock, and barrel. Every once in a while I get really down. I remember that I'm just a volunteer, and I'll be out of this soon, very soon. But for the people I'm working with, this is life.

Although such young volunteers leave their distant assignments and begin lives of their own, Coles says their experiences shape them for life. If citizens today could take on assignments to compensate for pollution harms to which they contribute, their efforts might also empower and enrich them in later life.[57]

Books like Coles's and Robert Bellah's *Habits of the Heart* tell the stories of many people whose lives have been ennobled and transformed by their service to others. They experience the sufferings of others, identify with them, and as a result live their lives differently. Many people have neighbors or friends whose lives have been shaped this way. Some of their stories are dramatic and well known, like that of singer Bono, of the Irish rock group U2. After he and his wife went to work in an Ethiopian refugee camp, their lives have never been the same. He founded an NGO to promote debt cancellation and international aid for Africa, and he has been perhaps the most visible spokesperson for the poor of the world. Actor-director Rob Reiner did something similar. He quit his job for 2 years to raise money to pass California's Proposition 10. This was a 1998 ballot initiative to raise the tax on cigarettes by 50 cents a pack, then use the proceeds for health and nutrition care for needy California preschoolers. And many people know how actor Martin Sheen has engaged in civil disobedience on behalf of U.S. farmworkers facing hazards in the fields. Winona La Duke has fought for land rights and environmental justice within her own Native-American Ojibwe Tribe.[58]

As goodwill ambassador for the United Nations Development Program, actor Danny Glover has traveled widely to promote reparations and debt relief for African nations. In the United States, he is an active board member of the Algebra Project, a math-empowerment program developed by civil-rights advocates. Trained at the Black Actors' Workshop of the American Conservatory, Glover says two events empowered him as an actor and a public citizen. They gave him vicarious experience of the sufferings of others and helped him realize what he needed to do about it. One experience was his appearance in a play about apartheid in South Africa. Another was his playing a homeless man in the movie *The Saint of Fort Washington*. Efforts like Glover's, helping protect lives and rights, often have a price. Because of his opposition to the death penalty and to the 2003 U.S. war in Iraq, people have boycotted Glover's films and labeled him "unpatriotic." [59] And NBC executives told actor Martin Sheen, formerly performing in the TV series, *West Wing*, that they were "very uncomfortable" with his social-justice activism. In 2002, prowar forces flooded the Burbank office of NBC. They tried to have Sheen fired from the series because he used his fame to draw attention to social-justice causes. Over the last 20 years, Sheen has been arrested more than 60 times for civil disobedience in connection with his fighting racism, homelessness, and nuclear testing. In response, he says simply: "I had to stand for something so I could stand to be me." Sheen says it doesn't matter whether people are Republicans or Democrats or Independents. Everyone "must make a contribution." Everyone "must accept responsibility for what goes down." Otherwise, he says, democracy will be "left to the wealthy and privileged." [60]

Such examples suggest there are many ways to accept the duties of the responsibility argument. Wayne Bauer of Campaign California, formerly the "Campaign for Economic Democracy," helps vulnerable renters, especially

Hispanics, join together in tenants' unions. Working with this egalitarian, grassroots organization, Bauer also has helped the Campaign promote government-sponsored daycare, environmental protection, and energy conservation. Another Californian, Mary Taylor, a member of the California Coastal Commission, is a housewife turned professor. She began community work with the League of Women Voters. Arguing that we all share a debt to society, she claims that her inspiration is her grandfather, who was in the Catholic Worker movement. For Mary Taylor, being a public citizen means living with generosity of spirit, caring for other people, and working with others to secure the public interest.[61] In Reno, Nevada, retired Air Force pilot Dennis Grover, active in the Libertarian Party, helps prevent public-health harms by funding and filming numerous videos for broadcast on public TV. These are on topics such as whether fluoride should be added to the drinking water and whether the mercury in vaccinations has added to the increase in autism.[62]

What is important about Bauer's, Taylor's, or Grover's service is not whether it springs from Democratic or Republican or some other roots. The crucial thing is that it contributes to the social way in which people learn. It is part of deliberative democracy. It comes from less powerful people, claiming their rights, who challenge more powerful institutions. It encourages debate and promotes respect for life and for human rights. Anita Roddick, the CEO who founded the cosmetics giant, Body Shop, believes almost everyone and every group can also promote respect for life and human rights. As Roddick sees it, there is no reason that corporations cannot both promote integrity and enjoy great financial success. She says the vast majority of the world's businesses are owned by local stakeholders, are fully responsible, and empower people in many good ways. Roddick herself provides a good example. She saw that Shell Oil cooperated with the Nigeria military dictatorship in 1995 to kill nonviolent environmental activists, like Ken Saro-Wiwa. They were protesting Shell's lax pollution control and destruction of indigenous Ogoni homelands. Roddick held Shell and fellow CEOs to a higher standard. If she had not orchestrated the international boycott against Shell, it might have gotten away with both the murders and the pollution. At Body Shop, Roddick established a regular executive position in social ethics. Her goal was not only that the company behave ethically but also that it promote ethics around the world. A doting grandmother, Roddick files dispatches from the Amazon rain forest, pillories warlike global leaders, and solicits spoofs of corporate logos. She even opened a publishing house to produce her books, *A Revolution in Kindness, Take It Personally,* and *Brave Hearts and Rebel Spirits.* The proceeds go to humanitarian work.[63]

Keeping in mind the example of Anita Roddick, citizens following the responsibility argument should be wary of any NGO involvement that is too neatly classified as pro-corporate or anti-corporate, right-wing or left-wing. Protestant theologian Richard Neuhaus claimed that many left-wing advocates vociferously advocate vegetarianism because they want to protect all life. Yet, he claims, they inconsistently defend abortion on demand. And writer Kurt Vonnegut warned that many right-wing advocates push the Ten Commandments on others, even in public places. Yet he claims they inconsistently fail to recognize the Beatitudes—especially its injunctions to be peacemakers and to be merciful.[64] As both sets of complaints suggest, the responsibility argument requires that people avoid ideology. Instead it requires empathy, education, interaction, and sustained, self-critical reflection. Public citizens—those who follow the responsibility argument—might even find themselves in a situation like that of Mairead Maguire, winner of the 1976 Nobel Peace Prize. Embraced by much of the world for her efforts to achieve peace in Ireland, she was rejected by both the Irish Republican Army and many fellow Irish as a British sympathizer. Left-wingers rejected her because of her religion; right-wingers rejected her because of her hunger strike at the jail of American peace activist Philip Berrigan. Fellow Roman Catholics criticized her for lobbying the pope for women's ordination as priests. Much the same has happened to Martin Sheen. The Right has rejected him because of his civil disobedience on behalf of farm workers. The Left has rejected him for his opposition to abortion on demand. Consistent with the earlier point about avoiding ideological "right" or "left" stances, the crucial point here is not whether Sheen's or Maguire's or any other positions are correct or incorrect. That is for the people to decide, case by case, using democratic deliberation and the methods outlined in this book. What is apparent is that Sheen and Maguire appear to have adopted reflective and self-critical positions. In so doing, they have contributed to deliberative democracy and promoted both life and human rights.[65]

For many people, the preceding examples of Roddick, Maguire, and Sheen are far removed from the ways they have chosen to live their lives. For them, following the responsibility argument is something they have chosen to do more in their personal, than in their political, lives. A good example is that of Jan and Damian Barthle of Louisville, Kentucky. They discovered, 30 years ago, that Damian's cancer would prevent their having children. Instead of worrying about their own future and a possible recurrence of Damian's cancer, they adopted a baby girl with severe cerebral palsy. She had been abandoned by her parents because of her extreme disabilities. When Jan and Damian took Melissa home, she was a total stranger, a four-year-old who could only lie in bed, too weak even to hold up her head. Despite their own full-time work as teachers, Jan and Damian spent many hours working with Melissa. They raised her as their own, never spoiled her, and did exercises to strengthen her muscles. They taught her and traveled around the country with her in their specially equipped van. Rather than self-centered or self-pitying, Melissa has become joyful, loving, and confident. She is able to use a wheelchair, and she graduated from high school. She is even able to hold a part-time library job and now lives on her own as an adult in a group home. Without Jan's and Damian's efforts, Melissa likely would have spent all her life lying in an institution, unable even to communicate.[66]

In the natural lottery of life, Melissa was disadvantaged. Jan and Damian—with their modest teachers' salaries—were advantaged. They decided to help level the playing field, to become responsible for a complete stranger. In the process, they not only loved and adopted Melissa, not only prevented further harm to her. They also dramatically helped her fulfill her life. Like the Polish workers discussed in the last chapter, they realized that they could not achieve big wins, massive change. Instead they became the change they sought. Their doing so empowered Melissa. It also helped create a more just and healthy society. For Robert Bellah, this is a society that takes a stand with the vulnerable, the poor, and the oppressed.

Bellah's community-based vision of a just social order is rooted firmly in the populism of Thomas Jefferson. When he visited France, Jefferson was appalled at the extremes of wealth and poverty that he found. He believed the United States had hope for the future only because it lacked such extremes. Following Jefferson, Bellah says crumbs from rich people's tables will not eliminate poverty. These crumbs also will not reduce life-threatening pollution. Instead, justice requires that extreme poverty and extreme pollution be eliminated. But how can anyone begin such a monumental task? One answer is that the task already has been begun by many, already moderately successful, NGOs. Others can join their efforts. Another answer is that people can try to become the change they seek—as the Barthles have done and as Gwen Pearson, Karen Silkwood, Reason Warehime, Adam Finkel, Adolph Coleman, and Juana Gutierrez have done. A third answer is given by Robert Bellah. He says people can begin the work of creating a just and healthy society by becoming less attached to the extrinsic rewards, like money, associated with work. Instead, he says, people can dedicate themselves to their own communities and to work that has intrinsic rewards.[67]

Princeton ethicist Peter Singer gives examples of many ordinary people whose lives show that they live by intrinsic, rather than extrinsic, rewards. He tells the story of a major donor to the Australian Conservation Foundation, a man who regularly sent the foundation checks for $1,000. When the head of the foundation went to the man's home, to thank him for his large donations over many years, he thought he must be at the wrong address. It was a small suburban home owned by an employee of the state department of public works, David Alsop. Despite his modest government salary and small home, Alsop donates 50 percent of his income to environmental causes. Whether or not people share Alsop's commitment, there is something ennobling about the way he lives his life.[68]

There also is something ennobling about the numbers of ordinary citizens—in Britain, for instance, roughly 6 percent of those eligible to donate—who repeatedly give blood to blood banks in Britain, Australia, Canada, Europe, and the Americas. This is the only supply of blood for medical purposes. Giving it requires about an hour of one's time, mostly from ordinary people who typically remain unknown and unheralded. In about 25 countries, there also are bone-marrow donor registries. There people offer to undergo anesthesia, stay overnight in a hospital, and donate their marrow to cancer victims—strangers—who need a match. In the United States, 650,000 donors are in the registry. In France, 63,000. In England, 180,000. Ordinary people also are often generous with their money. American surveys indicate that nearly 90 percent of Americans donate some money to charities. Indeed, at least 20 million families give at least 5 percent of their income to charity. And nearly half of all Americans donate their time to some charity. In addition, 82 percent of all Americans say they are willing to pay more for environmentally friendly products. This all suggests that many people are ready to take on the duties of the responsibility argument.[69]

Mandatory Service

If every citizen could have firsthand experiences of threats to health and to human rights, and of ways to alleviate them, accepting the demands of the responsibility argument would be easier. Such firsthand experiences would help people develop not only intellectual understanding but also the moral and empathetic understanding of fellow citizens that is necessary to make democracy work. The founding mothers and fathers of the United States recognized this need for moral education and understanding. As a result, they built it into the curriculum of most early educational institutions. Today, many high schools, colleges, and universities also try to develop moral understanding by requiring at least some public service or volunteer work of students. This is largely because they recognize that firsthand experience, serving those in need, is necessary both to personal moral education and to democracy.

Moreover, there are many precedents—like the military draft—for asking service of virtually all citizens. There obviously are some times when young people must be drafted, compelled to help defend—and die for—the nation. Surely also there are times when all young people ought to be asked to help prevent threats to the health and rights of fellow citizens. Chapter 4 argued for the *prima facie* duties of the responsibility argument, but such duties require implementation in a meaningful way. Working with NGOs is one form of implementation. But without universal implementation, through something like a national service program, moral education and deliberative democracy are likely to be incomplete. Many citizens are unlikely to learn all that is necessary to make them public citizens, dedicated to the common cause, understanding the needs of others. Otherwise, many citizens may remain free riders—people who enjoy the benefits of democratic citizenship, but who let others do its work and take its risks. Without something like a national service program, citizens will be saying something inconsistent. Although everyone ought to pay taxes for the good of the whole, not everyone ought to give time for the good of the whole. Yet neither democratic governments nor families will succeed if members merely give their monies but not their time, their talents, and their hearts.[70]

A meaningful national service program would be one way to carry out the suggestions of earlier chapters. The program might allow maximum choice regarding the types of efforts and the sorts of public or private institutions in which young people might serve. The key factor would be that public service is expected of virtually everyone, after high school. Indeed, if most people in democratic societies served for a year, full-time, in programs like Americorps, VISTA, or Big Brothers and Big Sisters, they would probably agree that such service should be part of everyone's education. It should be part of everyone's repayment of the debts of citizenship, part of the building blocks of democracy. A national service program could also be part of the compensation that citizens owe others who have been harmed by flawed institutions in which everyone participates. Besides, the benefits of such a program might be deep and long-lived. Psychiatrist Robert Coles argues that public service, "an idealism exerted, at one moment in life, sets in motion certain forces, crises, choices," that can change people forever, for the better. Many public-service veterans of "social and racial and economic struggles," says Coles, attribute the nature of their current lives to what happened "back then." Volunteers might have been uncertain of what they wanted to do with their lives. Nevertheless, says Coles, they became "sure of certain social convictions and ready to work to realize them." [71]

Many civil-rights or poverty workers do more than become ready to realize the convictions built during their service years. Coles says they also pass on their convictions and their dedication to service to their children. As one volunteer puts it:

> you see clearly what can be done, what you're doing, even with the disappointments, and you wish that more were being done, that more and more of us were 'sisters' and 'brothers' to each other. And so you look and look at the politics of the city, the state, the country, hoping that your service will get to be a part of a nation that is interested in being of service to its people: a nation that serves those in need of housing, food, and work, rather than lobbyists in need of favors by the million, and worth billions. . . . I am hoping for a different kind of morality in the nation, a morality informed by service [in which] we take responsibility for each other.

Coles says that service can be the light through which much of the darkness around us is defined. [72]

Conclusion

In showing the need for the responsibility argument and how we might implement it, these chapters are not calling for a "New Age" person committed only to personal growth. More important, they call for a recommitment to the classic traditions of ethics and democracy. They ask us to rise to the examples of everyday heroes all around us, to the challenges of Jefferson and Lincoln,

Coleman and Gutierrez. They ask that citizens not "retreat into professions and corporations . . . private pleasure and high consumption . . . abdication of responsibility, voluntary myopia." [73] We can be the change that life-sustaining democracies need. We can be the light that defines—and can often banish— the darkness around us.

Notes

Chapter 1

1. Indiana State Department of Health, "Testicular Cancer"; www.in.gov/isdh/factsfigures2003.pdf; accessed July 1, 2005. Facts about the Hammond childhood cancers are from J. Morris, "Small Time Polluter, Big-Time Problems," *US News and World Report* 128, no. 8 (2000): 57–58; Lauri Harvey, "Piecing Together a Cancer Puzzle," *Northwest Indiana Times* 92, no. 83 October 3, 1999, A1; http://nwitimes.com/articles/1999/10/03/export381839.txt; and the citizens' group IRATE; http://irateparents.org/index_files/aboutus.htm; all accessed July 1, 2005; hereafter cited as: IRATE. Information about IRATE and childhood cancers comes from Gwen Pearson, personal communication, by telephone, September 9, 2005.

2. See, e.g., T. Bowler, S. Gynsens, and C. Harney, "Neuropsychological Effects of Ethylene Dichloride (EDC) Exposure," *Neurotoxicology* 24, nos. 4–5 (2004): 553–562; EPA, "Vinyl Chloride"; www.epa.gov/OGWDW/dwh/t-voc/vinylchl.html; accessed July 1, 2005. ATSDR, "Vinyl Chloride: Analytic Methods"; www.atsdr.cdc.gov/toprofiles/tp20-c7.pdf; see also www.epa.gov/safewater/dwh/c-voc/vinylchl.html, both accessed July 1, 2005.

3. Morris, "Small Time Polluter," 57–58; Pearson, personal communication, September 9, 2005. After IRATE put pressure on Ferro, the company quickly moved to Port-de-Bouc, France. The company now releases no ethylene dichloride or vinyl chloride in the United States.

4. Agency for Toxic Substances and Disease Registry (ATSDR), *Petitioned Public Health Assessment, Keil Chemical, Hammond, Lake County, Indiana* (Washington, D.C.: ATSDR, 2001); www.atsdr.cdc.gov/HAC/PHA/keilchem/kei _toc.html and accessed July 1, 2006.

5. Morris, "Small Time Polluter," 57–58; Harvey, "Piecing Together a Cancer Puzzle."

6. EPA, "Vinyl Chloride"; ATSDR, "Vinyl Chloride: Analytic Methods"; see also www.epa.gov/safewater/dwh/c-voc/vinylchl.html; accessed July 1, 2005.

7. The label "Cancer Alley" is from Brett Hulsey, International Air Quality Board of the International Joint Commission, *Great Lakes Water Quality*

Agreement Public Forum (Niagara Falls, Ontario: International Joint Commission, November 1997). Toxics Release Inventory data, reported by industries to the US Environmental Protection Agency for all U.S. counties, are at www.epa .gov. The Health and Energy Company analyzed Toxics Release Inventory data in D. Ortman, *Great Lakes States, America's New Cancer Alley* (Omaha: Health and Energy Company, 2005). Because the Ferro Chemical Company was located in Hammond, Indiana, on the south shore of Lake Michigan, the wind patterns to and from the facility change with the seasons. During winter, the prevailing wind blows southward, from the lake and the Ferro plant, and toward the families. During summer, the prevailing winds blow northeast, toward the plant and the lake. Residences are one-quarter mile south of the chemical facility, which is near the lake.

8. Pearson, personal communication, September 9, 2005.

9. C. I. Jackson, *Honor in Science* (New Haven: Sigma Xi Society, 1986), 29. See also Kristin Shrader-Frechette, *Ethics of Scientific Research* (Lanham, Md.: Rowman and Littlefield, 1994), 42–44, 78–84.

10. American Association for the Advancement of Science, *Principles of Scientific Freedom and Responsibility* (Washington, D.C.: AAAS, 1980), 4.

11. Gwen Pearson, personal communication, by phone, July 2, 2005. Pearson, personal communication, September 9, 2005; see IRATE.

12. Quoted material is from APHA, *2004 Policy Statements* (Washington, D.C.: APHA, 2004), 12; www.apha.org/legislative/policy/2004/; accessed February 16, 2006. APHA recommendations from different years can be accessed at the foregoing website, by inserting the year desired into the web address, in the place of "2004." Thus 2003 recommendations are at www.apha.org/legislative/policy/2003/, and so on.

13. Iris Marion Young, "Activist Challenges to Deliberative Democracy," *Political Theory* 29, no. 5 (October 2001): 688; see also 670–690. See Young, *Inclusion and Democracy* (New York: Oxford University Press, 2000); Young, *Justice and the Politics of Difference* (Princeton: Princeton University Press, 1990); as well as James Bohman, *Public Deliberation* (Cambridge, Mass.: MIT Press, 1996). He emphasizes the importance of identifying the ways that structural inequalities block the political influence of some and magnify that of others, despite formal guarantees of political equality. See also Thomas Beitz, *Political Equality* (Princeton: Princeton University Press, 1990); John S. Dryzek, *Deliberative Democracy and Beyond* (New York: Oxford University Press, 2000); James Fishkin, *The Voice of the People* (New Haven: Yale University Press, 1995); Amy Gutmann and Dennis Thompson, *Democracy and Disagreement* (Cambridge, Mass.: Harvard University Press, 1996); A. Gutmann and D. Thompson, *Why Deliberative Democracy?* (Princeton: Princeton University Press, 2004); Stephen Macedo (ed.), *Deliberative Politics* (Oxford University Press, 1999); Jane Mansbridge, *Beyond Adversary Democracy* (New York: Basic Books, 1980); Onora O'Neill, *Towards Justice and Virtue* (Cambridge: Cambridge University Press, 1996); and Ian Shapiro, *Democratic Justice* (New Haven: Yale University Press, 1999).

14. Young, Justice and the Politics of Difference, 15–24, 26–28, 64–65.

15. Iris Marion Young, "Activist Challenges to Deliberative Democracy," *Philosophy of Education* 1 (2001): 42 of 41–55; hereafter cited as ACDD. Young, Inclusion and Democracy, 5. To emphasize the open and critical elements of deliberative democracy, Dryzek defends "discursive democracy": democracy that

is pluralistic, reflexive in examining established traditions, transnational, ecological, and dynamic. Young calls for "communicative democracy": seeing citizens' cultural and social differences as resources that enrich transformative deliberation, not something that must be overcome. To achieve the full participation that is characteristic of deliberative democracy, processes like "discourse ethics" must ensure that everyone competent to speak is allowed to speak, to question other assertions, to express desires and needs, to set the agenda, and to be free from coercion. Jurgen Habermas, "On Systematically Distorted Communication," *Inquiry* 13, no. 3 (1970): 205–218; see Habermas, *Between Facts and Norms* (Cambridge, Mass.: MIT Press, 1996; Habermas, *Moral Consciousness and Communicative Action* (Cambridge, Mass.: MIT Press, 1990); Habermas, *Justification and Application: Remarks on Discourse Ethics* (Cambridge, Mass.: MIT Press, 1993); see also James Fishkin, *Debating Deliberative Democracy* (Malden, Mass.: Blackwell, 2003); Gutmann and Thompson, Why Deliberative Democracy? and John Dryzek, *Democracy in Capitalist Times* (Oxford: Oxford University Press, 1996).

16. Quotations are from Young, "Activist Challenges to Deliberative Democracy," *Philosophy of Education* (2001), 42. Robert Dahl, *On Democracy* (New Haven: Yale University Press, 1998); Colin Farrelly, *An Introduction to Contemporary Political Theory* (London: Sage, 2004), esp. ch. 7.

17. Quotation is from Young, "Activist Challenges to Deliberative Democracy," *Philosophy of Education* (2001), 47; see 47–50; Dryzek, *Deliberative Democracy and Beyond*, ch. 4. See Bohman, *Public Deliberation*, and previous 4 notes plus Andrew Arato and Jean Cohen, *Civil Society and Political Theory* (Cambridge, Mass.: MIT Press, 1992).

18. Institute of Medicine, *Insuring America's Health* (Washington, D.C.: National Academy Press, 2004), 8, provides the 18,000 figure. Statistics on food-borne illness are from 1999 reports of the US Centers for Disease Control, as reported in Laurie Garrett, *Betrayal of Trust* (New York: Hyperion, 2000), 483.

19. CDC, *The State of the CDC, Fiscal Year 2003* (Atlanta: CDC, 2003), 4; www.cdccoalition.org/resources/StateofCDC.pdf; accessed February 19, 2006. For OTA citation, see note 31. For environmental justice, see Kristin Shrader-Frechette, *Environmental Justice: Creating Equality, Reclaiming Democracy* (New York: Oxford University Press, 2002).

20. Ludwig Wittgenstein, *Philosophical Investigations*, trans. G. E. M. Anscombe (Oxford: Blackwell, 1958), 4.

21. Don Eberly, "Building the Habitat of Character," in Don Eberly (ed.), *The Content of America's Character* (New York: Madison Books, 1995), 29; see also 25–46 and Lynn Schultz et al., "The Value of a Development Approach to Evaluating Character Development Programmes," *Journal of Moral Education* 30, no. 1 (March 2001): 3–27.

22. Sheldon Rampton and John Stauber, *Trust Us, We're Experts!* (New York: Penguin, 2002), 312–314.

23. National Institutes of Health, *Cancer Rates and Risks* (Washington, D.C.: NIH and NCI, 2000); http://seer.cancer.gov/publications/raterisk/ and accessed February 19, 2006.

24. Note 43 gives the "leading killer" statistic. S. Devesa et al., "Recent Cancer Trends in the United States," *Journal of the National Cancer Institute* 87, no. 3 (1995): 175–182; E. Steliarova-Foucher et al., "Geographical Patterns and Time Trends of Cancer Incidence and Survival among Children," *Lancet* 364, no. 9451

(2004): 2097–105; and SEER, *Cancer Statistics Review*, 1973–1997 (Washington, D.C.: NCI, NIH, 1998). See also notes 25–34; Samuel S. Epstein, "Reversing the Cancer Epidemic," *Tikkun* 17, no. 3 (May 2002): 56–66; Robert T. Greenlee, M. B. Hill-Harmon, Taylor Murray, and Michael Thun, "Cancer Statistics," *CA: A Cancer Journal for Clinicians* 1, no. 1 (2001): 15–36; Samuel Epstein, *The Politics of Cancer Revisited* (New York: East Ridge Press, 1998); Samuel Epstein, *Cancer-Gate* (Amityville, N.Y.: Baywood, 2005). Finally, see Devra Davis and David Hoel (eds.), "Trends in Cancer Mortality in Industrial Countries," *Annals of the New York Academy of Sciences* 609 (1990): 8877–8923.

25. APHA, *America's Health Rankings* (Washington, D.C.: APHA, 2005), 103.

26. Paul Lichtenstein, Niels Holm, Pia Verkasalo, Anastasia Iliadou, Jaakko Kaprio, Markku Koskenvuo, Eero Pukkala, Axel Skytthee, and Kari Hemminki, "Environmental and Heritable Factors in the Causation of Cancer," *New England Journal of Medicine* 343, no. 2 (2002): 78–85.

27. Institute of Medicine, Lovell Jones, John Paretto, and Christine Coussens (eds.), *Rebuilding the Unity of Health and the Environment* (Washington, D.C.: National Academy Press, 2005), esp. 2, 15, 43–44. The 6,000 estimate of annual U.S. children's deaths from cancer is from Institute of Medicine, *Making Better Drugs for Children with Cancer* (Washington, D.C.: National Academy Press, 2005), 18. See, for example, D. L. Davis and S. Webster, "The Social Context of Science: Cancer and the Environment," *Annals of the American Academy of Political and Social Science* 584, no. 1 (November 2002): 13–34. D. L. and H. L. Bradlow, "Can Environmental Estrogens Cause Breast Cancer?" *Scientific American* 273, no. 4 (October 1995): 166.

28. F. Valent, D. A. Little, R. Bertollini, L. E. Nemer, G. Barbonc, and G. Tamburlini, "Burden of Disease Attributable to Selected Environmental Factors and Injury among Children and Adolescents in Europe," *Lancet* 363, no. 9426 (2004): 2032–2039. Regarding the tumor-suppressor gene, see Anton Berns, "Tumour Suppressors: Timing Will Tell," *Nature* 424, no. 6945 (2003): 140.

29. Institute of Medicine, *Making Better Drugs,* 51. Stanford University Hospital and Clinics, *Cancer Overview*; http://cancer.stanfordhospital.com/healthInfo/cancerOverview/index.html; accessed July 6, 2005.

30. University of Iowa Comprehensive Cancer Center, *Viruses and Cancer*; www.vh.org/adult/patient/cancercenter/cancertips/viruses.html; accessed July 6, 2005. See note 29.

31. For the claim that 90 percent of cancers are "environmentally induced and theoretically preventable," see J. C. Lashof et al., Health and Life Sciences Division of the OTA, *Assessment of Technologies for Determining Cancer Risks from the Environment* (Washington, D.C.: OTA, 1981), 3, 6ff. Some scientists, however, disagree with the OTA; see Mike Mitka, "Disparity in Cancer Statistics Changing," *Journal of the American Medical Association,* 287, no. 6 (2002): 703–704; Susan S. Devesa, *Atlas of Cancer Morality in the U.S. 1950–1994* (Darby, PA: Diane, 2000). Other scientists (see note 26) attribute virtually all cancers to the environment (broadly understood to include factors like cigarette smoke, as well as industrial pollution).

32. D. D'Arrigo and C. Folkers, "All Levels of Radiation Confirmed to Cause Cancer," Nuclear Information and Resource Service June 30, 2005, Press Release; http://www.nirs.org/press/06-30-2005/ and accessed 10 October 2006. United Nations Scientific Committee on the Effects of Atomic Radiation, *Sources, Effects, and Risks of Ionizing Radiation* (New York: UN, 1994).

33. J. P. Leigh, S. B. Markowitz, M. Fahs, C. Shin, P. J. Landrigan, "Occupational Injury and Illness in the United States. Estimates of Costs, Morbidity, and Mortality," *Archives of Internal Medicine* 157, no. 14 (1997):1557–1568. E. M. Ward, P. A. Schulte, S. Bayard, A. Blair, P. Brandt-Rauf, M. A. Butler, D. Dankovic, A. F. Hubbs, C. Jones, M., Karstadt, G. L. Kedderis, R. Melnick, C. A. Redlich, N. Rothman, R. E. Savage, M. Sprinker, M. Toraason, A. Weston, A. F. Olshan, P. Stewart, S. H. Zahm, and National Occupational Research Agenda Team, "Priorities for Development of Research Methods in Occupational Cancer," *Environmental Health Perspectives* 111, no. 1 (2003): 1–12. J. Landrigan, "The Prevention of Occupational Cancer," *CA: A Cancer Journal for Clinicians* 46, no. 4 (1996): 254–255. J. Landrigan, "The Recognition and Control of Occupational Disease," *Journal of the American Medical Association* 266, no. 5 (1991): 676–680. J. Landrigan, "Commentary: Environmental Disease—A Preventable Epidemic," *American Journal of Public Health* 82, no. 7 (1992): 941–943. Paul Schulte, "Characterizing the Burden of Occupational Injury and Disease," *Journal of Occupational and Environmental Medicine* 47, no. 6 (2005): 607–622. A. Okun, T. J. Lentz, A. Schulte, and C. Stayner, "Identifying High-Risk Small Business Industries for Occupational Safety and Health Interventions," *American Journal of Industrial Medicine* 39, no. 3 (2001): 301–311. M. Toraason et al., "Applying New Biotechnologies to the Study of Occupational Cancer," *Environmental Health Perspectives* 112, no. 4 (2004): 413–416.

34. U.S. Department of Health and Human Services and National Cancer Institute (NCI), "Health Status Objectives," *Cancer* 16, no. 1 (1991): 416–440, and J. Michael McGinnis, "Attributable Risk in Practice," in Institute of Medicine, *Estimating the Contributions of Lifestyle-Related Factors to Preventable Death* (Washington, D.C.: National Academy Press, 2005), 17–19. J. M. McGinnis and W. H. Foege, "The Immediate vs. the Important," *Journal of the American Medical Association* 291, no. 10 (2004): 1263–1264. J. M. McGinnis and W. H. Foege, "Actual Causes of Death in the United States," *Journal of the American Medical Association* 270, no. 18 (1993): 2207–2212. See note 31 above.

35. Paul R. Ehrlich and Anne H. Ehrlich, *Betrayal of Science and Reason* (Washington, D.C.: Island Press, 1996), 154.

36. K. Bridbord et al., *Estimates of the Fraction of Cancer in the United States Related to Occupational Factors* (Bethesda, Md.: NCI, National Institute of Environmental Health Sciences, and National Institute for Occupational Safety and Health, 1978). S. S. Epstein, "The Politics of Cancer," *Multinational Monitor* 9, no. 3 (1988); www.multinationalmonitor.org/hyper/issues/1988/03/mm0388_05.html and accessed 23 October 2006.

37. E.g., J. Dich et al. "Pesticides and Cancer," *Cancer Causes Control* 8, no. 3 (1997): 420–443. D. Rall, "Laboratory Animal Toxicity and Carcinogenesis Testing," *Annals of the New York Academy of Sciences* 534, no. 1 (1988): 78–83. F. Falk et al., "Pesticides and PCB Residues in Human Breast Lipids and Their Relation to Breast Cancer," *Archives of Environmental Health* 47, no. 2 (1992): 143–146. J. B. Westin and E. Richter, "The Israeli Breast-Cancer Anomaly," *Annals of the New York Academy of Sciences* 609, no. 1 (1990): 269–279. Regarding chemicals' weakening the immune system see R. Sharma, "Evaluation of Pesticide Immunotoxicity," *Toxicology and Industrial Health* 4, no. 3 (1988): 373–380. Regarding radiation weakening the immune system see N. Sakaguchi, "Ionizing Radiation and Autoimmunity," *Journal of Immunology* 152, no. 5 (1994): 2586–95.

38. U.S. National Research Council, *Carcinogens and Anticarcinogens in the Human Diet* (Washington, D.C.: National Academy Press, 1996).

39. See earlier notes and Centers for Disease Control, "Cancer Fact Sheet"; www.cdc.gov/omh/AMH/factsheets/cancer.htm and accessed February 18, 2006.

40. NCI, ACS, North American Association of Central Cancer Registries, National Institute on Aging, and the CDC, including the National Center for Health Statistics and the National Center for Chronic Disease Prevention and Health Promotion, "Annual Report to the Nation on the Status of Cancer, 1973–1999," *Cancer* 94, no. 10 (May 15, 2002): 2766–92; see also www.nih.gov/news/pr/may2002/nci-14.htm and accessed February 18, 2006.

41. Quoted in NIH, *1987 Annual Cancer Statistics Review* (Bethesda, Md.: NCI, 1987), 1.4–1.8. NCI, *Surveillance, Epidemiology, and End Results, Cancer Statistics Review, 1973–1994* (Bethesda, Md.: NCI, 1994). See NIH, *Cancer Rates and Risks* (Bethesda: NCI, 2000); http://rex.nci.nin.gov/NCIPubInterface/rasterisk/; accessed February 18, 2006. See also *Rolodex—Cancer* (U.S. CDC, 2000); and American Cancer Society, *Cancer Facts and Figures, 2000* (Atlanta: ACS, 2000).

42. Elena Elkin, Clifford Hudis, Colin B. Begg, and Deborah Schrag, "The Effect of Changes in Tumor Size on Breast Carcinoma in the U.S.: 1975–1999," *Cancer* 104, no. 6 (2005): 1149–57.

43. ACS, *Cancer Facts and Figures, 2005* (Atlanta: ACS, 2005); www.cancer.org/downloads/STT/CAFF2005PWSecured4.pdf. Daniel DeNoon, "Cancer Now Top Killer of Americans," *WebMD,* January 19, 2005; http://my.webmd.com/content/article/99/105264.htm; accessed January 21, 2005 and accessed January 21, 2005.

44. APHA, APHA Policy Database; accessed February 17, 2006; www.apha.org/legislative/policy/policysearch/index.cfm?fuseaction=search_results; accessed January 21, 2005. Search terms "environment" and "cancer" used in APHA database. 2005 policy recommendations include 2005-LB-7, to increase funding for environmental and occupational health threats, and 2000 recommendations include PN-20008, to better regulate pesticide exposure.

45. Ibid. Search terms "environment" and "air pollution" used in APHA database. The APHA recommendations mentioned include those, respectively, from the years 2000, 2000, 1992, 1991, 1989, and 1985 and are policies numbers 200012, 200017, 9206, 9101, 8912, and 8511.

46. WHO, *Indoor Air Pollution and Health* (Bonn: WHO, 2005); www.who.int/mediacentre/factsheets/fs292/en/ and accessed February 20, 2005. Commonwealth Scientific and Industrial Research Organization, *Air Pollution* (Aspendale, Australia: Commonwealth Scientific and Industrial Research Organization, 1999); www.csiro.au/index.asp?id=AirPollution&type=mediaRelease; accessed February 20, 2005. Regarding ozone, see Steven N. Goodman, "The Methodologic Ozone Effect," *Epidemiology* 16, no. 4 (2005): 430–435.

47. Anna Gosline, "European Deaths from Air Pollution Set to Rise," *New Scientist* 17, no. 51 (September 2004); www.newscientist.com/article.ns?id=dn6364); accessed July 12, 2005.

48. APHA, "Policy Statements, 2000," *American Journal of Public Health* 91, no. 3 (March 2001): 21.

49. European Public Health Alliance, *Air, Water Pollution and Health Effects* (Brussels: European Public Health Alliance, 2006); www.epha.org/r/54 and accessed July 12, 2005.

50. William Haenzel, David B. Loveland, and Martin G. Sirken, "Lung Cancer Mortality as Related to Residence and Smoking Histories," *Journal of the National Cancer Institute* 28, no. 4 (1962): 947 of 947–1001. Warren Winkelstein, Edward Davis, Charles Maneri, and William Mosher, "The Relationship of Air Pollution and Economic Status to Total Mortality and Selected Respiratory System Morality," *Archives of Environmental Health* 14, no. 1 (1967): 162–171.

51. The Economist, *Pocket World in Figures, 2007 Edition* (London: Profile Books, 2006), pp. 104–105. Lester Lave and Eugene O. Seskin, "Air Pollution and Human Health," *Science* 169 (1970): 723–733, on air pollution; Jack Spengler et al., *Health Effects of Fossil Fuel Burning* (Cambridge Mass: Ballinger, 1980); Devra Davis, *When Smoke Ran Like Water* (New York: Basic Books, 2002), 103, 121. Regarding poor enforcement, see Michael Janofsky, "Study Ranks Bush Plan to Cut Air Pollution as Weakest of Three," *New York Times*, CLIII, no. 52876 (June 10, 2004): A16. www.nytimes.com/2004/06/10/politics/10air.html ?ex=1402200000&en=6d3a4a45d1e13015&ei=5007&partner=USERLAND.

52. Arden Pope, "Cardiovascular Mortality and Long-Term Exposure to Particulate Air Pollution," *Circulation* 109, no. 6 (January 2003): 71–77. R. Lall, M. Kendall, K. Ito, and G. Thurston, "Estimation of Historical Annual PM2.5 Exposures for Health Effects Assessment," *Atmospheric Environment* 38, no. 31 (2004): 5217–5226. C. A. Pope, R. T. Burnett, M. J. Thun, E. E. Calle, D. Krewski, K. Ito, and G. D. Thurston, "Lung Cancer, Cardiopulmonary Mortality, and Long-Term Exposure to Fine Particulate Air Pollution," *Journal of the American Medical Association* 287, no. 9 (2002): 1132–41. ABT Associates, *Particulate-Related Health Benefits of Reducing Power Emissions* (Bethesda, Md.: ABT Associates, 2000), is the Bush study. M. L. Bell, D. L. Davis, N. Gouveia, L. Cifuentes, and V. H. Borja-Aburto, "Mortality, Morbidity, and Economic Consequences of Fossil Fuel–Related Air Pollution in Three Latin American Cities," *Epidemiology* 15, no. 4 (July 2004): S44–S45; M. L. Bell and D. I. Davis, "Reassessment of the Lethal London Fog of 1952," *Environmental Health Perspectives* 109, no. 3 (June 2001): 389–394; D. L. Davis, L. Deck, H. Saldiva, and J. Correia, "The Selected Survivor Effect in Developed and Developing Countries Studies of Air Pollution," *Epidemiology* 10, no. 4 (July 1999): S107; L. Cifuentes, V. H. Borja-Aburto, N. Gouveia, G. Thurston, and D. L. Davis, "Assessing the Health Benefits of Urban Air Pollution Reductions Associated with Climate Change Mitigation (2000–2020)," *Environmental Health Perspectives* 109, no. 3 (June 2001): S419–S425; D. L. Davis, T. Kjellstrom, R. Slooff, A. McGartland, D. Atkinson, W. Barbour, W. Hohenstein, P. Nagelhout, T. Woodruff, F. Divita, J. Wilson, and J. Schwartz, "Short-Term Improvements in Public Health from Global-Climate Policies on Fossil-Fuel Combustion," *Lancet* 350, no. 9088 (1997): M. L. Bell, D. L. Davis, and G. Sun, "Analysis of the Health Effects of Severe Air Pollution in Developing Countries," *Epidemiology* 13, no. 4 (July 2002): 298; A. D. Kyle, T. J. Woodruff, A. Buffler, and D. L. Davis, "Use of an Index to Reflect the Aggregate Burden of Long-Term Exposure to Criteria Air Pollutants in the United States," *Environmental Health Perspectives* 110, no. 1 (February 2002): S95–S102; L. Cifuentes, V. H. Borja-Aburto, N. l Gouveia, G. Thurson, and D. L. Davis, "Climate Change: Hidden Health Benefits of Greenhouse Gas Mitigation," *Science* 293, no. 5533 (2001): 1257–59. See also U.S. Congress, *Implementation of the New Air Quality Standards for Particulate Matter and Ozone, S. HRG. 108–502* (Washington, D.C.: US Government Printing Office, 2004).

53. See CDC, *Cancer Health Statistics*; www.cdc.gov/nchs/fastats/cancer.htm; www.cdc.gov/nchs/fastats/heart.htm; all accessed February 19, 2005.

54. Heart statistics are from American Heart Association data at www.americanheart.org/presenter.jhtml?identifier=1200231&division=GMA001 and accessed February 19, 2005. Cancer statistics are from references in notes 19, 23–31, 33–43, 53. Chicago particulate releases are from EPA, *Toxics Release Inventory*; www.scorecard.org/env-releases/county.tcl?fips_county_code=17031 #data_summary and accessed February 19, 2005. Chicago cancer statistics are from Illinois Department of Public Health, *Illinois Cancer Statistics Review* (Springfield, Ill.: Illinois Department of Public Health, 2003), 2–21. The calculations are as follows. If NCI says 10 ug (micrograms) of particulate pollution causes a 0.18 increase in heart deaths, then Chicago's 17 ug average annual particulate pollution causes a (1.7) (0.18) annual increase in heart deaths, which total about 11,500 per year. If x = average annual Chicago heart deaths not from particulate pollution, then (1.7) (0.18) x = average annual deaths from Chicago's average particulates. Therefore $x + (1.7)$ (0.18) $x = 11,500$. This means $x + .306$ $x = 11,500$. This last equation means, in turn, that $1.31\ x = 11,500$, and thus that $x = 11,500/1.31$. But, if so, x (average annual Chicago heart deaths not from particulates) = 8,779. But $11,500 - 8,779 = 2,721$ average annual Chicago heart deaths, just from particulate pollutants.

55. World Health Organization, *Water for Life* (Geneva: WHO, 2005), 4; European Public Health Alliance, *Air, Water Pollution and Health Effects*; accessed June 15, 2006.

56. APHA, *Safe Drinking Water Act*, 7615 (Washington, D.C.: APHA, 1976); www.apha.org/legislative/policy/policysearch/index.cfm?fuseaction=view&id= 817; accessed February 18, 2006. K. P. Cantor, "Drinking Water and Cancer," *Cancer Causes Control* 8, no. 3 (1997): 292–308.

57. Quoted in B. Cohen et al., *Just Add Water: Violations of Federal Health Standards in Tap Water* (Washington, D.C.: Environmental Working Group of the Natural Resources Defense Council, 1996). D. S. Lantagne, "Engineering Inputs to the CDC Safe Water System Program," in *Frontiers of Engineering*, ed. National Research Council (Washington, D.C.: National Academy Press, 2006), p. 45.

58. EPA, *National Water Quality Inventory* (Washington, D.C.: EPA, 1998), ES-3; www.epa.gov/305b/98report/; accessed July 13, 2005.

59. CDC, *Blood Mercury Levels in Young Children and Childbearing-Aged Women* (Washington, D.C.: CDC, 2004), 7; www.cdc.gov/mmwr/preview/mmwr html/mm5343a5.htm. OMB Watch, "One in Five Women Carries Too Much Mercury," *OMB Watch* 7, no. 4 (February 2006); www.ombwatch.org/article/ articleview/3296/1/429; accessed March 10, 2006.

60. EPA, *National Listing of Fish Advisories* (Washington, D.C.: EPA, 2004), 2. Regarding weakened mercury regulations and enforcement, see Bridget Keuhn, "Medical Groups Sue over EPA Mercury Rule," *Journal of the American Medical Association* 294 (2005): 415–416. See Barton Reppert, "States, Congress, Environmental Groups Oppose New EPA Regulation," *Bioscience* 55, no. 6 (2005): 476.

61. R. Wiles et al., *Tap Water Blues* (Washington, D.C.: Environmental Working Group of the Natural Resources Defense Council, 1994), D. B. Baker et al., *Setting the Record Straight* (Washington, D.C.: Environmental Working Group of the Natural Resources Defense Council, 1995).

62. National Research Council, *Pesticides in the Diets of Infants and Children* (Washington, D.C.: National Academy Press, 1993), 228.

63. Environmental Working Group, 2005. U.S. E.P.A. 1990, *National Survey of Pesticides in Drinking Water Wells: Phase I Report.*

64. Wiles et al., *Tap Water Blues*, 2. Lantagne, 2006, p. 45.

65. EPA, *Pesticide Industry Sales and Usage* (Washington, D.C.: EPA, 1997), tables 10, 4. Regarding unnecessary pesticide use and replacement by Integrated Pest Management, see note 63, ch. 4 and David Pimental, et al., "Assessment of Environmental and Economic Impacts of Pesticide Use," in K. Shrader Frechette and L. Westra (eds.), *Technology and Values* (New York: Rowman and Littlefield, 1997), pp. 375–413.

66. A. Habibul, Y. Chen, F. Parvez, L. Zablotska, M. Argos, I. Hussain, H. Momotaj, D. Levy, Z. Cheng, V. Slavkovich, A. van Geen, G. R. Howe and J. H. Granziano, "Arsenic Exposure from Drinking Water and Risk of Premalignant Skin Lesions in Bangladesh: Baseline Results from the Health Effects of Arsenic Longitudinal Study," *American Journal of Epidemiology* 163, no. 12 (2006): 1138–1148. M. Bates et al., "Case-Control Study of Bladder Cancer and Arsenic in Drinking Water," *American Journal of Epidemiology* 141, no. 6 (1995): 523–530. M. Bates et al., "Arsenic Ingestion and Internal Cancers," *American Journal of Epidemiology* 135, no. 5 (March 1992): 462–476. H. Chiou et al., "Incidence of Internal Cancers and Ingested Inorganic Arsenic," *Cancer Research* 55, no. 6 (March 15, 1995): 1296–1300. M. Lai et al., "Ingested Inorganic Arsenic and Prevalence of Diabetes Mellitus," *American Journal of Epidemiology* 139, no. 5 (March 1994): 484–492. R. Engel and A. Smith, "Arsenic in Drinking Water and Mortality from Vascular Disease," *Archives of Environmental Health* 49, no. 5 (September/October 1994): 418–427.

67. A. Smith et al., "Cancer Risks from Arsenic in Drinking Water," *Environmental Health Perspectives* 97 (1992): 259–267. A. H. Smith, P. A. Lopipero, M. N. Bates, and C. M. Steinmaus, "Drinking Water Standards," *Science* 296, no. 5576 (2002): 2145–2146.

68. U.S. Environmental Protection Agency, *M/DBP Stage 2 Federal Advisory Committee DBP Cancer Health Effects Meeting #2 Summary* (Washington, DC: EPA 1999). Available from http://www.epa.gov/safewater/mdbp/st2may99.html and accessed on 24 October 2006. R. Morris et al., "Chlorination, Chlorination By-Products, and Cancer," *American Journal of Public Health* 82, no. 7 (July 1992): 955–963. M. McGeehin et al., "Case-Control Study of Bladder Cancer and Water Disinfection Methods in Colorado," *American Journal of Epidemiology* 138, no. 7 (October 1993): 492–501. K. P. Cantor, C. F. Lynch, M. E. Hildesheim, M. Dosemeci, J. Lubin, M. Alavanja, and G. Craun. "Drinking Water Source and Chlorination Byproducts in Iowa," *American Journal of Epidemiology* 150, no. 6 (1999): 552–560.

69. National Research Council, *Drinking Water and Health* (Washington, D.C.: National Academy Press, 1987). Natural Resources Defense Council, *Trouble on Tap* (Washington, D.C.: Natural Resources Defense Council, 1995).

70. EPA, *Report to the United States Congress on Radon in Drinking Water* (Washington, D.C.: EPA, 1994). EPA, *Understanding Radiation*; www.epa.gov/radiation/understand/health_effects.htm and accessed 22 October 2006.

71. National Research Council, *Health Effects of Exposure to Radon* (Washington, D.C.: National Academy Press, 1994).

72. APHA, *2003 Policy Statements;* www.apha.org/legislative; accessed February 18, 2006.

73. E. Olson and D. Cameron, *The Dirty Little Secret about Our Drinking Water* (Washington, D.C.: Natural Resources Defense Council, 1995). B. A. Cohen et al., *Just Add Water* (Washington, D.C., Environmental Working Group, 1996). Lantagne, 2006, p. 45.

74. P. Payment et al., "A Randomized Trial to Evaluate the Risk of Gastrointestinal Disease," *American Journal of Public Health* 81, no. 6 (June 1991): 703–708. J. M. Colford Jr., T. J. Wade, S. K. Sandhu, C. C. Wright, S. Lee, S. Shaw, K. Fox, S. Burns, A. Benker, M. A. Brookhart, M. van der Laan, and D. A. Levy, "A Randomized, Controlled Trial of In-Home Drinking Water Intervention to Reduce Gastrointestinal Illness," *American Journal of Epidemiology* 161, no. 5 (2005): 472–482.

75. M. LeChevallier et al., "Occurrence of Giardia and Cryptosporidiums in Surface Water Supplies," *Applied and Environmental Microbiology* 57, no. 9 (September 1991): 2610–2616. S. T. Goldstein, D. D. Juranek, O. Ravenholt, A. W. Hightower, D. G. Martin, J. L. Mesnik, S. D. Griffiths, A. J. Bryant, R. R. Reich, and B. L. Herwaldt, "Cryptosporidiosis: An Outbreak Associated with Drinking Water Despite State-of-the-Art Water Treatment," *Annals of Internal Medicine* 124, no. 5 (1996): 459–468.

76. International Bottled Water Association, *Twenty Questions about the Bottled Water Industry* (Alexandria, Va.: International Bottled Water Association, 1990), 1–4; see also Carol Potera, "The Price of Bottled Water," *Environmental Health Perspecttives* 110, no. 2 (February 2002): 76; Meirion R. Evans, C. Donald Ribeiro, and Eoland L. Salmon, "Hazards of Healthy Living: Bottled Water," *Emerging Infectious Diseases* 9, no. 10 (October 2003): 1219–1225; and Erik D. Olson, *Bottled Water: Pure Drink or Pure Hype?* (Washington, D.C.: National Resource Defense Council, 1999); www.nrdc.org/water/drinking/bw/bwinx.asp; accessed April 18, 2006.

77. UNICEF, *State of the World's Children*, 2005 (New York: UNICEF, 2005), and Natural Resources Defense Council, *Our Children at Risk* (Washington, D.C.: Natural Resources Defense Council, 1997).

78. APHA, *2000 Policy Statements*, "The Precautionary Principle and Children's Health"; www.apha.org/legislative/policy/Pols2000_rev.pdf accessed February 18, 2006. This is policy 200011.

79. WHO, *Effects of Air Pollution on Children's Health* (Bonn: WHO, 2005), 144.

80. WHO, *Effects of Air Pollution on Children's Health*, 155.

81. Cancer statistics are from Institute of Medicine, *Making Better Drugs*, 1, 5; also at U.S. National Childhood Cancer Foundation; www.curesearch.org/aboutcc/; accessed July 1, 2005. See U.S. National Research Council, *Offspring* (Washington, D.C.: National Academy Press, 2003), 237, and Institute of Medicine, *Infant Formula* (Washington, D.C.: National Academy Press, 2004).

82. APHA, "Protecting Human Milk from Persistent Toxic Chemical Contaminants," policy statement 2005-5; www.apha.org/legislative/policy/policysearch/index.cfm?fuseaction=view&id=1321; accessed February 19, 2006. Statistics on child-murder (about 1,400 annually) are from Department of Justice, Federal Bureau of Investigation, *Murder* (Washington, D.C.: Federal Bureau of Investigation, 2006), table 2.4; www.fbi.gov/ucr/cius_04/offenses_reported/violent_crime/murder.html; accessed August 18, 2006. Statistics on child abuse offenses

(about 1,100 per year) are from Tennyson Center for Children, *The Reality of Child Abuse and Neglect* (Denver: Tennyson Center, 2006); www.childabuse.org/about%20child%20abuse.html; accessed August 18, 2006.

83. Teresa Olle, *P is for Poison* (San Francisco: Calpirg, 2000), available at http://www.calpirg.org/reports/healthyschools.pdf and accessed December 12, 2006. Memorandum from Ann Katon to Ralph Lightstone, *Simplification of Adverse Effects Information for SB 950 Chemicals* (Sacramento: California Rural Legal Assistance Foundation, March 10, 1995). Natural Resources Defense Council, *Our Children at Risk.*

84. D. J. Ecobichon et al., "Neurotoxic Effects of Pesticides," in *The Effects of Pesticides on Human Health*, ed. S. R. Baker and Chris Wilkinson (Princeton: Princeton Scientific, 1990), 131–199. R. Repetto and S. Baliga, *Pesticides and the Immune System* (Washington, D.C.: World Resources Institute, 1996). J. Barnett and K. Rogers, "Pesticides," in *Immunotoxicity and Immunopharmacology*, ed. J. H. Dean et al. (New York: Raven Press, 1994), 191–213. T. Thomas et al., "Immunologic Effects of Pesticides," in Baker and Wilkinson, *The Effects of Pesticides on Human Health*, 261–295, esp. 266. R. McConnachie and A. C. Zahalsky, "Immunological Consequences of Exposure to Pentachlorophenol," *Archives of Environmental Health* 46 (July/August 1991): 249–253. F. M. Casares and K. J. Mantione, "Pesticides May Be Altering Constitutive Nitric Oxide Release, Thereby Compromising Health," *Medical Science Monitor* 12, no. 10 (2006): RA235–240.

85. U.S. National Research Council, *Pesticides in the Diets of Infants and Children*, 61.

86. J. M. Spyker, and D. L. Avery, "Neurobehavioral Effects of Prenatal Exposure to the Organophosphate Diazinon in Mice," *Journal of Toxicology and Environmental Health* (1977) 989–1002. See also notes 87–101 and J. S. Rotenberg and J. Newmark, "Nerve Agent Attacks on Children: Diagnosis and Management," *Pediatrics* 112, no. 3 (2003): 648–658.

87. L. Fenske et al., "Potential Exposure and Health Risks of Infants Following Indoor Residential Pesticide Applications," *American Journal of Public Health* 80, no. 6 (June 1990): 689–692.

88. X. Ma, P. A. Buffler, R. B. Gunier, G. Dahl, M. T. Smith, K. Reinier, and P. Reynolds, "Critical Windows of Exposure to Household Pesticides and Risk of Childhood Leukemia," *Environmental Health Perspectives* 110, no. 9 (2002): 955–960. R. Lowengart et al., "Childhood Leukemia and Parents' Occupational and Home Exposures," *Journal of the National Cancer Institute* 79, no. 1 (July 1987): 39–46. J. Buckley et al., "Occupational Exposures of Parents of Children with Acute Nonlymphocytic Leukemia," *Cancer Research* 49, no. 14 (1989): 4030–37.

89. E. Gold et al., "Risk Factors for Brain Tumors in Children," *American Journal of Epidemiology* 109, no. 3 (1979): 309–319. J. Leiss and D. Savitz, "Home Pesticide Use and Childhood Cancer," *American Journal of Public Health* 85, no. 2 (February 1995): 249–252. J. Davis et al., "Family Pesticide Use and Childhood Brain Cancer," *Archives of Environmental Contamination and Toxicology* 24, no. 1 (1993): 87–92.

90. E. Holly et al., "Ewing's Bone Sarcoma, Paternal Occupational Exposure, and Other Factors," *American Journal of Epidemiology* 135, no. 2 (1992): 22–129.

91. U.S. National Research Council, *Pesticides in the Diets of Infants and Children.*

92. American Public Health Association, "Poor Air Quality, Pollution Endanger Health of Children: Designing Healthier Communities for Kids," *The Nation's Health* 36, no. 2 (2006). California Air Resources Board, *Study of Children's Activity Patterns* (Sacramento: California Air Resources Board, September 1991), 66a–67. See note 92, and H. Needleman and P. Landrigan, *Raising Children Toxic Free* (New York: Farrar, Strauss, and Giroux, 1994). T. Woodruff, et al., "The Relationship between Selected Causes of Postneonatal Infant Mortality and Particulate Air Pollution in the United States," *Environmental Health Perspectives* 105, no. 6 (June 1997): 608–612. H. Saldiva et al., "Association between Air Pollution and Mortality Due to Respiratory Diseases in Children in São Paulo, Brazil," *Environmental Research* 65, no. 2 (1994): 218–225. M. Bobak, et al., "Air Pollution and Infant Mortality in the Czech Republic," *Lancet* 340, no. 8826 (1992): 1010–14. H. Knobel et al., "Sudden Infant Death Syndrome in Relation to Weather and Optimetrically Measured Air Pollution in Taiwan," *Pediatrics* 96, no. 6 (December 1995): 1106–10. D. L. Davis, *Urban Air Pollution Risks to Children, Environmental Health Indicator* (New York: World Resources Institute, October 1999). M. Lipsett and M. Bates, "The Hazards of Air Pollution to Children," in *Environmental Medicine*, ed. S. Brooks et al., (St. Louis: Mosby, 1995). R. Etzel, "Air Pollution Hazards to Children," *Otolaryngology—Head and Neck Surgery* 114, no. 2 (February 1996): 265–266.

93. U.S. CDC, "Populations at Risk from Air Pollution," *Morbidity and Mortality Weekly Report* 42, no. 16, April 30, 1993. N. Kulkarni, N. Pierse, L. Rushton, and J. Grigg, "Carbon in Airway Macrophages and Lung Function in Children," *New England Journal of Medicine* 355, no. 1 (2006): 21–30.

94. See, for example, Committee of the Environmental and Occupational Health Assembly of the American Thoracic Society, "Health Effects of Outdoor Air Pollution," *American Journal of Respiratory and Critical Care Medicine* 153, no. 1 (1996): 3–50. D. Bates, "The Effects of Air Pollution in Children," *Environmental Health Perspectives* 103, no. 6 (September 1995): 49–54. D. Spektor et al., "Effects of Concentration and Cumulative Exposure of Inhaled Sulfuric Acid on Trachea-Bronchial Particle Clearance in Healthy Humans," *Environmental Health Perspectives* 79, no. 1 (1989): 167–172. M. Lippman, "Health Effects of Ozone," *Journal of Air Pollution Control Associations* 39, no. 5 (1989): 672–695. J. Last, "Effects of Inhaled Acids on Lung Biochemistry," *Environmental Health Perspectives* 79, no. 1 (1989): 115–119. M. Utell and J. Samet, "Air Pollution in the Outdoor Environment," ed. S. Brooks et al., *Environmental Medicine* (St. Louis: Mosby, 1995) 462–469. C. A. Pope et al., "Health Effects of Particulate Air Pollution," *Environmental Health Perspectives* 103, no. 5 (May 1995): 472–448. L. Van Bree et al., "Lung Injury during Acute and Subchronic Exposure and Recovery," *American Review of Respiratory Disorders* 145, no. 4 (April 1992): A93. L. Van Bree, J. A. M. A. Dormans, A. J. F. Boere, P. J. A. Rombout, "Time Study on Development and Repair of Lung Injury Following Ozone Exposure in Rats," *Inhalation Toxicology* 13, no. 8 (2001): 703–718. P. Lioy et al., "Persistence of Peak Flow Decrement in Children Following Ozone Exposures Exceeding the National Ambient Air Quality Standard," *American Journal of Public Health* 81, no. 3 (1985): 350–359. R. Detels et al., "The UCLA Population Studies of CORD," *American Journal of Public Health* 81, no. 3 (1991): 350–359. K. Pinkerton et al., "Exposure to a Simulated 'Ambient' Pattern of Ozone Results in Significant Pulmonary Retention of Asbestos Fibers," *American Review of Respiratory Disease* 137, no. 4 (April 1988):

166. J. Raub et al., "Effects of Low Level Ozone Exposure on Pulmonary Function," *Advances in Modern Environmental Toxicology* 5 (1983): 363. Q. C. He et al., "Effects of Air Pollution on Children's Pulmonary Function," *Archives of Environmental Health* 48, no. 6 (1993): 382–391. G. Hoek and B. Brunekreef, "Acute Effects of a Winter Air Pollution Episode on Pulmonary Function and Respiratory Symptoms of Children," *Archives of Environmental Health* 48 (1993): 328–335. R. Schmitzberger et al., "Effects of Air Pollution on the Respiratory Tract of Children," *Pediatric Pulmonology* 15, no. 2 (1993): 68–74. C. A. Pope, "Respiratory Health and PM 10. Pollution," *American Review of Respiratory Disease* 144, no. 3 (1991): 668–674. M. Raizenne, "Health Effects of Acid Aerosols on North American Children," *Environmental Health Perspectives* 104, no. 5 (May 1996): 506–514. M. Studnicka et al., "Acidic Particles and Lung Function in Children," *American Journal of Respiratory and Critical Care Medicine* 151, no. 2 (1995): 423–430. L. Neas et al., "The Association of Ambient Air Pollution with Twice Daily Peak Expiratory Flow Rate Measurements in Children," *American Journal of Epidemiology* 141, no. 2 (1995): 111–222. L. Neas et al., "Fungus Spores, Air Pollutants, and Other Determinants of Peak Expiratory Flow Rate in Children," *American Journal of Epidemiology* 143, no. 8 (1996): 797–807. G. Hock et al., "Acute Effects of Ambient Ozone on Pulmonary Function of Children," *American Review of Respiratory Disease* 147, no. 1 (1993): 111–117. See also National Resources Defense Council and the Coalition for Clean Air, *No Breathing in the Aisles: Diesel Exhaust Inside School Buses* (Washington, DC: NRDC 2001). Available from http://www.nrdc.org/air/trans portation/schoolbus/schoolbus.pdf and accessed 29 October 2006.

95. M. Weitzman et al., "Recent Trends in the Prevalence and Severity of Childhood Asthma," *Journal of the American Medical Association*, 268, no. 19 (1992): 2673–77. E. Friebele, et al., "The Attack of Asthma," *Environmental Health Perspectives* 104, no. 1 (January 1996): 22–25. K. Weiss et al., "An Economic Evaluation of Asthma in the United States," *New England Journal of Medicine* 326, no. 13 (1992): 862–866. CDC, "Asthma Mortality and Hospitalization among Children and Young Adults—United States, 1980–1993," *Morbidity and Morality Weekly Report* 45, no. 17, May 3, 1996. George D. Thurston et al., "Summertime Haze Air Pollution and Children with Asthma," *American Journal of Respiratory and Critical Care Medicine* 155, no. 2 (February 1997): 654–660. M. White et al., "Exacerbations of Childhood Asthma and Ozone Pollution in Atlanta," *Environmental Research* 65, no. 1 (1994): 56–68. I. Romieu et al., "Effects of Air Pollution on the Respiratory Health of Asthmatic Children Living in Mexico City," *American Journal of Respiratory and Critical Care Medicine* 154, no. 2 (1996): 300–307. For the rule, proposed by the White House OMB in place of the Clean Air Scientific Advisory Committee recommendation, see www.epa.gov/air'particles'pdfs/anpr20060203.pdf (accessed February 20, 2006). For the state of California EPA comments, see Dr. Bart Ostro, "Comments for CASAC Meeting," www.epa.gov/sab/pdf/casac_pmrp_02-03-06_pub _statement_ostro_cal_epaoehha.pdf and accessed February 20, 2006. See also U.S. Senator Dianne Feinstein, "Feinstein Urges RPA to Adopt Toughter Air Quality Standards"; http://feinstein.senate.gov/06releases/r-epa-air0201.htm and accessed February 20, 2006.

96. European Public Health Alliance, *Air, Water Pollution and Health Effects*.

97. For U.S. ozone statistics, see note 51, The Economist. WHO, *Effects of Air Pollution on Children's Health*, 20, 23. See note 45 for APHA air-pollution

recommendations. American Lung Association, *Danger Zones* (Washington, D.C.: American Lung Association, 1995). U.S. CDC, "Asthma Mortality and Hospitalization." Ozone data are in preceding notes.

98. APHA, "The Precautionary Principle and Children's Health," and Environmental Defense Fund, *Legacy of Lead* (Washington, D.C.: Environmental Defense Fund, March 1990). U.S. Bureau of Mines, *Mineral Commodity Summaries* (Washington, D.C.: U.S. Department of the Interior, 1989), 90–91. (1988 data converted from metric tons to short tons; 1 metric ton equals about 2,200 pounds, while a U.S., or short, ton equals 2,000 pounds.) U.S. Department of the Interior, *US Geological Survey: Mineral Commodity Summaries, 2005* (Washington, DC: US Government Printing Office, 2005) pp. 94–95. Available from http://minerals.usgs.gov/minerals/pubs/mcs/2005/mcs2005.pdf and accessed 27 October, 2006.

99. U.S. National Research Council, *Measuring Lead Exposure in Infants, Children* (Washington, D.C.: National Academy Press, 1993), 187.

100. EPA, *Fact Sheet, National Primary Drinking Water Regulations for Lead and Copper* (Washington, D.C.: EPA, May 1991). U.S. Government Accountability Office, *Drinking Water: Safeguarding the District of Columbia's Supplies and Applying Lessons Learned to Other Systems (GAO-05-974T)* (Washington, DC: US Government Printing, 2004). Available from http://www.gao.gov/new.items/d04974t.pdf and accessed 27 October 2006.

101. U.S. Environmental Protection Agency, *America's Children and the Environment: Lead in the Blood of Children* (Washington, D.C.: U.S. EPA, 2006), available at www.epa.gov/envirhealth/children/body_burdens/b1.htm and accessed December 12, 2006. R. Stapleton, *Lead Is a Silent Hazard* (New York: Walker, 1994); "Is There Lead in Your Water?" *Consumer Reports* (February 1993): 73–82.

102. Regarding North American doses 300 times higher, see U.S. National Research Council, *Measuring Lead Exposure in Infants, Children* (Washington, D.C.: National Academy Press, 1993), 24. Agency for Toxic Substances and Disease Registry, *The Nature and Extent of Lead Poisoning in Children in the United States* (Washington, D.C.: U.S. Department of Health and Human Services, Public Health Service, 1988). J. L. Pirkle et al., "The Decline in Blood Lead Levels in the United States: The National Health and Nutrition Examination Surveys" (NHANES II, 1976 to 1980, and NHANES III, 1988 to 1991), *Journal of the American Medical Association* 272, no. 4 (1994): 284–291. U.S. CDC, *Preventing Lead Poisoning in Young Children* (Atlanta: CDC, 1991). D. Brody, "Blood Lead Levels in the U.S. Population," *Journal of the American Medical Association* 272, no. 4 (1994): 277–283. H. Needleman et al., "Low-Level Lead Exposure and the IQ of Children," *Journal of the American Medical Association* 263, no. 5 (1990): 673–678. H. Needleman et al., "Bone Lead Levels and Delinquent Behavior," *Journal of the American Medical Association* 275, no. 5 (1996): 363–369. J. Schwartz et al., "Relationship between Childhood Blood-Lead Levels and Stature," *Pediatrics* 77, no. 3 (1986): 281–288. J. Schwartz and D. Otto, "Blood Lead, Hearing Thresholds, and Neurobehavioral Development in Children and Youth," *Archives of Environmental Health* 42, no. 3 (1987): 153–160. R. Shukla et al., "Fetal and Infant Lead Exposure," *Pediatrics* 84, no. 4 (1989): 604–612. U.S. ATSDR, Toxicological Profile for Lead, 1992. A. Bhattacharya et al., "Postural Disequilibrium Quantification in Children with Chronic Lead Exposure," *Neurotoxicology* 9, no. 3 (1988): 327–340. P. Mushak et al.,

"Prenatal and Postnatal Effects of Low-Level Lead Exposure," *Environmental Research* 50, no. 1 (1989): 11–36. P. Baghurst et al., "Exposure to Environmental Lead and Visual-Motor Integration at Age Seven Years," *Epidemiology* 6, no. 2 (March 1995): 104–109. W. Sciarillo et al., "Lead Exposure and Child Behavior," *American Journal of Public Health* 82, no. 10 (October 1992): 1356–60.

103. American Academy of Pediatrics, Committee on Environmental Health, "Ambient Air Pollution: Respiratory Hazards to Children," *Pediatrics* 91, no. 6 (1993): 1210–13.

104. F. Perera, *Progress Report to the Colette Chuda Environmental Fund for the Molecular Epidemiological Study of Effects of Environmental Pollution on Women and the Developing Fetus* (New York: School of Public Health, Columbia University, 1994). J. H. Leem, B. M. Kaplan, Y. K. Shim, H. R. Pohl, C. A. Gotway, S. M. Bullard, J. F. Rogers, M. M. Smith, and C. A. Tylenda, "Exposures to Air Pollutants during Pregnancy and Preterm Delivery," *Environmental Health Perspectives* 114, no. 6 (2006): 906–910.

105. A. Pope, "Respiratory Hospital Admissions Associated with PM10 Pollution in Utah, Salt Lake, and Cache Valleys," *Archives of Environmental Health* 46 (1991): 90–97.

106. See note 105, and D. V. Bates and R. Sizto, "Hospital Admissions and Air Pollutants," *Environmental Research* 43, no. 2 (1987): 317–331. R. T. Burnett et al., "Effects of Low Ambient Levels of Ozone and Sulfates on the Frequency of Respiratory Admissions," *Environmental Research* 65, no. 2 (1994): 172–194. G. D. Thurston et al., "Respiratory Hospital Admissions and Summertime Haze Air Pollution," *Environmental Research* 65, no. 2 (1994): 271–290. C. Braun-Fahrlander et al., "Air Pollution and Respiratory Symptoms in Preschool Children," *American Review of Respiratory Disease* 145, no. 1 (1992): 42–47. J. Jaakkola et al., "Low Level Air Pollution and Upper Respiratory Infections in Children," *American Journal of Public Health* 81, no. 8 (August 1991): 1060–1063. E. von Mutius et al., "Air Pollution and Upper Respiratory Symptoms in Children," *European Respiratory Journal* 8, no. 5 (1995): 723–728. J. H. Ware et al., "Effects of Ambient Sulfur Oxides and Suspended Particles on Respiratory Health of Preadolescent Children," *American Review of Respiratory Disease* 133, no. 5 (1986): 834–842. D. Dockery et al., "Effects of Inhalable Particles on Respiratory Health of Children," *American Review of Respiratory Disease* 139, no. 3 (1989): 587–594. J. Schwartz et al., "Acute Effects of Summer Air Pollution on Respiratory Symptom Reporting in Children," *American Journal of Respiratory and Critical Care Medicine* 150, no. 5 (1994): 1234–42. EPA, Exhausted by Diesel: How America's Dependence on Diesel Engines Threatens Our Health (Washington, DC: EPA 1998). Available from http://www.nrdc.org/air/transportation/ebd/ebdinx.asp and accessed 28 October, 2006.

107. D. Bates, "Observations on Asthma," *Environmental Health Perspectives* 103, Suppl. 6 (September 1995): 243–252. White et al., "Exacerbations of Childhood Asthma and Ozone Pollution in Atlanta," *Environmental Research* 65, no. 5 (1994): 56–68. J. Schwartz et al., "An Association between Air Pollution and Mortality in Six U.S. Cities," *New England Journal of of Medicine* 329, no. 24 (1993): 1753–59. J. M. Samet, F. Dominici, F. C. Curriero, I. Coursac, S. L. Zeger, "Fine Particulate Air Pollution and Mortality in 20 US Cities, 1987–1994," *New England Journal of Medicine* 343, no. 24 (2000): 1742–1749.

108. L. Plunkett et al., "Differences between Adults and Children Affecting Exposure Assessment," in *Similarities and Differences between Children and*

Adults, ed. P. Guzelian (Washington, D.C.: International Life Sciences Institute, 1992).

109. EPA, *Fact Sheet, National Primary Drinking Water Regulations for Lead and Copper,* 3; *Fed. Reg.* 26, 470, June 7, 1991. See M. Shannon and J. Graef, "Lead Intoxication in Infancy," *Pediatrics* 89, no. 1 (January 1992): 87–90. M. Shannon and J. Graef, "Hazards of Lead in Infant Formula," *New England Journal of Medicine* 326, no. 9 (1992): 137.

110. WHO, *Water for Life.*

111. APHA Precautionary Principle (note 78). See also APHA, *Priority 2005 Issues: Fact Sheets, Health Disparities, Environmental Disparities, Racial/Ethnic Disparities,* 2005, 28–34; www.apha.org/legislative/legislative/index.htm; accessed February 19, 2006.Occupational fatalities are given in APHA, *Strengthening Worker/Community Right to Know*; www.apha.org/legislative/policy/policysearch/index.cfm?fuseaction=view&id=1143, and accessed March 16, 2006. APHA, *Increasing Worker and Community Awareness of Toxic Hazards in the Workplace*; www.apha.org/legislative/policy/policysearch/index.cfm? fuseaction=view&id=1078 and accessed March 16, 2006.

112. U.S. Census Bureau, *Low-Income Uninsured Children by State, 2003;* www.census.gov/hhes/hlthins/liuc03.html; accessed July 12, 2005.

113. See, for example, Shrader-Frechette, *Environmental Justice.* R. Calderon et al., "Health Risks from Contaminated Water," *Toxicology and Industrial Health* 9, no. 5 (September/October 1993): 879–900. Robert Bullard (ed.), *Unequal Protection* (San Francisco: Sierra Club Books, 1994). Bunyan Bryant (ed.), *Environmental Justice* (Washington, D.C.: Island Press, 1995). See note 116.

114. See earlier notes.

115. Environmental Defense Fund, *Scorecard* [Tabulation of industry reports to the US Environmental Protection Agency, Toxics Release Inventory data]; www.scorecard.org/community/ej-summary.tcl?fips_county_code=18089 #dist; accessed July 1, 2005.

116. Jack Griffith, R. C. Duncan, W. B. Riggan, and A. C. Pefforn, "Cancer Mortality in U.S. Counties with Hazardous Waste Sites and Ground Water Pollution," *Archives of Environmental Health* 44, no. 2 (1989): 69–74. P. Stretesky and M. J. Hogan, "Environmental Justice: An Analysis of Superfund Sites in Florida," *Social Problems* 45, no. 2 (1998): 268–287.

117. Quoted in Stuart Auerbach, "N.J.'s Chemical Belt Takes Its Toll: $4 Billion Industry Tied to Nation's Highest Cancer Death Rate," *Washington Post* 99, no. 65, February 8, 1976, A1. See also U.S. CDC, *2001 Incidence and Mortality Data, National Program of Cancer Registries, States. National* (Atlanta: CDC, 2001), 58–59; http://apps.nccd.cdc.gov/uscs/Table.aspx?Group=5f&Year=2002 &Display=n; accessed July 1, 2005. Cohen, "Waste Dumps Toxic Traps for Minorities," *The Chicago Reporter* April 1992, Available from http://www.chicago reporter.com/1992/04-92/0492WasteDumpsToxicTrapsforMinorities.htm and accessed 28 October 2006.

118. APHA, *Priority 2005 Issues: Fact Sheets, Health Disparities,* 26, 28, 34.

119. B. Goldman and L. Fitton, *Toxic Wastes and Race Revisited* (Washington D.C.: Center for Policy Alternatives, 1994). H. L. White, "Race, Class, and Environmental Hazards" in *Environmental Injustices, Political Struggles: Race Class and the Environment,* D. E. Camacho ed. (Durham, NC: Duke University Press, 1998).

120. Paul Farmer, *Pathologies of Power* (Berkeley: University of California Press, 2005). Air-pollution statistics are in D. R. Wennette and L. A. Nieves, "Breathing Polluted Air," *EPA Journal* 18, no. 1, March/April 1992, 16–17, and notes 44–46, 79–80, 92–97, 137. For European statistics, see European Public Health Alliance, *Air, Water Pollution and Health Effects*. Friends of the Earth, *Briefing: Incinerators and Deprivation* (London: Friends of the Earth 2004). Available from http://www.foe.co.uk/resource/briefings/incineration_deprivation .pdf and accessed 28 October 2006.

121. APHA, *Priority 2005 Issues: Fact Sheets, Health Disparities,* and M. White et al., "Exacerbations of Childhood Asthma and Ozone Pollution in Atlanta," *Environmental Reseach*, 65, no. 1 (1994): 56–68. M. Weitzman et al., "Racial, Social and Environmental Risks for Childhood Asthma," *American Journal of Diseases of Children* 144, no. 11 (November 1990): 1189–94. J. Schwartz et al., "Predictions of Asthma and Persistent Wheeze," *American Review of Respiratory Disease* 142, no. 3 (1990): 555–562. J. Cunningham et al., "Race, Asthma and Persistent Wheeze in Philadelphia School Children," *American Journal of Public Health* 86, no. 10 (October 1996): 1406–09. U.S. CDC, "Asthma Mortality and Hospitalization among Children and Young Adults," *Morbidity and Mortality Weekly Report,* May 3, 1996. R. S. Gupta, V. Carrion-Carire, and K. B. Weiss, "The Widening Black/White Gap in Asthma Hospitalizations and Mortality," *Journal of Allergy and Clinical Immunology* 117, no. 2 (2006): 351–358.

122. APHA, *Priority 2005 Issues: Fact Sheets, Health Disparities,* and D. Brody et al., "Blood Lead Levels in the U.S. Population: Phase 1 of the Third National Health and Nutrition Examination Survey (NHANES III, 1988 to 1991)," *Journal of the American Medical Association* 272, no. 4 (July 27, 1994): 277–283. See H. Needleman and D. Bellinger, "The Health Effects of Low-Level Exposure to Lead," *Annual Review of Public Health* 12 (1991): 111–140. U.S. CDC, "Update: Blood Lead Levels—United States, 1991–1994," *Morbidity and Mortality Weekly Report,* 46, no. 7 February 21, 1997. U.S. CDC, "Surveillance for Elevated Blood Lead Levels Among Children—United States, 1997–2001," *Morbidity and Mortality Weekly Report* 52, no. SS10 (September 12, 2003): 1–21, available from http://www.cdc.gov/MMWR/preview/mmwrhtml/ss5210a1.htm and accessed 28 October 2006.

123. Bruce Kennedy et al., "Income Distribution and Mortality," *British Medical Journal* 312, no. 7037 (1996): 1004–7. George A. Kaplan et al., "Inequality and Income and Mortality in the United States," *British Medical Journal* 312, no. 7037 (1996): 999–1003. See APHA, *Priority 2005 Issues: Fact Sheets, Health Disparities.* W. C. Holton, "Rich Map, Poor Map," *Environmental Health Perspectives* 112, no. 3 (2004): 176–179.

124. APHA, *Priority 2005 Issues: Fact Sheets, Health Disparities,* and Michael Wolff, Peter Rutten, Albert Bayers, and the World Bank Research Team, *Where We Stand* (New York: Bantam, 1992), 23, and U.S. Census Bureau, *Low-Income Uninsured Children by State, 2003;* Kevin Phillips, *Wealth and Democracy* (New York: Broadway, 2002), 151–155. Kevin Phillips, "The Progressive Interview," *The Progressive* 66, no. 9 (September 2002): 37 of 33–37; Lawrence Mishel, Jared Bernstein, and John Schmitt, *The State of Working America* (Ithaca, N.Y.: Economic Policy Institute, Cornell University Press, 2001). See also Thomas Piketty and Emmanuel Saez, *Income Inequality in the United States, 1913–1998,* working

paper no. W8467 (Washington, D.C.: National Bureau of Economic Research, September 2001).

125. Death rates of 1- to 15-year-olds are in Wolff et al., *Where We Stand,* 15–116. For infant-mortality data, see APHA, *Priority 2005 Issues: Fact Sheets, Health Disparities* 33, and U.S. Central Intelligence Agency, *The World Factbook* (Washington, D.C.: Central Intelligence Agency, 2004); www.cia.gov/cia/publications/factbook/rankorder2091rank.htm; accessed January 21, 2005. U.S. CDC, *Infant Mortality Fact Sheet* (Washington, D.C.: CDC, 2005); www.cdc.gov/omh/AMH/factsheets/infant.htm; accessed January 21, 2005. Wolff et al., *Where We Stand,* 112–113. Nicholas D. Kristof, "Health Care? Ask Cuba," *New York Times* CLIV, No. 53, 092, January 12, 2005), A23; nytimes.com/2005/01/12/opinion/12kris.htm?hp and accessed January 21, 2005.

126. S. L. Syme, and Berkman, "Social Class, Susceptibility, and Sickness," *American Journal of Epidemiology* 104, no. 1 (July 1976): 1–4; see also earlier notes; U.S. Institute of Medicine (notes 18, 27, 99, 102, 111, 127), and APHA, *Priority 2005 Issues: Fact Sheets, Health Disparities,* 34.

127. Note 111, and U.S. Institute of Medicine, *Hidden Costs, Value Lost* (Washington, D.C.: National Academy Press, 2003); U.S. Institute of Medicine, *Guidance for the National Healthcare Disparties Report* (Washington, D.C.: National Academy Press, 2002). U.S. Institute of Medicine, *A Shared Destiny* (Washington, D.C.: National Academy Press, 2003); U.S. Institute of Medicine, *The Unequal Burden of Cancer* (Washington, D.C.: National Academy Press, 1999). U.S. Institute of Medicine, *Unequal Treatment* (Washington, D.C.: National Academy Press, 2002). See also Melissa Marino, "Racial Disparity in Colorectal Cancer Deaths" (Nashville: Vanderbilt Medical Center, April 16, 2004). L. A. G. Ries, et al., *SEER Cancer Statistics Review, 1973–1991: Tables and Graphs,* NIH publ. no. 94–2789 (Bethesda, Md.: NCI, 1994), V. L. Freeman, Ramon Durazo-Arvizu, La Shon Keys, Marc Johnson, and Kristian Schofernak, "Racial Differences in Survival among Men with Prostate Cancer," *American Journal of Public Health* 94, no. 5 (May 2004): 803–809. Adam Wagstaff, Flavia Bustreo, Jennifer Bryce, and Marian Claeson, "Child Health," *American Journal of Public Health* 94, no. 5 (May 2004): 726–737. R. M. Campanelli, "Addressing Racial and Ethnic Health Disparities," *American Journal of Public Health* 93, no. 10 (October 2003): 1624–27. S. A. Ibrahim, S. B. Thomas, and M. J. Fine, "Archieving Heath Equity," *American Journal of Public Health* 93, no. 10 (October 2003): 1619–22. D. Mail, S. Lachenmayr, M. E. Auld, and K. Roe, "Eliminating Health Disparities," *American Journal of Public Health* 94, no. 4 (April 2004): 519–520; APHA, *Priority 2005 Issues: Fact Sheets, Health Disparities* 34.

128. For an overview of global public health, see Garrett, *Betrayal of Trust.* Poverty statistics in this paragraph are from Thomas Pogge, *World Poverty and Human Rights* (Cambridge, England: Polity, 2002). For other examples, see Shrader-Frechette, *Environmental Justice,* 163–184.

129. For the APHA statement on how flawed trade agreements harm health, see APHA policy statement 2001–21, Threats to Global Health and Equity: The General Agreement on Trade in Services (GATS) and the Free Trade Area of the Americas (FTAA), in APHA, "Policy Statements, 2001," *American Journal of Public Health* 92, no. 3 (March 2002): 472–474 of 451–483; www.apha.org/legislative/policy/2001/; accessed February 19, 2006.

130. As former US president Richard Nixon put it, the main purpose of American aid has been not to help other nations but to help ourselves. Of monies appropriated for direct, bilateral, U.S. assistance, 70 percent is spent in the United States, not overseas. United States laws require 90 percent of all military and food aid, plus half of all bilateral development assistance, to be spent on U.S. goods and services. As a result, U.S. foreign aid is mainly a subsidy for U.S. businesses—sometimes, U.S. polluters seeking to put dangerous and substandard facilities abroad. Rather than promoting life-saving medical and public-health projects, more than three-quarters of U.S. foreign-aid economic loans have gone to pay debt service on old loans, usually to U.S. or multinational banks. Half of all U.S. foreign aid is to U.S. military contractors, and 88 percent of all U.S. military aid, plus 36 percent of all U.S. foreign aid, goes to only two nations, Israel and Egypt. Partly as a result, Africa's total debt now exceeds the annual value of all its products. During 1980–90, when the United States cut bilateral aid to Africa by more than a third, more than 3.5 million Africans died of hunger. Patrick M. Regan, "U.S. Economic Aid and Political Repression," *Political Research Quarterly* 48, no. 3 (September 1995): 613–628. Michael E. O'Hanlon, *Enhancing U.S. Security through Foreign Aid* Darby, PA: Diane, 1994. John McCain, "A World Safe for the U.S.," *Freedom Review* 26, no. 3 (May 1995): 12. Ian Vasquez, "U.S. Aid," *Human Events* 51, no. 16 (1995): 18–20. N. M. Khilji and E. M. Zampelli, "The Fungibility of U.S. Military and Non-military Assistance and the Impacts on Expenditures of Major Aid Recipients," *Journal of Development Economics* 43, no. 2 (April 1994): 345–362. Sheila Kaplan, "Porkbarrel Politics at U.S. AID," *Multinational Monitor* 14, no. 9 (September 1993): 10–15. See also Peter H. Koehn and Olatunde J. B. Ojo (eds.), *Making Aid Work* (Lanham, Md.: University Press of America, 1999). WHO pesticide statistics are from J. T. Mathews et al., *World Resources 1986* (New York: Basic Books, 1986), 48–49; R. Repetto, *Paying the Price* (Washington, D.C.: World Resources Institute, 1985); 3, and John Leslie, *The End of the World* (New York: Routledge, 1998). See also notes 131 and 132. Regarding clinical trials, see National Bioethics Advisory Commission, *Ethical and Policy Issues in International Research: Clinical Trials in Developing Countries*, vols. 1 and 2 (Bethesda, Md.: National Bioethics Advisory Commission, 2001); Marcia Angell, "The Ethics of Clinical Research in the Third World," *New England Journal of Medicine* 337, no. 337 (1997): 847–849; H. Varmus and D. Satcher, "Ethical Complexities of Conducting Research in Developing Countries," *New England Journal of Medicine* 337, no. 337 (1997): 1003–5; Hepeng Jia, "China Beckons to Clinical Trial Sponsors," *Nature Biotechnology* 23, no. 768 (June 30, 2005); www.nature.com/nbt/journal/v23/n7/full/nbt0705–768.html; accessed Feburary 17, 2006; Susan Bull, *Ethics of Research* (London: Science and Development Network, 2002); www.scidev.net/dossiers/index.cfm?fuseaction=dossierItem &Dossier=5; accessed February 17, 2006. See also WHO, *International Clinical Trials Registry Newsletter* 1, no. 1 (November 2005); www.who.int/ictrp/news/ICTRP_Newsletter_November_2005_No1.pdf; accessed February 17, 2006; U.S. National Research Council, *Intentional Human Dosing Studies* (Washington, D.C.: National Academy Press, 2004). F. R. Wolf, "Helping Enhance the Livelihood of People (HELP) Around the Globe Commission Act," Introduction of the HELP Commission Act to become Public Law, October 9, 2003. Available from http://helpcommission.gov/Mission/tabid/53/Default.aspx and accessed 29 October 2006.

131. Barbara Briggs, David Cook, Jack McKay, and Charles Kernaghan, *Paying to Lose Our Jobs* (New York: National Labor Committee, 1992), 17–18; www.nlcnet.org/campaigns/archive/haiti/Haiticoup.shtml; accessed March 10, 2006. National Labor Committee data were confirmed by US GAO, *Foreign Assistance: AID's Private Sector Assistance Program at a Crossroads*, GAO/NSAID-93-55 (Washington, D.C.: Government Printing Office, 1993), 2, 27. Maquiladora and Carribean wage statistics are from Ellen Rosen, *Making Sweatshops* (Berkeley: University of California Press, 2002), 150–176, esp. 155, 167; quotation is from 151. Studies showing less safe working conditions, lower pages, worker coercion, and sweatshop conditions abroad, respectively, are in US GAO, *Foreign Assistance: AID's Private Sector Assistance Program at a Crossroads*, and Rosen, *Making Sweatshops*, 238; 53, 241, 246; 241; and 129–152, 242–246. For resulting U.S. job losses, lower U.S. wages, but U.S. consumer savings, see 225–235 and note 132. See also United Nations Commission on Human Rights, "Forced Labour and Exploitation of Indonesian Migrant Workers," *Sub-Commission on the Promotion and Protection of Human Rights Working Group on Contemporary Forms of Slavery* 28th Session, Geneva, (June 16–20, 2003); http://www.antislavery.org/archive/submission/submission2003-indonesia.htm and accessed on 29 October 2006.

132. See chapter 6, and Robert Watson, "U.S. Aid to the Third World," *Journal of Third World Studies* 11, no. 2 (fall 1994): 202–239. M. Bhattacharya, "USAID," *Economic and Political Weekly* 29, no. 37 (1994): 2401. Andrew Cohen, "The Help That Hurts," *Progressive* 58, no. 1 (January 1994): 27. Joseph R. Biden Jr., "The Environment and World Trade," *Environmental Law* 23, no. 2 (1993): 687–696; for criticisms of the World Bank, International Monetary Fund, OPIC, NAFTA, and WTO, see Rosen, *Making Sweatshops*, 5, 8, 19–22, 132–135, 149–176.

133. APHA, *America's Health Rankings*, 17, 86, 98, 103; see earlier statistics.

134. APHA, *America's Health Rankings*, 18. Nicholas Freudenberg, "Time for a National Agenda to Improve the Health of Urban Populations," *American Journal of Public Health* 90, no. 6 (June 2000): 837–840.

135. Economist, *Pocket World 2007*, 102–105.

136. US EPA, *Toxics Release Inventory*; wwws.epa.gov/tri/; and Juliet Eilperin, "Toxic Emissions Rising, EPA Says," *Washington Post,* June 23, 2004, A-2; www.washingtonpost.com/wp-dyn/articles/A61795-2004Jun22.html; both accessed February 16, 2006.

137. U.S. EPA, Office of Inspector General, *EPA's Method for Calculating Air Toxics Emissions for Reporting Results Needs Improvement*, 2004-P-00012 (Washington, D.C.: EPA, 2004); GAO, *Air Pollution: EPA Should Improve Oversight of Emissions Reporting*, GAO-01-46 (Washington, D.C.: EPA, 2001); U.S. House of Representatives, Committee on Government Reform, *Oil Refineries Fail to Report Millions of Pounds of Harmful Emissions* (Washington, D.C.: U.S. Congress, 1999); Environmental Integrity Project and Galveston-Houston Association for Smog Prevention, *Who's Counting? The Systematic Underreporting of Toxic Air Emissions* (Washington, D.C.: Environmental Integrity Project, 2004).

138. EPA, Toxics Release Inventory *Data Release* (May 11, 2005), 2; www.epa.gov/tri/tridata/tri03/index.htm; accessed February 16, 2006.

139. See notes 136–138, and Environmental Working Group, *Strengthening the TRI* (Washington, D.C.: Environmental Working Group, 2006); www.ewg

.org/reports/cheminventory/execsumm.php?print_version=1; accessed February 16, 2006.

140. APHA, *Priority 2005 Issues: Fact Sheets, Health Disparities* 28.

141. For variants of this argument, see chapter 3, and R. Doll and R. Peto, "The Causes of Cancer," *Journal of the National Cancer Institute* 66, no. 6 (1981): 1191–1308. However, Doll and Peto excluded the data on many of the highest-cancer-risk subgroups, e.g., blacks. See R. Clapp and M. Lefevre, Environmental and Occupational Causes of Cancer (University of Massachusetts: Lowell Center for Sustainable Production, 2005); www.sustainableproduction.org/downloads/causes%20of%20cancer.pdf and accessed 28 October, 2006.

142. APHA, *Priority 2005 Issues: Fact Sheets, Health Disparities*; www.apha .org/legislative/policy/2005/; accessed February 19, 2006.

143. See note 42.

144. The Economist, *Pocket World 2007*, 80, 86. WHO, *World Health Report 2004, Statistical Annex* (Geneva: WHO, 2004), 132–135, 144–147; www .who.int/shr/2004; accessed July 20, 2005.

145. Frances Rosenbluth and Michael Thies, "The Political Economy of Japanese Pollution Regulation," paper presented at the 1999 American Political Science Association meetings, available from Rosenbluth at Yale University and at www.yale.edu/leitner/pdf/199–01/pdf; accessed June 20, 2006. See Jeffrey Broadbent, *Environmental Politics in Japan* (Cambridge: Cambridge University Press, 1998), and note 146.

146. The Economist, *Pocket World 2007*, 75. Wolff et al., *Where We Stand*, 6, and U.S. Energy Information Agency, *Japan: Environmental Issue* (Washington, D.C.: DOE, 2004); www.eia.doe.gov/emeu/cabs/japanenv.html; accessed August 15, 2006.

147. John Robbins, *The Food Revolution* (Boston: Conari, 2001), 366.

148. WHO, *World Health Report 2004*, 132–135, 144–147; at www.who .int/shr/2004; accessed July 12, 2005.

149. U.S. CDC, *The State of the CDC, Fiscal Year 2003*, 4.

150. Susmita Dasgupta, Hua Wanf, and David Wheeler, *Is Stricter Regulation Worthwhile?* (New York: World Bank, 1997); www.worldbank.org/nipr/work_paper/survive/china-htmp6.htm; accessed July 13, 2005. Hemamala Hettige, Muthukumara Mani, and David Wheeler, *Industrial Pollution in Economic Development* (New York: World Bank, 1997); www.worldbank.org/nipr/work_paper/kuznet/kuznetsp5.htm#11; accessed July 13, 2005. U.S. CDC 2005 report on asthma is L.Y. Ward et al., "Direct and Indirect Costs of Asthma in School-Age Children"; www.cdc.gov/pcd/issues/2005/jan/04_0053.htm and accessed 29 October, 2006.

151. Harvard Law School, "Harvard Study Finds Medical Bills Push Many into Bankruptcy" (Cambridge, Mass.: Harvard Law School, February 3, 2005); www.law.harvard.edu/news/2005/02/03_bankruptcy.php.

152. Wendell Berry, *A Continuous Harmony* (Emeryville, Calif.: Shoemaker and Hoard, 1972), 79.

Chapter 2

1. Janet Raloff, "Silkwood: The Legal Fallout," *Science News*, 125 no. 5 (February 4, 1984): 74–75, 79; Howard Kohn, *Who Killed Karen Silkwood?* (New York: Summit Books, 1981), 29, 126–127, 141, 357, 359, 372; and

Richard Rashke, *The Killing of Karen Silkwood* (Boston: Houghton Mifflin, 1981), 78–80, 91–98, 380. See also Joyce Hannam, *The Death of Karen Silkwood* (Oxford: Oxford University Press, 2000), and Ronald Hardert, "Harassment of Nuclear Scientists, Nuclear Plant Workers and Grassroots Anti-nuclear Activists," *International Journal of Humanities and Peace* 17, no. 1 (2001): 80. A. Bale, "The American Compensation Phenomenon," *International Journal of Health Services* 20, no. 2 (1990): 253–275.

2. See note 1.

3. Jeffrey Stein, "Karen Silkwood: The Deepening Mystery," *Progressive* 45, no. 1 (January 1981): 14–21; Rashke, *The Killing*, 5; see also Richard L. Rashke, *The Killing of Karen Silkwood* (Ithaca, N.Y.: Cornell University Press, 2000).

4. Hans Baer, "Kerr-McGee and the NRC," *Social Science and Medicine* 30, no. 2 (1990): 239–240; see also 237–248.

5. See the beginning of chapter 3, note 8 here, and, for example, U.S. Office of Human Radiation Experiments, *Report of the Advisory Committee on Human Radiation Experiments* (Washington, D.C.: US Government Printing Office, 1994); http://ris.eh.doe.gov.ohre/roadmap/achre/; accessed June 15, 2005. U.S. Congress, *American Nuclear Guinea Pigs* (Washington, D.C.: U.S. Government Printing Office, 1986); U.S. Congress, *Government Liability for Atomic Weapons Testing Program* (Washington, D.C.: U.S. Government Printing Office, 1987); U.S. Congress, *The Radiation Protection Act of 1991* (Washington, D.C.: U.S. Government Printing Office, 1992).

6. For discussion of nuclear history, the AEC, the Brookhaven Report, and the Price-Anderson Act, see Kristin Shrader-Frechette, *Nuclear Power and Public Policy* (Boston: Kluwer, 1983), 1–24, 73–109, and Kristin Shrader-Frechette, *Environmental Justice: Creating Equality, Reclaiming Democracy* (New York: Oxford University Press, 2002), 152–162. C. Folkers, "Price-Anderson Act," *Nuclear Information and Resource Services*, October 2001; www.nirs.org/factsheets/priceandpersonactfactsheet1001.htm and accessed 29 October, 2006.

7. Chernobyl cost and mortality statistics are from Shrader-Frechette, *Environmental Justice*, 40, 85–88, 112, 188–191, 201, and UN Development Programme and the UN Childrens Fund, *The Human Consequences of the Chernobyl Nuclear Accident* (New York: UN, January 25, 2002), 63; UN General Assembly, *Report of the Secretary, Optimizing the International Effort to Study, Mitigate and Minimize the Consequences of the Chernobyl Disaster* (New York: UN, October 8, 2001). These documents say Chernobyl damages in Belarus are between $235 and $260 billion, and in Ukraine, $148 billion. Because contamination spread all over the world, because Russian Chernobyl costs are close to those of Belarus and Ukraine, and since half of all Chernobyl-related deaths will occur outside the former USSR, Chernobyl costs likely will be over $500 billion. Hurricane Katrina costs are from John D. Mckinnon et al., "First Estimates on Katrina Costs for Washington Hit $200 Billion," *Wall Street Journal* 246, no. 47 (September 7, 2005): A1–A4. Hurricane Katrina mortality data are from Genevieve Roberts, "Final Katrina Death Toll Put at 972 as Search Is Called Off," *Independent (London)*, October 5, 2005, 29.

8. See preceding notes and U.S. Congress, *Worker Safety at DOE Nuclear Facilities* (Washington, D.C.: US Government Printing Office, 1999). U.S. Congress, *Worker Safety at DOE Nuclear Sites* (Washington, D.C.: US Government Printing Office, 1994). US General Accounting Office (GAO), *DOE: DOE's Nuclear Safety Program Should Be Strengthened* (Washington, D.C.: US

Government Printing Office, 1999). US GAO, *DOE: Clear Strategy on External Regulation Needed* (Washington, D.C.: US Government Printing Office, 1998). US Office of Technology Assessment (OTA), *Complex Cleanup* (Washington, D.C.: U.S. Government Printing Office, 1991). The one-in-five lifetime-core-melt probability for all U.S. reactors is from U.S. Nuclear Regulatory Commission, *Reactor Safety Study*, WASH 1400 (Washington: U.S. Nuclear Regulatory Commission, 1975), 175ff. Shrader-Frechette, *Nuclear Power and Public Policy*, 73–109, shows why the American Physical Society criticizes the U.S. Nuclear Regulatory Commission estimates as too low.

9. See note 8, and Frederick Upton, U.S. Rep., Michigan, in U.S. Congress, *Worker Safety at DOE Nuclear Facilities*, 98–99.

10. John Dingell, in U.S. Congress, *Worker Safety at DOE Nuclear Sites*, 159.

11. U.S. GAO, *DOE: Clear Strategy*, 4. G. Sawyer, *Report of the State of Nevada Commission on Nuclear Projects* (Carson City: Commission on Nuclear Projects, 1988), 8–9, 13.

12. James Wells, in U.S. Congress, *Worker Safety at DOE Nuclear Sites*, 15–22, 25.

13. U.S. Congress, *Worker Safety at DOE Nuclear Facilities*; U.S. Congress, *Worker Safety at DOE Nuclear Sites*.

14. Gary Jones, in U.S. Congress, *Worker Safety at DOE Nuclear Facilities*, 5, 43–49.

15. U.S. GAO, *DOE: Clear Strategy*, 3; John Dingell, "Testimony," in U.S. Congress, *Worker Safety at DOE Nuclear Sites*, James Well, US GAO, in U.S. Congress, *Worker Safety at DOE Nuclear Sites*, 3–15; and Tara O'Toole, in U.S. Congress, *Worker Safety at DOE Nuclear Sites*, 70. U.S. OTA, *Complex Cleanup*, 8, 77, 80, 84, 99–100, 111, 138–143.

16. Quotations are from "The Nuclear Answer?" *Economist.com*, July 7, 2005; available only at www.economist.com/opinion/displayStory.cfm?story_id =4151435; accessed July 23, 2005. MIT study is E. Moniz and J. Deutsch, *The Future of Nuclear Power* (Cambridge, Mass.: MIT Laboratory for Energy and the Environment, 2003). Friends of the Earth, *Why Nuclear Power Is Not An Achievable and Safe Answer to Climate Change* (London: FOE, 2005).

17. See, for instance, U. R. Fritsche, *Comparing Greenhouse-Gas Emissions and Abatement Costs of Nuclear and Alternative Energy Options* (Berlin: Institute for Applied Ecology, 1997). Data showing that a majority of scientists claim that nuclear energy will not help global warming are from Sheldon Rampton and John Stauber, *Trust Us, We're Experts!* (New York: Penguin, 2002), 311.

18. "The Nuclear Answer?" Economist. For statistics on nuclear, solar, and all other costs of electricity, see U.S. DOE and U.S. EPA data in G. T. Miller, *Living in the Environment* (New York: Brooks/Cole, 2000), 392. For the falsification of 1998–2000 Yucca data, see Naomi Lubick, "Falsification Alleged at Yucca Mountain," *Geotimes* 50, no. 5 (Alexandria, Va.: American Geological Institute, 2005); www.geotimes.org/may05/NN_YuccaFraud.html; accessed July 23, 2005. For Chernobyl statistics, see note 7.

19. U.S. National Research Council, *Building Consensus through Risk Assessment and Management* (Washington, D.C.: National Academy Press, 1994). See also R. E. Dunlap, M. E. Kraft, and E. A. Rosa (eds.), *Public Relations to Nuclear Waste* (Durham, N.C.: Duke University Press, 1993); D. A. Bella, C. D. Mosher, and S. N. Calvo, "Establishing Trust: Nuclear Waste Disposal," *Journal of Professional Issues in Engineering* 114, no. 1 (1988): 40–50. See prior notes

for Congress, GAO, and OTA claims. U.S. Board on Life Sciences, National Research Council, *Reopening Public Facilities After a Biological Attack* (Washington D.C.: National Academy Press, 2005).

20. See notes 5, 21–24, and Public Law 97–144.

21. U.S. NCI, *Estimated Exposures and Thyroid Doses Received by the American People from Iodine-131 in Fallout Following Nevada Atmospheric Nuclear Bomb Tests*, NIH publication 97-4264 (Washington, D.C.: U.S. NIH, 1997).

22. U.S. Institute of Medicine. *Exposure of the American People to Iodine 131 from Nevada Nuclear-Bomb Tests* (Washington, D.C.: National Academy Press, 1998). D. Rush and J. Geiger, "NCI Study on I-131 Exposure from Nuclear Testing," *Physicians for Social Responsibility* 4, no. 3 (Winter 1997–98): 1–5.

23. Institute of Medicine, *Exposure of the American People to Iodine 131*, 42; NCI, *Estimated Exposures and Thyroid Doses Received by the American People from Iodine-131*, 8.5–8.31; U.S. Advisory Committee on Energy-Related Epidemiologic Research (ACERER) Report in U.S. *Centers for Disease Control* (CDC), *Feasibility of Determining the Health Consequences of Nuclear Weapons Testing* (Washington, D.C.: CDC, 2006); www.cdc.gov/search.do?action =search&queryText=acerer and accessed December 12, 2006. U.S. Congress, *National Cancer Institute's Management of Radiation Studies* (Washington, D.C.: Government Printing Office, 1998). For fallout cancer estimates, see Steven Simon, Andre Bouville, and Charles Land, "Fallout from Nuclear Weapons Tests and Cancer Risks," *American Scientist* 94, no. 801 (January/February 2005): 48–57. For citizen loss of trust in government handling of fallout exposures, see F. Owen Hoffman, A. Iulian Apostoaei, and Brian Thomas, "A Perspective on Public Concerns about Exposure to Fallout from the Production and Testing and Nuclear Weapons," *Health Physics* 82, no. 5 (2002): 736–748.

24. V. Kiernan, "Radiation Doctors Abused Trust," *New Scientist* 148, no. 1999 (1995): 8. R. Faden, Chair, Advisory Committee on Human Radiation Experiments, *Final Report*, 1995; www.eh.doe.gov/ohre/roadmap/achre/report .html and accessed December 12, 2006.

25. Jerome Kassirer, *On the Take* (New York: Oxford University Press, 2005), 155, 165; Marcia Angell, *The Truth about the Drug Companies* (New York: Random House, 2005), 69–72.

26. Angell, *The Truth about the Drug Companies*, ix, xii–xiv, xv, 219; see also 37–93, 206–210. See Susan Ehringhaus and David Korn, "Conflicts of Interest in Human Subjects Research," *Issues in Science and Technology* 19, no. 2 (2002): 79–82, and the US National Academy of Sciences discussion on conflicts of interest; www.nationalacademies.org/coi/bi-coi_form-0.pdf; accessed October 26, 2005. Also see Kassirer, *On the Take*, 50–62, 164–169.

27. Kassirer, *On the Take*, 157–159; see 160–167. Quotation is from 165. See the next section of the chapter for a definition of conflicts of interest.

28. For coverage of the U.S. Food and Drug Administration (FDA) study and predicted deaths from Vioxx, see APHA, "2005 APHA Award for Excellence"; www.apha.org/sections/awards/06_awards/winner_apha.htm; accessed March 13, 2006; Emma Marris, "Suppressed Study Raises Spectre of Flawed Drug Regulation in U.S.," *Nature* 432, no. 537 (December 2004): 537–538; and Angell, *The Truth about the Drug Companies*, 265–276. See also Snigda Prakash, "Did Merck Try to Censor Vioxx Critics?" National Public Radio, June 9, 2005; www.npr.org/ templates/story/story.php?storyId=4696711 [and 4696609]; accessed July 23, 2005.

29. Gardiner Harris and Alex Berenson, "Ten Voters on Panel Backing Pain Pills Had Industry Ties," *New York Times* CLV, no. 53, 137 (February 25, 2005): A1; for information on federal advisory panels, see Sheldon Krimsky, *Science in the Private Interest* (Savage, Md.: Rowman and Littlefield, 2003), 91–106. Regarding problems in the drug industry, see Angell, *The Truth about the Drug Companies*; Merrill Goozner, *The $800-Million Pill* (Berkeley: University of California Press, 2004); and Katharine Greider, *The Big Fix* (New York: Public Affairs, 2003).

30. Krimsky, *Science in the Private Interest*, 95–97; Robert Musil, "Political Science on Federal Advisory Panels," *Physicians for Social Responsibility Reports* 924, no. 25 (2003): 3. See subsequent notes and, for instance, J. C. Grubman, "Science and the Bush Administration," *Science* 307, no. 5709 (January 2005): 519; C. Hadley, "Science Policy in the USA; Bush Administration May Have Caused Long-Term Damage, Scientists Fear," *Embo Reports* 5, no. 10 (October 2004): 932–935; A. C. Revkin, "Bush vs. the Laureates," *New York Times* CLIV, no. 53,007 (October 19, 2004): F1. D. Baltimore, "Science and the Bush Administration," *Science* 305, no. 5692 (September 2004): 1873; A. Lawler and J. Kaiser, "Report Accuses Bush Administration, Again, of 'Politicizing' Science," *Science* 305, no. 5688 (August 2004): 1240; D. Wilkie, "Bush and Science at Loggerheads," *Scientist* 18, no. 15 (August 2004): 50–51; "Bush 'Science,' " *New Scientist* 183, no. 2456 (July 2004): 4; G. Markowitz and D. Rosner, "Politicizing Science," *Journal of Public Health Policy* 24, no. 2 (2003): 105–129; J. Dawson and P. Guinnessy, "Bush Administration Accused of Misusing Science," *Physics Today* 57, no. 4 (April 2004): 30–31; W. Sweet, "Bush Administration's 'Science' Is under Fire," *IEEE Spectrum* 41, no. 4 (April 2004): 12–13; J. Block, "Science Gets Sacked," *International Journal of Health Services* 34, no. 1 (2004): 177–179; M. McKee and T. E. Novotny, "Political Interference in American Science," *European Journal of Public Health* 13, no. 4 (December 2003): 289–291; E. Check, "Bush Accused of Power Abuse over Science," *Nature* 424, no. 6950 (August 2003): 715; J. Glanz, "At the Center of the Storm over Bush and Science," *New York Times* CLIII, no. 52,804 (March 2004): F1.

31. Philip Hilts, *Protecting America's Health* (New York: Knopf, 2003), 295, 314, 322.

32. See, for instance, Geoff Brumfiel, "U.S. Science Policy: Mission Impossible?" *Nature* 428, no. 9 (2004): 250 of 250–251. The 6,000-plus scientists' statement is called "Restoring Scientific Integrity in Policymaking," available on the website of the Union of Concerned Scientists; www.ucsusa.org/global_environment/rsi/page.cfm?pageID=1320; accessed July 23, 2005. See also U.S. Congress, House of Representatives, *Politics and Science in the Bush Administration* (Washington, D.C.: U.S. Government Printing Office, 2003). For Bush administration responses to these criticisms, see John H. Marburger, "On Scientific Integrity in the Bush Administration," April 2, 2004, available from the U.S. Office of Science and Technology Policy; www.ostp.gov/htm/ucs/ResonsetoCongressonUCSDocument April2004.pdf; accessed March 13, 2006.

33. C. Moore, "Rethinking the Think Tanks," *Sierra* 87, no. 4 (2002): 58.

34. Sharon Beder, *Global Spin* (Glasgow: Green Books, 2002), 118–199, 267ff. U.S. Congress, House of Representatives, *Politics and Science in the Bush Administration.* E. Shaeffer, "Power Plants and Public Health," *Physicians for Social Responsibility Reports* 34 (2002): 3. Musil, "Political Science on Federal Advisory Panels," 3.

35. For conflicts of interest, see Kassirer, *On the Take*, 50–62; previous 10 notes; and U.S. Congress, House of Representatives, *Politics and Science in the Bush Administration*. Shaeffer, "Power Plants and Public Health." Musil, "Political Science on Federal Advisory Panels."

36. *Economist*, "The Uncorrupt," *Economist* 373, no. 8398 (October 23–29, 2004), 106.

37. U.S. Congress, Committee on Government Operations, *The Agent Orange Coverup* (Washington, D.C.: U.S. Government Printing Office, 1990); see also U.S. GAO, *Agent Orange* (Washington, D.C.: U.S. Government Printing Office, 1999); APHA, "Recognizing and Addressing the Environmental and Occupational Health Problems Posed by Chlorinated Organic Chemicals," resolution 9304, January 1, 1993; www.apha.org/legislative/policy/policysearch/index .cfm?fuseaction=view&id=88; and APHA, "Prevention of Dioxin Generation," resolution 9607, 1996; www.apha.org/legislative/policy/policysearch/index.cfm ?fuseaction=view&id=125; both accessed March 13, 2006. U.S. National Research Council, *Veterans and Agent Orange* (Washington, D.C.: National Academy Press, 2001, 2003); U.S. National Research Council, *Hormonally Active Agents in the Environment* (Washington, D.C.: National Academy Press, 1999); U.S. National Research Council, *Dioxins and Dioxin-Like Compounds in the Food Supply* (Washington, D.C.: National Academy Press, 2003); American Medical Association, *The Health Effects of Agent Orange* (Chicago: American Medical Association, 1994); Michael Gough, *Agent Orange, Dioxin* (New York: Plenum, 1986); U.S. Congress, *Agent Orange Studies* (Washington, D.C.: U.S. Government Printing Office, 1986); J. Bailar, "How Dangerous Is Dioxin?" *New England Journal of Medicine* 324, no. 4 (1991): 260–262. M. Fingerhut, W. Halperin, and D. Marlow, "Cancer Mortality in Workers Exposed to 2,3,7, 8-tetrochlorodibenzo-p-dioxin," *New England Journal of Medicine* 324, no. 4 (1991): 212–218. M. DeVito, L. Birnbaum et al., "Comparisons of Estimated Body Burdens of Dioxinlike Chemicals," *Environmental Health Perspectives* 103, no. 9 (1995): 827. International Joint Commission, *Sixth Biennial Report on Great Lakes Water Quality* (Ottawa and Washington, D.C.: International Joint Commission, 1992); Paul Ehrlich and Anne Ehrlich, *Betrayal of Science and Reason* (Washington, D.C.: Island Press, 1996), 167–170. Beder, *Global Spin*, 141–146. See also Lois Gibbs and Stephen Lester, *Dying from Dioxin* (Boston: South End Press, 1995). Devra Davis, *When Smoke Ran Like Water* (New York: Basic Books, 2002), 178. For dioxin debates, see Rampton and Stauber, *Trust Us, We're Experts*, 135–141. For U.S. EPA coverup, see *Jenkins v. U.S. Environmental Protection Agency*, 92-CAA-6, *American Law Journal* (December 14, 1992); www.whistleblowers.org/ 92caa06a.htm; accessed March 13, 2006; and *Tozzi v. U.S. Environmental Protection Agency*, Civ. No. 00–0173, Ruling Case Law, June 29, 2001; www.thecre .com/regbylit/20010702_paperwork.html; accessed March 13, 2006.

38. Richard T. DeGeorge, "Ethics and Automobile Technology," in *Technology and Values*, ed. Kristin Shrader-Frechette and Laura Westra (Lanham, Md.: Rowman and Littlefield, 1997), 279–294. OMB Watch, "Is Cost-Benefit Analysis Needed?" *The Watcher: OMB Watcher* 6, no. 6 (2005): 18–21.

39. Quoted in Beder, *Global Spin* 143; see 141–146. Jeff Johnson, "Dioxin Risk," *Environmental Science and Technology* 29, no. 1 (1995): 24A–25A. David Lapp, "Defenders of Dioxin," *Multinational Monitor* 12, no. 10 (October 1991): 8–12. Jeff Bailey, "Dueling Studies," *Wall Street Journal* CCXIX, no. 35 (February 20, 1992): 1, A4. Leslie Roberts, "Dioxin Risks Revisited," *Science* 251,

no. 4994 (February 8, 1991): 624–626, and "Flap Erupts over Dioxin," *Science* 251, no. 4996 (February 22, 1991): 866–867. U.S. National Research Council, *Health Risks from Dioxin and Related Compounds* (Washington, D.C.: National Academies Press, 2006).

40. For those who deny obvious harm from breast implants, despite some manufacturer information suppression, see U.S. Institute of Medicine, *Safety of Silicone Breast Implants* (Washington, D.C.: National Academy Press, 2000), and Marcia Angell, *Science on Trial* (New York: Norton, 1996). For information about these alleged cases of information suppression and crime, see Beder, *Global Spin*, 141–160, 213–220; Samuel Epstein, Nicholas Ashford, Brent Blackwelder, Barry Castleman, Gary Cohen, Edward Goldsmith, Anthony Mazzocchi, and Quentin Young, "The Crisis in U.S. and International Cancer Policy," *International Journal of Health Services* 32, no. 4 (2002): 669–707; Samuel Epstein, *Cancer-Gate* (Amityville, N.Y.: Baywood, 2005), 106–109,175; Rampton and Stauber, *Trust Us, We're Experts*, esp. 164–168.

41. Alex Berenson, "At Vioxx Trial, a Discrepancy Appears to Undercut Merck's Defense," *New York Times*, CLIV, no. 53, 281 (July 20, 2005): C1, C9. For other Vioxx information, see note 28.

42. See, for instance, Barry Meier, "Faulty Heart Devices Force Some Scary Decisions," *New York Times* CLIV, no. 53, 251 (Monday June 20, 2005): A1, A12; and Stacy Horn, "Counting Corporate Crooks," *New York Times CLIV, no. 53, 276* (July 16, 2005): A27.

43. Krimsky, *Science in the Private Interest*, 41–47.

44. For the Olivieri case, see Krimsky, *Science in the Private Interest*, 45–47, and Kassirer, *On the Take*, 59–60.

45. P. A. Rochon, J. H. Gurwitz, R. W. Simms, P. R. Fortin, D. T. Felson, K. L. Minaker, and T. C. Chalmers, "A Study of Manufacturer-Supported Trials of Nonsteroidal Anti-inflammatory Drugs in the Treatment of Arthritis," *Archives of Internal Medicine* 154, no. 2 (1994): 157–163. Natural Resources Defense Council, "Science Under Attack," August 15, 2005; www.nrdc.org/health/science/ijscience.asp and accessed 29 October 2006.

46. E. G. Campbell, K. S. Louis, and D. Blumenthal, "Looking a Gift Horse in the Mouth," *Journal of the American Medical Association* 279, no. 13 (1998): 995–999. Regarding Brown University see David G. Kern, "The Unexpected Result of an Investigation of an Outbreak of Occupational Lung Disease," *International Journal of Occupational Environmental Health* 4, no. 1 (1998): 19–32; David G. Kern et al., "Flock Workers' Lung," *Annals of Internal Medicine* 129, no. 4 (15 August 1998): 261–272; and Donna R. Euben, "Corporate Interference in Research," *Academe* 86, no. 6 (2000). Regarding corporate-sponsored research showing 98 percent success, see Mildred K. Cho and Lisa A. Bero, "The Quality of Drug Studies Published in Symposium Proceedings," *Annals of Internal Medicine* 124, no. 5 (1 March 1996): 485–489. Finally see Sheldon Krimsky and L. S. Rothenberg, "Financial Interest and Its Disclosure in Scientific Publications," *Journal of the American Medical Association* 280, no. 3 (1998): 225–226. For *Journal of the American Medical Association* data, see Eval Press and Jennifer Washburn, "The Kept University," pt. 2, *Atlantic Monthly* (March 2000); www.theatlantic.com/issues/2000/03/ press2.htm and accessed February 10, 2005. See also Rampton and Stauber, *Trust Us, We're Experts*, 216–217; Catherine DeAngelis et al.; J. Kassirer, "Financial Conflict of Interest," *American Journal of Law and Medicine* 27, no. 2 (2001): 149–162.

238   NOTES TO PAGES 55–60

47. Beder, *Global Spin,* 63–74. Monsanto SLAPP is covered at 143, and in text earlier. Persecution of Needleman, Amdur, Molina, and Byers is in Davis, *When Smoke Ran Like Water,* 273–276. Winfrey case is in Rampton and Stauber, *Trust Us, We're Experts,* 260.

48. For Nestlé information, see World Health Organization (WHO), *Feeding Infants and Young Children* (Geneva: WHO-UNICEF, 1979) and APHA, "Nestle Boycott," policy 8126, 1-1-1981; www.apha.org/legislative/policy/policysearch/index.cfm?fuseaction=view&id=998; accessed March 13, 2006. See also note 47. Information on the Nader SLAPP is in Charles McCarrey, *Citizen Nader* (New York: Saturday Review Press, 1972), 28, 44, 196. The MDB case is in Rampton and Stauber, *Trust Us, We're Experts,* 131–135; Nestlé quotations are from 131, and Davis and Puztai material is from pp. 142–143 and 152–163. M. Carter, "Mongoven, Briscoe, and Duchin: Destroying Tobacco Control Activism from the Inside," *Tobacco Control* 11, no. 2 (2002): 112–118.

49. Joel Brinkley, "Out of Spotlight, Bush Overhauls U.S. Regulations," *New York Times,* CLII, no. 52,941 (August 14, 2004): A1, A10. Regarding the proposed change in the Toxics Release Inventory, see U.S. EPA, "EPA Proposed Burden Reduction Rule for the Toxics Release Inventory," September 21, 2005; http://yosemite.epa.gov/opa/admpress.nsf/d9bf8d9315e942578525701c005e573c/ed5dcfbbd6f58e7e852570830048f830!OpenDocument. For APHA criticism of alleged "paperwork reduction," as justification for weakening public health and environmental protections, see APHA, "OMB Abuse of the Paperwork Reduction Act," policy 8716; www.apha.org/legislative/policy/policysearch/index.cfm?fuseaction=view&id=1145; all accessed March 13, 2006.

50. See note 49 and Rampton and Stauber, *Trust Us, We're Experts,* 84, for occupational-death statistics from the 1997 *Archives of Internal Medicine.* See chapter 1, esp. note 33, for journal citations on occupational health.

51. Regarding consent, see R. R. Faden and T. L. Beauchamp, *A History and Theory of Informed Consent* (New York: Oxford University Press, 1987), and T. L. Beauchamp and J. L. Childress, *Principles of Biomedical Ethics* (New York: Oxford University Press, 1994). See also Kristin Shrader-Frechette, *Risk and Rationality* (Berkeley: University of California Press, 1991), 72–73, 86–87, 153–156, 206–214, and Shrader-Frechette, *Environmental Justice,* 17–20, 73–83, 105–113, 121–133, 164–175. For genetically-engineered-food statistic, see Rampton and Stauber, *Trust Us, We're Experts,* 170, also 169–189.

52. Vanessa Blum, "Blackballing the Blacklist," *Corporate Counsel* 8, no. 10 (October 2001): 115–116. See Douglas A. Schuler, Kathleen Rehbein, and Roxy Cramer, "Pursuing Strategic Advantage through Political Means," *Academy of Management Journal* 45, no. 4 (2002): 659–672.

53. See note 54.

54. Quoted in Epstein, *Cancer-Gate,* 106, including second quotation from Ralph Nader.

55. Beder, *Global Spin,* 222. Don Hazen, "Who Owns the Media and How It Works," in *Spin Works,* ed. Robert Bray (San Francisco: Independent Media Institute, 2002), 7.

56. Mark Crispin Miller, "Free the Media," in *We the Media,* ed. Don Hazen and Julie Winokur (New York: Norton, 1997), 5 of 4–5. Free Press, "Who Owns the Media? (2005); http://freepress.net/ownership/chart.php?chart-cable and accessed 28 betaken 2006.

57. Don Hazen, "Defining the Paradox," in Hazen and Winokur, *We the Media*, 27 of 27–28. E. Joyce, "Three Movie Studios Hit with Lawsuit," *Ecommerce* (September 24, 2002); www.internetnews.com/ec-news/article.php/1469311 and accessed 28 October 2006.

58. Hazen, 28. See note 60.

59. Martin Lee and Norman Solomon, *Unreliable Sources* (New York: Carol, 1990), 77–81. Jim Naureckas, "Corporate Ownership Matters," *Extra!* 18, no. 6 (November/December 1995): 13. See note 59, and Beder, *Global Spin*, 195–212. For Westinghouse and General Electric nuclear-contractor monies, see U.S. Congress, 1999 (note 8), and US GAO, *DOE: DOE's Nuclear Safety Program Should Be Strengthened*; Shrader-Frechette, *Environmental Justice*, 152–161. Fairness and Accuracy in Reporting, "Some Critical Media Voices Face Censorship," *Extra* 16, no. 6 (April 3, 2003).

60. Marc Gunther, "All in the Family," *American Journalism Review* 21, no. 11 (October 1995): 40. Richard Stapleton, "Green vs. Green," *National Parks* 66, no. 6 (November/December 1992): 34. Kate O'Callahan, "Whose Agenda for America?" *Audubon* 94, no. 5 (September/October 1992): 86. Erwin Knoll, "Conflict of Interest?" *Progressive* 57, no. 3 (1993): 4. Karl Grossman, "Three Mile Island," *Extra!* 6, no. 4 (July/August 1993): 6. Todd Putnam, "The GE Boycott," *Extra!* 4, no. 1 (January/February 1991): 4–5. FAIR, "GE Irrelevancies," *Extra!* (January/February 1991): 4. Lee and Solomon, *Unreliable Sources*, 78. Beder, *Global Spin*, 134–136, 224–225. For media problems generally, see Beder, 195–213 and note 58 above. In February 2006, Toshiba of Japan bought Westinghouse from Viacom (the TV-syndication division of CBS that bought its parent CBS in 2000), although global Westinghouse headquarters remains in Pittsburgh; see Toshiba Corporation, "Toshiba Acquires Westinghouse from BNFL"; www .toshiba.co.jp/about/press/2006_02/pr0601.htm; accessed March 13, 2006. When Viacom bought CBS, it was thereby controlling both 35 percent of the TV market (the largest television group in the country, with the CBS network and stations in 18 of the top 20 markets in the United States) and Paramount Pictures, one of the top four U.S. film studios, as well as Simon & Schuster, a major U.S. publishing house; Blockbuster, the top video rental outlet; cable channels like MTV, Nickelodeon, the Nashville Network, and Showtime; a majority interest in Infinity Broadcasting Corporation, the nation's largest radio and outdoor advertising company; popular internet sites like marketwatch.com; and five parks. FAIR, "Action Alert: The Viacom-CBS Merger," September 10, 1999; www.fair.org/ activism/cbs-viacom-alert.html; accessed May 1, 2006. J. Hollar et al., "Fear and Favor 2005, Influence on the News," *Extra!* 19, no. 2 (March April, 2006).

61. Hazen, "Defining the Paradox," 8.

62. Beder, *Global Spin*, 161.

63. Donald Collins, "Dictating Content," in Hazen and Winokur, *We the Media*, 57. Beder, *Global Spin*, 180–182.

64. Kim Deterline, "How to Detect and Fight Bias in News Media," in Bray, *Spin Works*, 88–90. Beder, *Global Spin*, 198, 209; see 191–212.

65. Makani Themba, "Holding the CEOs Accountable," in Hazen and Winokur, *We the Media*, 89–90. *New England Journal of Medicine* quotation is from Stacey Eidson, "We've Come a Long Way, Baby?" in Hazen and Winokur, *We the Media*, 93. For information on the powerful tobacco industry and its lobbyists and PR see Rampton and Stauber, *Trust Us, We're Experts*, 229–247.

The APHA recommendations for curbs on advertising include, for instance, APHA, "Encourage Health Behavior by Adolescents," policy statement 200027; www.apha.org/legislative/policy/policysearch/index.cfm?fuseaction=view&id=234; "Regulation of Tobacco Products," policy 9412; www.apha.org/legislative/policy/policysearch/index.cfm?fuseaction=view&id=78 both accessed May 1, 2006.

66. Dan Bischoff, "Corporate Money Dominates Issue Advertising," *St. Louis Journalism Review* 26, no. 188 (July/August 1996): 11–12. Rhoda Karpatkin and Anita Holmes, "Making Schools Ad-Free Zones," *Educational Leadership* 53, no. 1 (1995): 72–76. James Fallows, *Breaking the News* (New York: Pantheon, 1995). Michael Jacobson and Laurie Mazur, *Marketing Madness* (Boulder: Westview, 1995), 23–54. James Twitchell, "But First, a Word from Our Sponsor," *Wilson Quarterly* 20, no. 3 (1996): 68–77. Lee and Solomon, *Unreliable Sources,* 67–85. Tom Riley, *The Price of Life* (Bethesda, Md.: Adler and Adler, 1986). Alecia Swasy, *Soap Opera* (New York: Random House, 1993). Joyce Nelson, *Sultans of Sleaze* (Toronto: Between the Lines, 1989). Prakash Sethi, *Advocacy Advertising* (Lexington, Mass.: Lexington, 1977). Beder, *Global Spin,* 166–172, 186–194. A. Wohl, "The School Marketplace," *American Education* 25, no. 3 (Fall 2001): 16–21, 46.

67. Quotation is from Beder, *Global Spin,* 164. Roy Fox, "Manipulated Kids," *Educational Leadership* 53, no. 1 (1995): 77–79. Amy Aidman, *Advertising in Schools* (Carbondale: University of Illinois, ERIC Clearinghouse on Early Childhood and Elementary Education, 1995). Beder, *Global Spin,* 164–165, 188. Sethi, *Advocacy Advertising.* For discussion of the ethics of vulnerability, and the ethics of benevolence, see Joseph Butler, *Fifteen Sermons* (London: Bell, 1953); J. S. Mill, *Utilitarianism* (Indianapolis: Hackett, 1979); Nel Noddings, *Caring* (Berkeley: University of California Press, 1984); T. A. Roberts, "The Concept of Benevolence," *Social Philosophy and Policy* 4, no. 2 (1987); Richard Taylor, *Good and Evil* (London: MacMillan, 1970). See note 66 and M. Dittmann, "Protecting Children from Advertising," *Monitor on Psychology* 35, no. 6 (2004): 58.

68. All quotations are from Don Hazen and Julie Winokur, "Scary but True," in Hazen and Winokur, *We the Media,* 73. See Rampton and Stauber, *Trust Us, We're Experts,* 22–24.

69. Paul Krugman, *The Great Unraveling* (New York: Norton, 2003), 280, 384. Other PR labels are from Rampton and Stauber, *Trust Us, We're Experts,* 55.

70. Greenhouse and air-pollution information are from Krugman, *The Great Unraveling,* 336–337, 342–343. For the educational-plan information, see Sam Dillon, "Connecticut to Sue the U.S., Saying 'Left Behind' Law Leaves State in Debt," *New York Times* CLIV, no. 53,176, April 6, 2005, A21. For the distinction between the demands of law and the demands of ethics, see David Lyons, *Ethics and the Rule of Law* (Cambridge: Cambridge University Press, 1984), and Joel Feinberg and Hyman Gross (eds.), *Philosophy of Law* (Belmont, Calif.: Wadsworth, 1986). See also Alan Goldman, *Moral Foundations of Professional Ethics* (Totowa, N.J.: Rowman and Allanheld, 1980); David Luban, *Lawyers and Justice* (Princeton: Princeton University Press, 1988); Gerald Postema, "Moral Responsibility in Professional Ethics," *New York University Law Review* 55 (1980): 63–89, Jeffrie Murphy and Jules Coleman, *The Philosophy of Law* (Boulder, Colo.: Westview, 1990).

71. See note 70. For propaganda labels, see Rampton and Stauber, *Trust Us, We're Experts*, 291–297.

72. Danielle Nierenberg, "U.S. Environmental Policy," *World Watch* 14, no. 4 (2001): 12–21. See Ariana Huffington, "What Are They Thinking in Washington?" *Sierra* 87, no. 5 (2002): 41–42.

73. GAO, *Media Contracts*, GAO-6-305 (Washington, D.C.: U.S. Government Printing Office, 2006). Quotation is from Robert Pear, "Buying of News by Bush's Aides Is Ruled Illegal," *New York Times*, CLV, no. 53,354 (October 1, 2005): front page A1.

74. Beder, *Global Spin*, 107–111, 269–270; Rampton and Stauber, *Trust Us, We're Experts*, 13, 102–104, 112–119; quotations are from 117, 103.

75. Christopher Plant and Judith Plant, *Green Business* (Devon, England: Green Books, 1991). Joseph LaCovey, "Business Changes Its Ways," *Public Relations Journal* 47, no. 4 (April 1991): 23. Douglas Kellner, *Television and the Crisis of American Democracy* (Boulder, Colo.: Westview, 1990). Alan Durning, *How Much Is Enough?* (London: Earthscan, 1992), 125. Quotations are from Beder, *Global Spin*, 178–179; see also 129–130, 180, 228–229, and Rampton and Stauber, *Trust Us, We're Experts*, 46–49. S. Beder, "Environmentalists Help Manage Corporate Reputations," *Ecopolitics* 1, no. 4 (2002): 60–72.

76. Beder, *Global Spin*, 34–35, 40–41, 102.

77. "The Clean-Air Wars," *New York Times*, CLIV, no. 53,282 (July 21, 2005): A26.

78. For Three-Mile-Island cancers, see Steve Wing, David Richardson, Donna Armstrong, and Douglas Crawford-Brown, "A Reevaluation of Cancer Incidence Near the Three-Mile-Island Nuclear Plant," *Environmental Health Perspectives* 105, no. 1 (January 1997): 138–143. For the Health Tracking Act, see Nancy Pelosi, *National Health Tracking Act* (Washington, D.C.: U.S. House, 2002); www.house.gov/pelosi/prNationwideHealthTrackingAct.HTM and accessed May 1, 2006. Regarding avoiding epidemiological studies of weapons testing, see Kristin Shrader-Frechette, *Burying Uncertainty* (Berkeley: University of California Press, 1993), 26, 155. For "statistical casualties," deaths not traceable individually to particular events, see Kristin Shrader-Frechette, *Risk Analysis and Scientific Method* (Boston: Kluwer, 1985), 145ff. For discussion of problems with causality, see Kristin Shrader-Frechette, *Risk and Rationality* (Berkeley: University of California Press, 1991), 60–63, 200–205. For nuclear weapons cancers, see previous 6 notes and Shrader-Frechette, *Ethics of Scientific Research*, 5, and chapter 1.

79. Thomas Kerns, *Environmentally Induced Illnesses* (London: McFarland, 2001), 11–16. For Toxics Release Inventory information, see the last chapter.

80. State of California, Office of Environmental Health Hazard Assessment, *Proposition 65*; www.oehha.ca.gov/prop65.html; accessed November 27, 2005. See Epstein, *Cancer-Gate*, 106–109.

81. See Kassirer, *On the Take*.

82. Angell, *The Truth about the Drug Companies*, 198, 200, 206–207; see earlier Angell citations in chapter 1, note 130; chapter 2, notes 25, 40.

83. Seeta Gangadharan, "Grassroots or Astroturf?" in Bray, *Spin Works*, 100–101. Dixy Lee Ray and Lou Guzzo, *Environmental Overkill* (Washington, D.C.: Regnery, 1993), 149, 186. Elizabeth Whelan, *Toxic Terror* (Buffalo, N.Y.: Prometheus, 1993), 7, 10. For these and more such examples, see Beder, *Global Spin*, 17, 18, 23, 24 ff. See earlier notes for the distinction between ethics and

law. S. Beder, "Ecos Corp's 'Win-Win' Spin for Corporate Environmentalism," *PR Watch* 9, no. 2 (2002): 9–11.

84. Information on 2004 lobbying statistics is from Matthew Continetti, "Contract Killers," *New York Times* CLV, No. 53,354 (October 1, 2005): A29. Dick Armey statistics are from Dick Armey, "Washington's Lobbying Industry," www.flattax.gov; accessed May 1, 2006; and D. Stout, "Tab for Washington Lobbying," *New York Times* CXLVIII, no. 51598, July 29, 1999. See Center for Responsive Politics; www.opensecrets.org/lobbyists/index.asp (accessed May 1, 2006) for lobbying dollars. Legislative data on the effects of lobbyists, campaign contributions, and political-action committees (PACs) are from Janet M. Box-Steffensmeier and J. Tobin Grant, "All in a Day's Work," *Legislative Studies Quarterly* 25, no. 4 (1999): 511–524. See also "Why People Who Value Families Should Care about Campaign Finance Reform," *Common Cause*; www.commoncause .org; accessed May 1, 2006. See previous notes and Kevin Phillips, *Wealth and Democracy* (New York: Broadway, 2002), 326–327. See also Paul Starr, "Democracy versus Dollars," *American Prospect* vol. 8, no. 31 (March/April 1997): 6–9; Patricia O'Toole, *Money and Morals* (New York: Clarkson Potter, 1998); Venetia Murray, *An Elegant Madness* (New York: Penguin Putnam, 1999); Elizabeth Drew, *The Corruption of American Politics* (Woodstock, N.Y.: Peter Meyers, 1999); Vance Packard, *The Ultra-Rich* (Boston: Little, Brown, 1989); William Kreml, *America's Middle Class* (Durham, N.C.: Carolina Academic Press, 1997); Center for Public Integrity, *The Cheating of America* (New York: Center for Public Integrity, 2001), 13–15; and Stephen Ansolabehere, James Snyder Jr., and Micky Tripathi, "Are PAC Contributions and Lobbying Linked?" *Politics* 4, no. 2 (2002): 131–156.

85. Al Wilhite and Chris Paul, "Corporate Campaign Contributions and Legislative Voting," *Quarterly Review of Economics and Business* 29, no. 3 (22 September 1989). D. E. Apollonio and R. J. La Raja, "Who Gave Soft Money," *Journal of Politics* 66, no. 4 (November 2004): 1134–54. T. J. Rudolph, "Corporate and Labor PAC Contributions. Measuring the Effects," *Journal of Politics* 61, no. 1 (November 1999): 195–206. R. A. Smith, "Interest-Group Influence in the U.S. Congress," *Legislative Studies Quarterly* 20, no. 1 (February 1995); 89–139. See next notes, and D. A. Luke, "Where There's Smoke, There's Money," *American Journal of Preventive Medicine* 27, no. 5 (2004): 363–372. Center for Responsive Politics, *2004 Presidential Campaign Contributions by Industry*; http:// usgovingo.about.com/od/thepoliticalsystem/a/industrybucks.htm; Center for Responsive Politics, *Pharmaceuticals/Health Products*; www.opensecrets.org/indus tries/indus.asp?Ind=H04; and Center for Responsive Politics, *Finance/Credit Companies: Long-Term Contribution Trends*; all at (Washington, D.C.: Center for Responsive Politics, 2004) and all accessed March 20, 2005. For Abramoff lobbying claim, see Philip Shenon, "Lobbyist Sought $9 Million to Set Bush Meeting," *New York Times, CLV, no 53, 394* (November 10, 2005), A1, A21.

86. See previous notes and information from the website of the Campaign Finance Information Center at the University of Missouri; www.campaignfinance .org.; accessed May 1, 2006. Quotation is from Phillips, *Wealth and Democracy*, 323–325; see 293–316, and Alan Brinkley, *Voices of Protest* (New York: Random House, 1982), 326, as well as the previous notes. See also Shaeffer, "Power Plants and Public Health," 3. M. Hertsgaard, "Trashing the Environment," *The Nation* 276, no. 4 (2003): 15–19; Slater, 42.

87. Center for Responsive Politics, *2004 Presidential Election* (Washington, D.C.: Center for Responsive Politics, 2004); http://usgovingo.about.com/gi/dynamic/offsite.htm; accessed March 20, 2005. See U.S. Department of State, *The Decline of Union Power*; http://economic.about.com/od/laborinamerica/a/union_decline.htm; accessed March 20, 2005. C. T. Koeller, "Union Activity and the Decline in American Trade-Union Membership," *Journal of Labor Research* 15, no. 1(1994): 19–32. W. T. Dickens and J. S. Leonard, "Accounting for the Decline in Union Membership," *Industrial and Labor Relations Review* 38, no. 3 (1985): 323–334. See 3 previous notes.

88. Plato, *Complete Works*, trans. Benjamin Jowett (New York: Vintage, 1991), 253–261.

Chapter 3

1. Personal communications with Reason Warehime, 1996–2000, at his home in Gibsonton, Florida (hereafter cited as Warehime interviews). See Carole Gallagher, *American Ground Zero* (Cambridge, Mass.: MIT Press, 1993).

2. Gallagher, *American Ground Zero*, 73–74.

3. Warehime interviews.

4. Warehime interviews.

5. Nancy Hogan, "Shielded from Liability," *ABA Journal* 80, no. 5 (May 1994): 56–60.

6. I witnessed these accusations against Warehime at the Notre Dame lecture.

7. International Commission on Radiological Protection, *Draft 2005 Recommendations* (Stockholm: International Commission on Radiological Protection, 2005), 33: "any effect on IQ following in utero doses of a few tens of mGy would be undetectable and therefore of no practical significance." U.S. CDC, *Mortality and Morbidity Weekly Report* 39, no. SS 2 (1990): 7, states: "illnesses occurring after years of exposure to low-level toxins are not detectable." For the Hawk's Nest silicosis, and other coverups, see Sheldon Rampton and John Stauber, *Trust Us, We're Experts* (New York: Penguin, 2001), 75–90.

8. World Health Organization (WHO), *Report of the Committee of Experts on Tobacco Industry Documents: Tobacco Company Strategies to Undermine Tobacco Control Activities at the World Health Organization* (Geneva: WHO, 2000).

9. Regarding front groups and ghostwriting, see Sharon Beder, *Global Spin* (Glasgow: Green Books, 2002), 28–31, 237; Rampton and Stauber, *Trust Us, We're Experts,* pp. 12–16, 132. Common Cause Education Fund, *Wolves in Sheep's Clothing: Telecom Industry Front Groups and Astroturf* (Washington, DC: Common Cause, March 2006); available from http://www.commoncause.org/atf/cf/{FB3C17E2-CDD1-4DF6-92BE-BD4429893665}/WOLVESREPORT.PDF and accessed 29 October 2006. Common Cause Education Fund, *Wolves in Sheep's Clothing, Part II* (Washington, DC: Common Cause, August 2006); available from http://www.commoncause.org/atf/cf/{FB3C17E2-CDD1-4DF6-92BE-BD4429893665}/WOLVESPART2.PDF and accessed 29 October 2006. Jerome Kassirer, *On the Take* (New York: Oxford University Press, 2005), 31–35. Marcia Angell, *The Truth about the Drug Companies* (New York: Random House, 2005), esp. 201; see also 173–216. Watchdog groups (ExxonSecrets.org, *Fact Sheet: The Advancement of Sound Science Coalition*; www.exxonsecrets.org/html/orgfactsheet.php?id=6; accessed May 1, 2006) claim that the TASSC coalition,

founded in 1993 as a Philip Morris front group, received negative exposure in 1998 from a *New York Times* article revealing its funders. As a consequence, they say the TASSC label was dropped and the group continues to operate instead as the Advancement of Sound Science Center, housed at Steve Milloy's home. Milloy was the TASCC director at the time of the 1998 exposé.

10. Kassirer, *On the Take,* 97–100. For health-related conflicts of interest, see 50–60.

11. "Corporate America's Woes," *Economist* 365, no. 8301 (November 30, 2002): 59. TV percentages are from Beder, *Global Spin,* 75–76. Fortune-500 and top-ten listings are from "Fortune 500, 2005"; http://money.cnn.com/magazines/fortune/fortune500/; accessed March 15, 2006.

12. Danny Schechter, "The Fourth Estate," in *We the Media*, ed. Don Hazen and Julie Winokur (New York: Norton, 1997), 155 of 152–155. For think tanks and industry dollars, see Rampton and Stauber, *Trust Us, We're Experts,* 302–307, 211.

13. See the American Enterprise Institute website for Sunstein's 20 "working papers"; www.aei-brookings.org/ta_search.php and accessed March 15, 2006. For industry-think-tank citations, see Cass Sunstein, *Risk and Reason* (New York: Cambridge University Press, 2002), 5, 27, 40, 138. See also Kristin Shrader-Frechette, "Flawed Attacks on Contemporary Human Rights," *Human Rights Review* 7, no. 2 (2005). Shrader-Frechette, "Review of *Risk and Reason* by Cass Sunstein," *Ethics* 114, no. 2 (2004): 376. For free-market environmentalism, see Cass Sunstein, *Laws of Fear* (New York: Cambridge University Press, 2005), esp. 152–155, and *Risk and Reason*. For criticism of this stance, see chapter 2 here, and Shrader-Frechette, Review of *Laws of Fear* by Cass Sunstein, *Ethics and International Affairs* 20, no. 1 (spring 2006): 123–125.

14. Beder, *Global Spin,* 75–79. See Sharon Beder, *Suiting Themselves* (London: Earthscan, 2006).

15. Kassirer, *On the Take,* 60–61, 116–117, 120–122; see also 102–115, 118–119, 123–128.

16. Kassirer, OTT, 94–95, 34–35.

17. J. T. Bennett and T. J. Di Lorenzo, *Unhealthy Charities:* (New York: Basic Books, 1994). H. Hall and G. Williams, "Professor vs. Cancer Society," *Chronicle of Philanthropy*, IV, no. 7 (January 28, 1992), 26. T. J. Di Lorenzo, "One Charity's Uneconomic War on Cancer," *Wall Street Journal* CCXIX no. 51 (March 15, 1992): A10. S.S. Epstein, "American Cancer Society: The World's Wealthiest 'Non-Profit' Institution," *Journal of Health Services* 29, no. 3 (1999): 565–78. Samuel Epstein, *Cancer-Gate* (Amityville, N.Y.: Baywood, 2005), 80–81.

18. Ralph Moss, *The Cancer Industry* (Brooklyn: Equinox Press, 1996), and Epstein, *Cancer-Gate,* 287. For ACS criticisms see Rampton and Stauber, *Trust Us, We're Experts,* 16; G. Edward Griffin, *World without Cancer* (Westlake Village, Calif.: American Media, 1997), 146–152, 330–331; Marcus Cohen, "The Impact of Medical Censorship on Patient Care," *Townsend Letter for Doctors and Patients* (December 2004); www.findarticles.com/p/articles/mi_m0ISW/is_257/ai_n763803. Samuel Epstein, "American Cancer Society," *International Journal of Health Services* 29, no. 3 (1999): 565–578, and Samuel Epstein, Nicholas Ashford, Brent Blackwelderr, Barry Castleman, Gary Cohen, Edward Goldsmith, Anthony Mazzocchi, and Quentin Young, "The Crisis in U.S. and International Cancer Policy," *International Journal of Health Services* 32, no. 4

(2002): 669–707. B. Lerner, "No Shrinking Violet," *Western Journal of Medicine* 174, no. 5 (2001): 362–65.

19. "ACS-Led Cancer Dialogue Beset by Mistrust, Lack of Openness," *Cancer Letter* 26, no. 3 (2000): 1–12; Epstein, *Cancer-Gate*, 139.

20. Moss, *The Cancer Industry*; B. Cohen et al., *Just Add Water: Violations of Federal Health Standards in Tap Water* (Washington, D.C.: Environmental Working Group of the Natural Resources Defense Council, 1996); Epstein, *Cancer-Gate*, 293.

21. S. Kaplan, "PR Giant Makes Hay from Client Cross-Pollination," *PR Watch* 1, no. 1 (1994): 4.

22. J. F. Viel et al., "Soft-Tissue Sarcoma and Non-Hodgkins Lymphoma Clusters around a Municipal Solid Waste Incinerator with High Dioxin Emission Levels," *American Journal of Epidemiology* 152, no. 1 (2000): 13–19. N. Floret et al., "Dioxin Emissions from a Solid-Waste Incinerator and Risks of Non-Hodgkins Lymphoma," *Epidemiology* 14, no. 4 (2003): 392–398. NIH, *Atlas of Cancer Mortality* (Bethesda, Md.: NIH, 1995). S. S. Epstein, *The Politics of Cancer, Revisited* (Hankins, N.Y.: East Ridge Press, 1998). L. Kohlmeier, J. Rehn, and H. Hoffmeister, "Lifestyle and Trends in Worldwide Breast Cancer Rates," *Annals of the New York Academy of Sciences* 609 (1990): 259–268. For these charges, see notes 18 and 23.

23. These charges are made by Moss, *The Cancer Industry*; by B. Cohen et al., *Just Add Water*; and by Epstein, *Cancer-Gate*, 13–14, 81–91, 138–139, among others. See chapter 1 and note 18 above. International Agency for Research on Cancer, *Occupational Exposures of Hair-Dressers and Barbers and Personal Use of Hair Colourants* 57 (1993): 43–118. For ACS change, see American Lung Association, *Breath Matters,* May 1, 2003; www.californialung.org/ALAC/enews0304.html; accessed November 29, 2005.

24. Kei Koizumi, *R &D Trends and Special Analyses, AAAS Report XXIX, XXVII* (Washington, D.C.: American Association for the Advancement of Science, 2005, 2004), and Koizumi remarks, spring 2005, 2004, to the US EPA Science Advisory Board. Beder, *Global Spin*, esp. 75–80, 114–118. D. Barnes and L. Bero, "Why Review Articles on the Health Effects of Passive Smoking Reach Different Conclusions," *Journal of the American Medical Association* 279, no. 19 (1998): 1566–1570.

25. Kassirer, *On the Take,* 42–44.

26. Cases are from Krimsky, *Science in the Private Interest* (Savage, Md.: Rowman and Littlefield, 2003), 51, 115–120, and Catherine D. DeAngelis, Phil B. Fontanarosa, and Annette Flanagin, "Reporting Financial Conflicts of Interest and Relationships between Investigators and Research Sponsors," *Journal of the American Medical Association* 286, no. 1 (2001): 89–92. See Kassirer, *On the Take,* 31–35, for ghostwriting, and 27–28, for off-label promotion, particularly for Neurontin and Provigil. For the Zoloft data, see Carl Elliott, "Pharma Goes to the Laundry," *Hastings Center Reports* 34, no. 5 (September/October 2004): 18–23.

27. Christopher Oleskey, Alan Fleischman, Lynn Goldman, Kurt Hirschhorn, Philip J. Landrigan, Marc Lappe, Mary Faith Marshall, Herbert Needleman, Rosamond Rhodes, and Michael McCally, "Pesticide Testing in Humans," *Environmental Health Perspectives* 112, no. 8 (June 2004): 914–919. For Dow prisoner studies, see Beder, *Global Spin*, 143, and Elizabeth Shogren, "Testing Pesticides on Humans," National Public Radio, June 17, 2005; www.npr.org/templates/story/story.php?storyId=4707438; accessed October 28, 2005. See

also Science Advisory Board, US Environmental Protection Agency, *Comments on the Use of Data from the Testing of Human Subjects*, EPA-SAB-EC-00-017 (Washington, D.C.: EPA, 2000), and Michael Janofsky, "Limits Sought on Testing for Pesticides," *New York Times* CLIV, no. 53,261 (June 30, 2005): A17. The California tests on college students are discussed in Senator Barbara Boxer, "Senate Passes Boxer Amendment Imposing One-Year Moratorium on EPA Use of Human Pesticide Testing," June 29, 2005; http://boxer.senate.gov/news/record .cfm?id=239845; accessed March 13, 2006, and in U.S. House of Representatives, Committee on Government Reform, *Human Pesticide Experiments* (Washington, D.C.: US Government Printing Office, June 2005); www.democrats .reform.house.gov/Documents/20050617123506-17998.pdf; accessed March 13, 2006.

28. Beder, *Global Spin*, 116; see 114–118. See Beder, *Suiting Themselves*.

29. The educational statistics are from Sam Dillon, "At Public Universities, Warnings of Privatization," *New York Times*, CLV, no. 53,369 (October 16, 2005): A12.

30. Krimsky, *Science in the Private Interest*, esp. 35–45. Rampton and Stauber, *Trust Us, We're Experts*, 212–213. Kassirer, *On the Take*, 179–180. Eval Press and Jennifer Washburn, "The Kept University," pt. 1, *Atlantic Monthly* 285, no. 3 (March 2000), 39–54; www.theatlantic.com/issues/2000/03/press.htm and accessed March 13, 2005. See also Campbell, "Declaration of Financial Interests," *Nature* 412, no. 6849 (2003): 751.

31. Re university-corporate funding, see previous note. Re benzene, see R. B. Hayes et al., "Benzene and the Dose-Related Incidence of Hematologic Neoplasms in China," *Journal of the National Cancer Institute* 89, no. 14 (1997): 1065–71; Qing Lan et al., "Hematotoxicity in Workers Exposed to Low Levels of Benzene," *Science* 306, no. 5702 (2004): 1774–76; Rampton and Stauber, *Trust Us, We're Experts*, 85; and Wendy Benjaminson, "Petroleum Industry Funds Challenge to Benzene Study," *Associated Press Online*, April 28, 2005, 1, abstract at http://pqasb.pqarchiver.com/ap/833567471.html?did=833567471&FMT=ABS &FMTS=FT&date=Apr+28%2C+2005&author=WENDY+BENJAMINSON &pub=Associated+Press&desc=Petroleum+industry+funds+challenge+to+ benzene+study; accessed October 30, 2005.

32. Kassirer, *On the Take*, 7–11, 26–27.

33. Ibid., 44–46. Rampton and Stauber, *Trust Us, We're Experts*, 195–221.

34. Asaf Bitton et al., "The p53 Tumor Suppressor Gene and the Tobacco Industry," *Lancet* 365, no. 9458 (2005): 531–540. David Cooper, "p53 Mutations, Benzo[a]pyrene and Lung Cancer," *Mutagenesis* 13, no. 4 (July 1998): 319–320. Thilo Paschke, "Analysis of Different Versions of the IARC p53 Database," *Mutagenesis* 15, no. 6 (November 2000): 457–458. See Alex Barnum, "How Big Tobacco Reneged on Pledge," *San Francisco Chronicle* 364 (January 14, 2005), A1, and David Nicholson, "Nottingham's Smoking Gun," *the -scientist.com*, May 18, 2001, available only online; www.the-scientist.com/news/ 20010518/04 and accessed March 13, 2006. See Krimsky, *Science in the Private Interest*, 73, 80–85, and Kristin Shrader-Frechette, *Ethics of Scientific Research* (Lanham, Md.: Rowman and Littlefield, 1994), 9. For "junk science" and TASSC, see Rampton and Stauber, *Trust Us, We're Experts*, 234–265 and 195–221.

35. Kristin Shrader-Frechette, *Burying Uncertainty* (Berkeley: University of California Press, 1993), 50–59.

36. Oleskey et al., "Pesticide Testing in Humans," 916.

37. International Commission on Radiological Protection, *Draft 2005 Recommendations*. Past-President remarks are in Richard Clarke, "Control of Low-Level Radiation Exposure," *Journal of Radiological Protection* 19, no. 2 (1999): 107–108. Re International Commission on Radiological Protection problems, see Kristin Shrader-Frechette, "Models in Panther Biology and Radiobiology," *Philosophy Today* 48, no. 5 (2004): 96–108, and "Radiobiology and Gray Science," *Science and Engineering Ethics* 11, no. 2 (2005): 167–169.

38. See previous note.

39. The Dutch results are in R. M. Cooke, "Risk Assessment and Rational Decision Theory," *Dialectica* 36, no. 4 (1982): 330–351. See R. Cooke, *Subjective Probability and Expert Opinion* (New York: Oxford University Press, 1991), ch. 9. See US Nuclear Regulatory Commission, *Reactor Safety Study*, NUREG75/014, WASH-1400 (Washington, D.C.: U.S. Government Printing Office, 1975), 15, 40, 96–97, 108–109, 118, 186, 224, 239, 245–246. N. C. Rasmussen, "Methods of Hazard Analysis and Nuclear Safety Engineering," in *The Three Mile Island Nuclear Accident*, ed. T. Moss and D. Sill (New York: New York Academy of Sciences, 1981), 29. See also Kristin Shrader-Frechette, *Risk and Rationality* (Berkeley: University of California Press, 1991), 5ff., 55ff., 83ff., 95–96, 189ff. For overconfidence biases and error ranges, see D. Kahnemann, Paul Slovic, and A. Tversky, *Judgment under Uncertainty* (Cambridge: Cambridge University Press, 1982).

40. International Atomic Energy Agency, *An International Peer Review of the Yucca Mountain Site Characterization Project* (Vienna: International Atomic Energy Agency, 2001). See also Richard A. Kerr, "Nuclear Waste Disposal," *Science* 288, no. 5466 (2000): 602; Colin Macilwain, "Out of Sight, Out of Mind," *Nature* 412, no. 6850 (2001): 850–852. Rodney C. Ewing and Allison Macfarlane, "Yucca Mountain," *Science* 296, no. 5568 (2002): 659–660; and United States General Accounting Office (GAO), *Nuclear Waste*, GAO-02-539T (Washington, D.C.: US Government Printing Office, 2002); www.gao.gov and accessed March 13, 2006. See also US National Academy of Sciences, *Rethinking High-Level Radioactive Waste Disposal* (Washington, D.C.: National Academy Press, 1990); U.S. National Research Council, *Building Consensus through Risk Assessment and Management* (Washington, D.C.: U.S. National Academy Press, 1994). Regarding verification-validation, see Shrader-Frechette, *Burying Uncertainty*, 145–149.

41. Bruce Ames and Lois Gold, "Pesticides, Risk, and Applesauce," *Science* 244, no. 4096 (1989): 757 of 755–57. Bruce Ames and Lois Gold, "The Causes and Prevention of Cancer," *Environmental Health Perspectives* 105, supp. 4 (June 1997): 865–874. Elizabeth Whelan, "Who Says PCBs Cause Cancer?" *Wall Street Journal*, December 12, 2000; Michael Gough, *"Environmental Cancer" Isn't What We Thought or Were Told*; available at the Cato Institute website; www.cato .org/tetimony/ct-mg030697.html; accessed May 28, 2005; Rampton and Stauber, *Trust Us, We're Experts*, 222–266; Paul and Anne Ehrlich, *Betrayal of Science and Reason* (Washington, D.C.: Island, 1996), 153–187. S. Lichter and S. Rothman, *Environmental Cancer* (New Haven, CT: Yale University Press, 1999).

42. Ames and Gold, "Pesticides, Risk, and Applesauce," 757; Ames and Gold, "The Causes and Prevention of Cancer." Elizabeth Whelan claims animal tests should be used to regulate chemicals more strictly only when two or more species exhibit "highly lethal" cancers that do not also occur spontaneously, that have short latency, and that arise at low doses. Whelan, "Stop Banning Products

at the Drop of a Rat," *Insight* 10, no. 50 (December 1994): 18–20. Whelan, *Ratty Test Rationale* (New York: American Council on Science and Health, 2005); www.acsh.org/healthissues/newsID.1035/healthissue_detail.asp; accessed November 29, 2005.

43. See Thomas Beauchamp and James Childress, *Principles of Biomedical Ethics* (New York: Oxford University Press, 1989); Charles Culver and Bernard Gert, *Philosophy in Medicine* (New York: Oxford University Press, 1982); Norman Daniels, *Just Health Care* (New York: Oxford University Press, 1985). Warren Reich, *Encyclopedia of Bioethics* (New York: Free Press, 1978); Robert Veatch, *A Theory of Medical Ethics* (New York: Basic Books, 1981).

44. Re: ethics and burdens of proof, see Shrader-Frechette, *Risk and Rationality*, pp. 100–145; Carl Cranor, *Toxic Torts* (Cambridge: Cambridge University Press, 2006), and *Regulating Toxic Substances* (New York: Oxford University Press, 1993). Re: virtue and protecting the vulnerable, see Philippa Foot, *Virtues and Vices and Other Essays in Moral Philosophy* (Berkeley: University of California Press, 1978); Peter Geach, *The Virtues* (Cambridge: Cambridge University Press, 1977); Robert Kruschwitz and Robert Roberts (eds.), *The Virtues* (Belmont, Calif.: Wadsworth, 1987); Edmund Pincoffs, *Quandaries and Virtues* (Lawrence: University of Kansas Press, 1986); G. H. von Wright, *The Varieties of Goodness* (London: Routledge, 1963).

45. Regarding ethical responsibility, classic works include Aristotle, *Nicomachean Ethics*, esp. books I–II; Joel Feinberg, *Doing and Deserving* (Princeton: Princeton University Press, 1970); Peter French, *Collective and Corporate Responsibility* (New York: Columbia University Press, 1984); Jonathan Glover, *Responsibility* (London: Routledge, 1970); and Michael Zimmerrman, *An Essay on Moral Responsibility* (Savage, Md.: Rowman and Littlefield, 1988). Regarding deontological and contractarian ethics, classic works include Ernest Barker (ed.), *Social Contract* (Westport, Conn.: Greenwood, 1980); James Buchanan and Gordon Tullock, *The Calculus of Consent* (Chicago: University of Chicago Press, 1975); Ronald Dworkin, *Taking Rights Seriously* (Cambridge, Mass.: Harvard University Press, 1977); John Locke, *Two Treatises of Government* (Cambridge: Cambridge University Press, 1977); John Rawls, *A Theory of Justice* (Cambridge, Mass.: Harvard University Press, 1971); and John Simmons, *Moral Principle and Political Obligations* (Princeton: Princeton University Press, 1979).

46. Regarding utilitarianism, see Shrader-Frechette, *Risk and Rationality*, 100–130; Richard Brandt, *Ethical Theory* (Englewood Cliffs, N.J.: Prentice-Hall, 1959), esp. chs. 12–19; John Stuart Mill, *Utilitarianism*, ed. J. M. Robson (Toronto: University of Toronto Press, 1969); Samuel Scheffler (ed.), *Consequentialism and Its Critics* (New York: Oxford University Press, 1988); J. J. C. Smart, *Utilitarianism* (Cambridge: Cambridge University Press, 1973); Amartya Sen and Bernard Williams (eds.), *Utilitarianism and Beyond* (Cambridge: Cambridge University Press, 1982).

47. Regarding the reasonable-person test, see Alan Gewirth, "The Rationality of Reasonableness," *Synthese* 57, no. 2 (1983): 225–247; Virginia Held, "Rationality and Reasonable Cooperation," *Social Research* 44, no. 4 (1977): 708–744; John Rawls, "Kantian Constructivism in Moral Theory," *Journal of Philosophy* 77, no. 9 (1980): 515–572; David Richards, *A Theory of Reasons for Actions* (Oxford: Clarendon Press, 1971). Adam Finkel, "Rodent Tests Continue to Save Human Lives," *Insight* 10, no. 50 (December 1994): 20–22. See Whelan, "Stop Banning Products at the Drop of a Rat," Whelan, *Ratty Test Rationale*,

and T. Still, "Animal Testing," *Wisconsin Technology Network* (November 21, 2005); http://wistechnology.com/article.php?id=2489 and accessed November 12, 2006.

48. Whelan, "Stop Banning Products at the Drop of a Rat," Whelan, *Ratty Test Rationale*. Bruce Ames, Lois Gold, and Walter Willett, "The Causes and Prevention of Cancer," *Proceedings of the National Academy of Sciences* 92, no. 12 (June 1995): 5261, 5262 of 5258–5265. See following note and Epstein, *Cancer-Gate*, 12–16. American Council on Science and Health quotation is from Rampton and Stauber, *Trust Us, We're Experts*, 247.

49. G. E. Moore, *Principia Ethica* (Cambridge: Cambridge University Press, 1951), 23–41, 60–63, 108, 146. For various senses of the naturalistic fallacy, see K. S. Shrader-Frechette, *Nuclear Power and Public Policy* (Boston: Kluwer, 1983), ch. 6, and Kevin Elliott, "Biomedical Ethics, Public-Health Risk Assessment, and the Naturalistic Fallacy," *Public Affairs Quarterly* 16, no. 4 (2002): 351–376. Philosophers generally refer to the naturalistic fallacy as consisting of the second error, not the first. Thanks to Kevin Elliott for clarification of this issue; remaining errors are my own.

50. Kristin Shrader-Frechette, *Environmental Justice: Creating Equality, Reclaiming Democracy* (New York: Oxford University Press, 2002), 3–116, 135–162. For consent, see preceding notes and preceding chapter, esp. note 51.

51. The ACS uses the "cure frame" at www.cancer.org/docroot/home/index.asp; accessed November 18, 2005.

52. H. L. Bradlow, D. L. Davis, G. Lin, D. Sepkovic, and R. Tiwari, "Effects of Pesticides on the Ratio of 16-Alpha/2-Hydroxyestrone—A Biological Marker of Breast-Cancer Risk," *Environmental Health Perspectives* 103, no. 1 (October 1995): S147–S150. D. L. Davis, M. J. Pongsiri, and M. Wolff, "Recent Developments on the Avoidable Causes of Breast Cancer," *Annals of the New York Academy of Sciences* 837 (1997): 513–523; D. L. Davis, D. Axelrod, M. Osborne, N. Telang, H. L. Bradlow, and E. Sittner, "Avoidable Causes of Breast Cancer," *Cancer Annals of the New York Academy of Sciences* 883 (1997): 112–128; H. Mussalo-Rauhamaa et al., "Occurrence of Beta-hexachloro-cyclohexane in Breast Cancer Patients," *Cancer* 66, no. 10 (1990): 2124–28. T. Dao, "The Role of Ovarian Hormones in Initiating the Induction of Mammary Cancer in Rats by Polynuclear Hydrocarbons," *Cancer Research* 22 (1962): 973–984. National Toxicology Program, *Carcinogenicity Studies of 1,2 Dichloropropane in F344/N Rats and B6C3F1 Mice*, technical report 263 (Research Triangle Park, N.C.: US Department of Health and Human Services, 1989). NCI and National Toxicology Program, "Bioassay of 1, 2 Bibromoethane for Possible Carcinogenicity," NIH 80–1766 (Washington, D.C.: U.S. Department of Health, Education and Welfare, 1980). International Agency for Research on Cancer, *Occupational Exposures in Insecticide Applications* 53 (1991): 441–466. A. Donna et al., "Triazine Herbicides and Ovarian Epithelial Neoplasms," *Scandinavian Journal of Work and Environmental Health* 15, no. 1 (1989): 47–53. P. Lichtenstein et al., "Environmental and Heritable Factors in the Causation of Cancer," *New England Journal of Medicine* 343, no. 2 (2000): 78–85. E. V. Kliewer and K. R. Smith, "Breast Cancer Mortality among Immigrants in Australia and Canada," *Journal of the National Cancer Institute* 87, no. 15 (1995): 1154–61. C. Willett, "Balancing Lifestyle and Genomics Research for Disease Prevention," *Science* 296, no. 5568 (2002): 695–698. Heiko Becher et al., "Quantitative Cancer Risk Assessment for Dioxins," *Environmental Health Perspectives* 106,

supp. 2 (1998): 663–670. B. E. Henderson, R. K. Ross, and M. C. Pike, "Toward the Primary Prevention of Cancer," *Science* 254, no. 5035 (1991): 1131–38. U.S. GAO, *Breast Cancer* (Washington, D.C.: U.S. Government Printing Office, 1991). J. Harris et al., "Breast Cancer," *New England Journal of Medicine* 327, no. 5 (1992): 319–328. O. G. Fitzhugh et al., "Chronic Oral Toxicity of Aldrin and Dieldrin in Rats and Dogs," *Food, Cosmetics, and Toxicology* 2 (1964): 551–562. NCI, *Bioassay of Chlordane for Possible Carcinogenicity* (Bethesda, Md.: NCI, 1977). David Rall, "Laboratory Animal Toxicity and Carcinogenesis," *Annals of the NY Academy of Sciences* 534 (1988): 78–83. J. D. Scribner and N. K. Mottet, "DDT Acceleration of Mammary-Gland Tumors," *Carcinogenesis* 2, no. 12 (1981): 1236–39. M. Wasserman et al., Organochlorine Compounds in Neoplastic and Adjacenty Apparently Normal Breast Tissue," *Bulletin of Environmental Contaminants and Toxicology* 15, no. 4 (1976): 478–484. F. Falck et al., "Pesticides and Their Relation to Breast Cancer," *Archives of Environmental Health* 47, no. 2 (1992): 143–146. D. L. Davis et al., "Medical Hypothesis: Xeno-estrogens as Preventable Causes of Breast Cancer," *Environmental Health Perspectives* 101, no. 5 (1993): 372–377. A Segaloff and W. S. Maxfield, "The Synergism between Radiation and Estrogen in the Production of Mammary Cancer," *Cancer Research* 31, no. 2 (1971): 166–168; Kohlmeier et al., "Lifestyle and Trends in Worldwide Breast Cancer Rates." J. Brody et al., "Breast Cancer Risk and Historical Exposure to Pesticides," *Environmental Health Perspectives* 112, no. 8 (2004): 889–97. See also notes 53–57.

53. For absence of material on chemicals, see "Breast Cancer News," at the website of National Breast Cancer Awareness Month; www.nbcam.org/newsroom_news.cfm; accessed November 29, 2005. Quoted material is from Epstein, *Cancer-Gate*, 137; see also 83, 119, 138, and John Robbins, *The Food Revolution* (York Beach, Me.: Conari, 2001), 40–43.

54. John Cairns, "The Treatment of Diseases and the War against Cancer," *Scientific American* 253, no. 5 (November 1985): 51–59. S. Batt and L. Gross, "Cancer Inc.," *Sierra* 84, no. 5 (Sept/Oct 1999); www.sierradub.org/sierra/199909/cancer.asp and accessed 13 November 2006.

55. J. C. Bailar et al., "Progress against Cancer?" *New England Journal of Medicine* 314, no. 19 (May 29, 1997): 1226–1232; T. J. Smith et al., "Efficacy and Cost-Effectiveness of Cancer Treatment," *Journal of the National Cancer Institute* 85, no. 18 (September 1993): 1460–74.

56. P. Greaves et al., "Two-Year Carcinogenicity Study of Tamoxifen," *Cancer Research* 53, no. 17 (1993): 3919–24. W. A. Fugh-Berman and S. S. Epstein, "Tamoxifen," *Lancet* 340, no. 8828 (1992): 1143–45. K. Smigel, "Breast Cancer Prevention Trial Takes Off," *Journal of the National Cancer Institute* 84, no. 9 (1992): 669–670; see previous 4 notes.

57. Regarding the tamoxifen controversy, see "Studies Spark Tamoxifen Controversy," *Science News*, 145, no. 9 (February, 26, 1994): 133. X. Han and J. G. Liehr, "Induction of Covalent DNA Adducts in Rodents by Tamoxifen," *Cancer Research* 52, no. 2 (1992): 1360–63. Imperial Chemical Industries Group, *Data Presented at the FDA Oncology Drugs Advisory Committee Meeting* (Bethesda, Md.: NCI, June 29, 1990). S. G. Nayfield et al., "Potential Role of Tamoxifen in Prevention of Breast Cancer," *Journal of the National Cancer Institute* 83, no. 20 (1991): 1450–59. "Tamoxifen Trial Controversy," *Lancet* 339, no. 8795 (1992): 735. L. E. Rutqvist et al., "Contralateral Primary Tumors

in Breast Cancer Patients," *Journal of the National Cancer Institute* 83, no. 18 (1991): 1299–1306. S. B. Gusberg, "Tamoxifen for Breast Cancer," *Cancer* 65, no. 7 (1990): 1463–64. S. S. Epstein, D. Steinman, and S. LeVert, *The Breast Cancer Prevention Program* (New York: MacMillan, 1997). Epstein, *Cancer-Gate*, 2005, 67, 83–87, 145–161; Robbins, *The Food Revolution*, 40. See previous 5 notes and L. Bergman et al., "Risk and Prognosis of Endometrial Cancer after Tamoxifen," *Lancet* 356, no. 9233 (2000): 881–87.

58. See R. Doll and R. Peto, "The Causes of Cancer," *Journal of the National Cancer Institute* 66 (1981): 1191–1308, for their claims. For charges against Doll and Peto, see Richard Clapp, Genevieve Howe, Molly Lefevre, *Environmental and Occupational Causes of Cancer* (Lowell, Mass.: Lowell Center for Sustainable Production, 2005); Epstein, *Cancer-Gate*, 2005, 15. P. J. Landrigan and D. B. Baker, "Clinical Recognition of Occupational and Environmental Disease," *Mt. Sinai Journal of Medicine* 62, no. 5 (1995): 406–411. P. J. Landrigan, S. B. Marsowitz, W. J. Nicholson, and D. B. Baker, "Cancer Prevention in the Workplace," in *Cancer Prevention and Control*, ed. P. Greenwald, B. S. Kramer, and D. L. Weed (New York: Marcel Dekker, 1995), 393–410. J. Siemiatycki, et al., "Listing Occupational Carcinogens," *Environmental Health Perspectives* 112, no. 15 (2004): 1447–1459. S. H. Zahm and A. Blair, "Occupational Cancer among Women," *American Journal of Industrial Medicine* 44, no. 6 (2003): 565–575. Regarding weapons testing, see U.S. Congress, *American Nuclear Guinea Pigs* (Washington, D.C.: Government Printing Office, 1986); U.S. Congress, *Government Liability for Atomic Weapons Testing Program* (Washington, D.C.: Government Printing Office, 1987); U.S. Congress, *The Radiation Protection Act of 1991* (Washington, D.C.: Government Printing Office, 1992). For industry estimates, see R. A. Stallones and T. A. Downes, *A Critical Review of Estimates of the Fraction of Cancers in the U.S. Related to Environmental Factors: Report to the American Industrial Health Council* (Houston: University of Texas School of Public Health, 1979).

59. Regarding the mammography controversy, see "The Mammography Screening Controversy: Questions and Answers October, 2002," National Breast Cancer Controversy (Washington D.C.; 2006); www.natlbcc.org/bin/index.asp ?strid=498&depid=9&btnid=2 X. Han and J. G. Liehr, "Induction of Covalent DNA Adducts in Rodents by Tamoxifen," *Cancer Research* 52, no. 2 (1992): 1360–1363. Imperial Chemical Industries Group, *Data Presented at the FDA Oncology Drugs Advisory Committee Meeting* (Bethesda, Md.: NCI, June 29, 1990). S. G. Nayfield et al., "Potential Role of Tamoxifen in Prevention of Breast Cancer," *Journal of the National Cancer Institute* 83, no. 20 (1991): 1450–59. "Tamoxifen Trial Controversy," *Lancet* 339, no. 8795 (1992): 735. L. E. Rutqvist et al., "Contralateral Primary Tumors in Breast Cancer Patients," *Journal of the National Cancer Institute* 83, no. 18 (1991): 1299–1306. S. B. Gusberg, "Tamoxifen for Breast Cancer," *Cancer* 65, no. 7 (1990): 1463–64. S. S. Epstein, D. Steinman, and S. LeVert, *The Breast Cancer Prevention Program* (New York: MacMillan, 1997). Epstein, *Cancer-Gate*, 2005, 67, 83–87, 145–161; Robbins, *The Food Revolution*, p 40. See previous 5 notes.

60. See, for instance, Ames and Gold, "The Causes and Prevention of Cancer." Doll and Peto, "The Causes of Cancer." Peto, "Saturated Fat Avoidance," *Science* 235 (1987): 1562. R. Doll, "Health and the Environment in the 1990s," *American Journal of Public Health* 82, no. 7 (1992): 933–941. B. Ames and

L. Gold, "Misconcepcions on Pollution and the Causes of Cancer," *Angewandte Chemie International Edition English* 29, no. 11 (1990): 1197–1208. See Epstein, *Cancer-Gate*, 2005, 117, 134, for criticism of these claims.

61. The "trivial" claim is from Bruce Ames, "Chemicals, Cancers, Causalities, and Cautions," *Chemtech* 29, no. 10 (October 1989): 591 of 590–598. The "low concern" claim is from Bruce Ames et al., "Ranking Possible Carcinogenic Hazards," *Science* 235, no. 4796 (1987): 271 of 271–280. The "tiny" claim is from Ames, Gold, and Willett, "The Causes and Prevention of Cancer," 5262. See following note; Epstein, *Cancer-Gate*, 2005, 12–16; and note 41 (Rampton and Stauber, *Trust Us, We're Experts,* 247) for criticisms of these claims.

62. Re human rights, compensation, and paternalism, see notes 43–50; Shrader-Frechette, *Environmental Justice*, 117–162; Shrader-Frechette, "Flawed Attacks on Contemporary Human Rights," *Human Rights Review* 7, no. 1 (2005): 92–110; Shrader-Frechette, "MacIntyre on Human Rights," *Modern Schoolman* LXXIX, no. 1 (Nov. 2001): 1–21; Shrader-Frechette, "Natural Rights and Human Vulnerability: Aquinas, MacIntyre, and Rawls," *Public Affairs Quarterly* 16, no. 2 (April 2002): 99–124; and Alan Gewirth, *Human Rights* (Chicago: University of Chicago Press, 1982), Richard Brandt (ed.), *Social Justice* (Englewood Cliffs, N.J.: Prentice-Hall, 1962), and Rawls, *A Theory of Justice.*

63. For instance, Institute of Medicine, *Infant Formula* (Washington, D.C.: National Academy Press, 2004), 85–124, esp. 123–124; Devra Davis, *When Smoke Ran Like Water* (New York: Basic Books, 2002), esp. ch. 6; John Wargo, *Our Children's Toxic Legacy* (New Haven: Yale University Press, 1998); S. M. Snedeker, "Pesticides and Breast Cancer Risk," *Environmental Health Perspectives* 109, supp. 1 (2001): 35–47; T. Colborn, D. Dumanoski, and J. Myers, *Our Stolen Future* (New York: Dutton, 1996), 68–86.

64. E.g., Lovell Jones, John Parretto, and Christine Coussens (eds.), Institute of Medicine, *Rebuilding the Unity of Health and the Environment* (Washington, D.C.: National Academy Press, 2005), and Clapp, Landrigan, and Zahm references in note 58.

65. E.g., Clapp, Landrigan, and Zahm references in note 58, and S. S. Epstein and J. B. Swartz, "Carcinogenic Risk Estimation," *Science* 240, no. 4855 (1988): 1043–45.

66. Richard Peto and M. A. Schneiderman, "Afterword," in Richard Peto and M. A. Schneiderman (eds.), *Quantification of Occupational Cancer* (New York: Cold Spring Harbor, 1981), 695–697.

67. All these assumptions and claims are made in the references cited in notes 60, 61, and 71, esp. in Ames and Gold, "The Causes and Prevention of Cancer."

68. Ames and Gold, "The Causes and Prevention of Cancer," 868–69.

69. Institute of Medicine and National Research Council, *Making Better Drugs for Children with Cancer* (Washington, D.C.: National Academy Press, 2005), esp. 51. G. E. Dinse, D. M. Umbach, A. J. Sasco, D. G. Hoel, and D. I. Davis, "Unexplained Increases in Cancer Incidence in the United States from 1975 to 1994," *Annual Review of Public Health* 20, no. 1 (1999): 173–209.

70. The 60,000 figure is from J. Michael McGinnis, "Attributable Risk in Practice," in Institute of Medicine, *Estimating the Contributions of Lifestyle-Related Factors to Preventable Death* (Washington, D.C.: National Academy Press, 2005), 17–19. J. M. McGinnis and W. H. Foege, "The Immediate vs. the Important," *Journal of the American Medical Association* 291, no. 10 (2004):

1263–64. J. M. McGinnis and W. H. Foege, "Actual Causes of Death in the United States," *Journal of the American Medical Association* 270, no. 18 (1993): 2207–12. Other sources say virtually all cancers are environmentally induced, where environment includes factors like cigarette smoke, as well as industrial pollution (Paul Lichtenstein, Niels Holm, Pia Verkasalo, Anastasia Iliadou, Jaakko Kaprio, Markku Koskenvuo, Eero Pukkala, Axel Skytthee, and Kari Hemminki, "Environmental and Heritable Factors in the Causation of Cancer," *New England Journal of Medicine* 343, no. 2 (2002): 78–85; see chapter 1 statistics). For the pesticide figure, see chapter 1. The OTA, WHO, and other sources are also cited in chapter 1.

71. Ames and Gold, "The Causes and Prevention of Cancer"; for Ames's attack on Proposition 65, see Cristine Russell, "Proposition 65: California's Controversial Gift," *Alicia Patterson Foundation Reporter* 12, no. 1 (1989); www .aliciapatterson.org/APF1201/Russell/Russell.html; accessed November 29, 2005; Russell is a *Washington Post* reporter.

72. Quoted in Beder, *Global Spin,* 97. See William Freudenburg, Robert Gramling, and Debra Davidson, "Scientific Certainty Argumentation Methods," *Sociological Inquiry* 77, no. 2 (2007), in press.

73. Quotation from Beder, Global Spin, 98; see 97–99. For the flawed claim of public irrationality, see Rampton and Stauber, *Trust Us, We're Experts,* 208, 310. See note 13 for free-market environmentalism and the cost-benefit rule.

74. National Research Council, *Valuing Ecosystems Services* (Washington, D.C.: National Academy Press, 2005), 2. Re CBA, see Shrader-Frechette, *Risk and Rationality,* 169–196, and Shrader-Frechette, "Review of Sunstein's *Risk and Reason,*" Ethics. See also the discussion in chapter 2 of free-market environmentalism.

75. See K. Shrader-Frechette, *Risk and Rationality,* 46.

Chapter 4

1. John Carey, "Beryllium Exposure," *Business Week,* no. 3931 (May 2, 2005), 40. Clarification of Finkel case information comes from Adam Finkel, personal communication, email, October 11, 2005; hereafter cited as: Finkel, PCE. With a Harvard doctorate in human-health risk assessment, Finkel also holds a master's degree in public policy from Harvard's Kennedy School of Government. From 1995 to 2000, Finkel was director of health standards for all of the U.S. Occupational Safety and Health Administration (OSHA). As OSHA regional administrator, he supervised 100 inspectors and worried that they were not being told of a test (for beryllium sensitization) that could reveal whether they were already in the early stages of beryllium disease. While strengthening the beryllium standard is one issue, Finkel says OSHA's not screening its employees is more egregious. Why? Because the federal government has covertly "dropped the ball" on many chemical standards, people are less likely to be disturbed about not screening, even when they should be. If OSHA cannot protect the people whose salaries it pays, it is less likely to protect the larger population it is charged with protecting.

2. Finkel, PCE.

3. PEER salary-test comparison; www.peer.org/news/news_id.php?row_id =461; accessed March 15, 2006. Finkel, PCE. James J. Nash, "Whistleblower Asks: Is OSHA Failing to Protect Its Own Employees," *Occupational Hazards*

65, no. 11 (November 2003): 69–70. Cindy Skrzycki, "OSHA Slow to Act on Beryllium Exposure," *Washington Post*, February 1, 2005, E1. Charles Offutt, *Beryllium Effects on OSHA Inspectors Wider Than Feared* (Washington, D.C.: PEER, March 28, 2005). L. M. Sixel, "OSHA May Be Falling Short on Protecting Its Inspectors," *Houston Chronicle*, April 6, 2005; Im.sixel@chron.com, and *Houston Chronicle* website; accessed March 15, 2006.

4. Second quotation is from Skrzycki, "OSHA Slow to Act on Beryllium Exposure." First quotation is from Finkel, PCE. Adam Finkel, interview, "OSHA Inspectors: Left Twisting in the Wind," in Jordan Barab (former special assistant to the assistant secretary of OSHA), ed., *Confined Space: News and Commentary on Workplace Health and Safety* (Philadelphia: American Federation of State, County and Municipal Employees (AFSCME), January 19, 2005); http://spewingforth.blogspot,com/2005/01/osha-inspectors-left-twisting-in-wind.html; accessed September 7, 2005. See Terance D. Miethe, *Whistleblowing at Work* (Boulder, Colo.: Westview, 1999).

5. Sixel, "OSHA May Be Falling Short." Jeffrey Young, "Dems Press to Strengthen Standards on Inspectors' Exposure to Beryllium" *The Hill* 12, no. 51 (June 9, 2005), 14. Quotation is from Finkel, PCE. After Finkel was removed from his directorship, his only OSHA assignment in Washington was "to help plan a conference that was to be held three years later—work that a competent college student could have done as an intern." On the day the first article appeared, emails from Henshaw's personal press secretary revealed she called the reporter's boss. She "complained that 'you and Finkel colluded to leak this story.'" "The same day," says Finkel, "Henshaw held up the newsletter containing the story in front of the 20 senior executives at OSHA and said 'one of you in this room' leaked the story.'" Nevertheless, Finkel claims, "Henshaw and the press secretary both claimed that although the former was mad about the leak, and the latter 'fingered' me as the source, the two of them never spoke to each other about the issue." The upshot? "[Worker] protection laws are supposed to be interpreted in the employee's favor.... [Yet] only a day elapsed and the boss did everything but jab his finger in my eye when he went after 'the leaker.'" Finkel notes that the U.S. Office of the Special Counsel (OSC) ultimatey sided with OSHA against him because the OSC claimed that it "could not prove that the adverse action taken against me was directly connected to my 'protected disclosure.'" Note, however, that between January and September, they did grant me three separate 'stays' (injunctions) blocking the forced move to [Washington] D.C. [from Denver] until they could render a decision." Finkel, PCE.

6. Thomas Beauchamp and James Childress, *Principles of Biomedical Ethics* (New York: Oxford, 1992); see discussion of disclosure and consent in chapters 2 and 3.

7. Skrzycki, "OSHA Slow to Act on Beryllium Exposure," E1; Young, "Dems Press to Strengthen Standards"; Sixel, "OSHA May Be Falling Short"; and Jordan Barab, "Wednesday, April 28, 2004, OSHA to Test for Beryllium Disease," in Barab, *Confined Space*. Newman claims are from Sam Roe, "OSHA Offers Tests for Staff Exposed to Deadly Beryllium," *Chicago Tribune*, April 24, 2004, sec. 1, 13. Quotations are from Finkel, PCE. OSHA also "did not target the offer of testing at those with the highest exposures" or even warn them. Instead, OSHA "simply told every inspector" about eligibility. It ignored the fact that some inspectors had received 50 times the beryllium dose necessary to cause disease.

According to the *Chicago Tribune*, Newman also faulted the OSHA letters. He claimed the agency downplayed the risks and did not encourage testing. He said OSHA failed to note that simply walking through a beryllium area for a few minutes might be enough to cause disease.

8. The PEER material is from Charles Offutt, "More Than a Thousand Whistleblower Cases Dumped," February 23, 2005; www.peer.org/news/news_id.php?row_id=483; accessed November 30, 2005. According to court documents (www.peer.org/news/news_id.php?row_id=600; see www.peer.org/news/news_id.php?row_id=600; accessed November 30, 2005), the U.S. OSC has championed one federal employee who has claimed retaliation against him. This was a Smithsonian worker who claimed he was harassed for supporting creationism instead of evolution. The U.S. OSC wrote him a supportive 11-page legal brief even though it concluded it had no jurisdiction over his case. Quotations are from Finkel, PCE, except for one from Jeff Ruch, email to Kristin Shrader-Frechette, November 29, 2005.

9. Sixel, "OSHA May Be Falling Short." Carey, "Beryllium Exposure." U.S. Freedom of Information Act (FOIA) information is from Finkel, PCE. Finkel PCE, adds: "Whether it was out of fear, apathy, disagreement over the facts, or antipathy" to him personally, he "got essentially no help over the years from anyone who might have been expected to help [exposed workers]," including fellow OSHA officials. One fellow regional administrator said: "If any of my inspectors breathed too much beryllium, it was their own damn fault." Finkel also says he received help neither from "the medical staff at OSHA" nor "the union that represents the inspectors themselves. The union president, Ron Yarman, immediately called Davis Layne to complain that Finkel had called him to offer to help further in providing testing to all his constituents."

10. First Finkel quotation is from Carey, "Beryllium Exposure." Second (long) quotation is from Finkel, PCE. Remaining Finkel statements are from Adam Finkel, PCE, "Email to Kristin Shrader-Frechette," September 9, 2005.

11. Finkel, PCE.

12. Finkel, PCE.

13. Devra Davis, *When Smoke Ran Like Water* (New York: Basic Books, 2002), 272.

14. See, for instance, Peter Singer, *One World* (New Haven, CT: Yale University Press, 2002), and Peter Unger, *Living High and Letting Die* (New York: Oxford University Press, 1996).

15. Quoted material is from APHA, "Human Rights in the Curricula for Health Professionals"; www.apha.org/legislative/policy/policysearch/index.cfm?fuseaction=view&id=165, policy 9813. See APHA, "Public Health Code of Ethics"; www.apha.org/codeofethics/ethics.htm; and "APHA's Principles on Public Health and Human Rights"; www.apha.org/wfpha?PrincPH1.htm; as well as policies 2000314, 2000323, 2002-5, and 9924 from 2000, 2000, 2002, and 1999, respectively, at www.apha.org/legislative/policy/policysearch/index.cfm?fuseaction=search_results; all accessed March 17, 2005. For discussion of the APHA statement, see A. W. Nichols, "Amending the United States Constitution to Include Environmental Rights," *Nation's Health* 27, no. 8 (September 1997): 18–19.

16. Ronald Dworkin, *Taking Rights Seriously* (Cambridge, Mass.: Harvard University Press, 1977). For APHA statements on rights to know, for instance, see APHA policies 8714 and 8416; www.apha.org/legislative/policy/policysearch/index.cfm?fuseaction=view&id=1143, 1078; accessed March 16, 2006. For

similar rights-based approaches in public health, see R. P. Claude and B. H. Weston (eds.), *Human Rights in the World Community* (Philadelphia: University of Pennsylvania Press, 1992). J. Mann, et al., "Health and Human Rights," *Health and Human Rights* 1, no. 1 (1994): 7–23. S. R. Benatar, "Global Disparities in Health and Human Rights," *American Journal of Public Health* 88, no. 2 (1998): 295–300. Paul Farmer, "Pathologies of Power: Rethinking Health and Human Rights," *American Journal of Public Health* 89, no. 10 (1999): 1486–96. A. Ugalde and J. T. Jackson, "The World Bank and International Health Policy: A Critical Review," *Journal of International Development* 7, no. 3 (1995): 525–541. B. I. Hamm, "A Human Rights Approach to Development," *Human Rights Quarterly* 23, no. 4 (2001): 1005–31. P. Braveman and S. Gruskin, "Poverty, Equity, Human Rights and Health," *Bulletin of the World Health Organization* 81, no. 7 (2003): 1–13. N. Kass, "An Ethics Framework for Public Health," *American Journal of Public Health* 91, no. 11 (2001): 1776–82. L. Gostin and J. Mann, "Towards the Development of a Human Rights Impact Assessment for the Formulation and Evaluation of Public Health Policies," *Human Rights and Health* 1, no. 1 (1994): 58–80. A. E. Yamin, "The Right to Health under International Law and its Relevance to the United States," *American Journal of Public Health* 95, no. 7(2005): 1156–61. By definition, the discussion here of human rights applies only to humans. For discussion of the larger question of duties to other beings, see Peter Singer (ed.), *In Defense of Animals* (Oxford: Blackwell, 2006); Singer, *Animal Liberation* (New York: HarperCollins, 2002); Singer, *Writings on an Ethical Life* (New York: HarperCollins, 2000); and Singer, *How Are We to Live?* (Amherst, Mass.: Prometheus, 1995).

17. Dworkin, *Taking Rights Seriously*, 267–279; Jeremy Bentham, "A Critical Examination of the Declaration of Rights," in *Bentham's Political Thought*, ed. Bhiku Parekh (New York: Barnes and Noble, 1973); see next note.

18. Dworkin, *Taking Rights Seriously*. Henry Shue, *Basic Rights* (Princeton: Princeton University Press), 1980. See previous note and Ian Brownlie (ed.), *Basic Documents on Human Rights* (Oxford: Clarendon Press, 1981). Alan Gewirth, *Human Rights* (Chicago: University of Chicago Press, 1982). David Lyons (ed.), *Rights* (Belmont, Calif.: Wadsworth, 1979). Rex Martin, *Rawls and Rights* (Lawrence: University Press of Kansas, 1986). James Nickel, *Making Sense of Human Rights* (Berkeley: University of California Press, 1987). John Rawls, *A Theory of Justice* (Cambridge, Mass.: Harvard University Press, 1971). Kristin Shrader-Frechette, "Natural Rights and Human Vulnerability: Aquinas, MacIntyre, and Rawls," *Public Affairs Quarterly* 16, no. 2 (April 2002): 99–124. Kristin Shrader-Frechette, "MacIntyre on Human Rights," *The Modern Schoolman* LXXIX no. 1 (November 2001): 1–21. United Nations materials on rights are at United Nations, Universal Declaration of Human Rights; www1.umn.edu/humanrts/instree/b1udhr.htm; accessed March 15, 2006. For codes of medical ethics, see World Medical Association, "World Medical Association Declaration of Helsinki: Ethical Principles for Medical Research Involving Human Subjects," *Journal of the American Medical Association* 284, no. 23 (2000): 3043–45. P. Riis, "Perspectives on the Fifth Declaration of Helsinki," *Journal of the American Medical Association* 284, no. 23 (2000): 3045–46. *The Declaration of Helsinki;* www.wma.net/e/policy/b3.htm. *The Nuremberg Code;* www.ushmm.org/research/doctors/Nuremberg_Code.htm. *The Declaration of Geneva;* www.wma.net/e/policy/c8.htm. *The International Code of Medical Ethics;* www

.wma.net/e/policy/c8.htm, all accessed March 15, 2006. See also Ludwig Edelstein, *The Hippocratic Oath* (Baltimore: Johns Hopkins University Press, 1943).

19. See previous note. Much of this rights account is from Dworkin, *Taking Rights Seriously*, and Thomas Pogge, *World Poverty and Human Rights* (Cambridge: Polity, 2002), 56ff.; quotation is from 64. For dissenters to human rights, see A. S. Preis, "Human Rights as Cultural Practice," *Human Rights Quarterly* 18, no. 2 (1986): 286–315.

20. This rights account relies on Dworkin, *Taking Rights Seriously*, and Pogge, *World Poverty and Human Rights*, 47–48, 70, 214. See previous two notes and UNICEF, *State of the World's Children, 2005* (New York: UNICEF, 2005); Natural Resources Defense Council, *Our Children at Risk* (Washington, D.C.: Natural Resources Defense Council, 1997). United Nations, *Convention on the Rights of the Child*; www1.umn.edu/humanrts/instree/k2crc.htm; both accessed March 15, 2006. Children's Defense Fund, *Key Facts about American Children*, August 2004; www.childrensdefense.org/data/keyfacts.asp; accessed March 16, 2006. Children's Defense Fund, *Where America Stands*, August 2004; www .childrensdefense.org/data/america.asp; accessed March 16, 2006.

21. Although they do not concern environmental injustice, Pogge, *World Poverty and Human Rights*, 208–210, and Rawls, *A Theory of Justice*, 54–60, 258–284, 453–462, make similar arguments.

22. The 40 percent figure is from David Pimentel, "Ecology of Increasing Disease," *BioScience* 48, no. 10 (October 1998): 817–827. The APHA statements on the millions at risk and on 100,000 workplace-related deaths are APHA policies 8714, 8416, and 9606; www.apha.org/legislative/policy/policysearch/index.cfm?fuseaction=view&id=1143, 1078, 124; accessed March 16, 2006. The U.S. regulation of annual risks, whose proability exceeds one in a million, is substantiated in Kristin Shrader-Frechette, *Risk and Rationality* (Berkeley: University of California Press, 1991), 71–72.

23. In turn, as the APHA noted in 1998, "human-rights violations have direct effects on people's health and quality of life." (APHA, "Human Rights in the Curricula for Health Professionals," policy 9813; www.apha.org/legislative/policy/policysearch/index.cfm?fuseaction=view&id=165; accessed March 15, 2006.)

24. Pogge, *World Poverty and Human Rights*, 21; see also 15–20, 96–117. See Joel Feinberg, *Doing and Deserving* (Princeton: Princeton University Press, 1970); Peter French, *Collective and Corporate Responsibility* (New York: Columbia University Press, 1984); Jonathan Glover, *Responsibility* (London: Routledge, 1970); Michael Zimmerman, *An Essay on Moral Responsibility* (Savage, Md.: Rowman and Littlefield, 1987).

25. U. S. Environmental Protection Agency, *Automobiles and Ozone*, EPA 400-F-92-006 (Washington, DC: EPA, 1992).

26. California Air Resources Board, *California's Air Quality History*; http://www.arb.ca.gov/html/brochure/history.htm and accessed 11-6-06.

27. European Environment Agency, *Air Quality and Ancillary Benefits of Climate-Change Policies* (Copenhagen: EEA, 2006), p. 16.

28. Peter Wahlin and Finn Palmgren, *Source Apportionment of Particles and Particulates (PM10) Measured by DMA and TEOM in a Copenhagen Street Canyon* (Roskilde, Denmark: National Environmental Research Institute, 2000).

29. California Air Resources Board, *50 Things You Can Do*; http://www.arb .ca.gov/html/brochure/50things.htm and accessed 11-7-06.

30. "Automakers Sue California over Auto Emissions," *Daily Auto Insider*, December 9, 2004; http://www.caranddriver.com/dailyautoinsider/8976/auto makers-sue-california-over-auto-emissions.html and accessed 11-6-06. Union of Concerned Scientists, *Automaker Lobbyists Seek to Keep Oregon Autos Polluting*, August 17, 2005; www.ucsusa.org/clean_vehicles/avp/automaker-v-the-people-oregon-response.html and accessed November 7, 2006.

31. U. S. Environmental Protection Agency. *Pesticide Industry Sales and Usage* (Washington, DC: U. S. EPA, 1997), Tables 10, 4.

32. Whole Foods Market, *One Year after USDA Organic Standards are Enacted More Americans are Consuming Organic Food* (Austin, TX: Whole Foods Market, 2006); http://www.wholefoodsmarket.com/company/pr_10-14-03 .html and accessed December 14, 2006.

33. See notes 92–97 in chapter 1. American Public Health Association, Precautionary Principle, and Environmental Defense Fund, *Legacy of Lead* (Washington, DC: EDF, March 1990). Bureau of Mines, *Mineral Commodity Summaries*, (Washington, DC: US Department of the Interior, 1989), pp. 90–91. (1988 data are converted from metric tons to short tons; one metric ton equals about 2,200 pounds, while a US or short ton equals 2,000 pounds.) Clean Air Council, Children's Environmental Health (Washington, DC: CAC, 2006); http://www.cleanair.org/CEH/CEHHazards.html#lead and accessed November 6, 2006.

34. Keith E. Forrester and Richard W. Goodwin, "Engineering Management of Msw Ashes: Field Empirical Observations of Concrete-like Characteristics." In Theodore G. Brna and Raymond Klicius, eds., Vol. I, *Proceedings of International Conference on Municipal Waste Combustion*, Hollywood, FL, April 11–14, 1989, En 40-11/14-1989e (Ottawa, Canada: Minister of Supply and Services Canada, 1989), 5b–16b.

35. For Chicago pollution data see chapter 1, and Kristin Shrader-Frechette, *Environmental Justice: Creating Equality, Reclaiming Democracy* (New York: Oxford University Press, 2002), 71–74.

36. Pogge, *World Poverty and Human Rights*, 50, 197, makes similar points. For Wal-Mart abuses, see N. Lichtenstein, *Wal-Mart* (New York: New Press, 2006), J. Norman, *The Case Against Wal-Mart* (Atlantic City, N.J.: Raphael, 2004), and Anthony Bianco and Wendy Zeller, "Is Wal-Mart Too Powerful?" *Business Week*, no. 3852 (October 10, 2003), 100–110. Liza Featherstone, "Wal-Mart Values," *Nation* 275, no. 21 (December 16, 2002), 11. Bob Ortega, "Ban the Bargains," *Wall Street Journal* 224, no. 71 (October 11, 1994), A1. David M. Halbfinger, "Taking On a Giant," *New York Times* 154, no. 53232 (June 6, 2005): E1–E7. APHA echoes this citizen responsibility in APHA, "The Role of Public Health in Ensuring Healthy Communities," policy 9521; www.apha.org/ legislative/policy/policysearch/index.cfm?fuseaction=view&id=116; accessed March 15, 2006; and APHA, "Reforming the Health-Care Delivery System"; www .apha.org/legislative/issues/reform.htm; accessed March 15, 2006.

37. Sweatshop, clothing, and economic data are from Ellen Rosen, *Making Sweatshops* (Berkeley: University of California Press, 2002), 2–3, 226–227, 224–235; see 1–12. See also J. V. Millen and T. H. Holtz, "Transnational Corporations and the Health of the Poor," in J. Y. Kim, J. V. Millen, A. Irwin, and J. Gershman (eds.), *Dying for Growth: Global Inequality and the Health of the Poor* (Monroe, ME: Common Courage Press, 2000), 177–223. D. M. Shilling and R. Rosenbaum, "Principles for Global Corporate Responsibility," *Business*

and Society Review 95, no. 94 (summer 1995): 55–56. R. Labonte, "Global-ization, Trade, and Health," in *Health and Social Justice*, ed. Richard Hofrichter (Hoboken, N.J.: Wiley, 2003), 469–500.

38. David Roodman, *How Much Does the U.S. Help?* (Washington, D.C.: Center for Global Development, 2005); www.cgdev.org/content/opinion/detail/2959/; accessed May 10, 2006.

39. W. Boyd, "Death of a Writer," *New Yorker* 71, no. 38 (November 27, 1995), 51–55. A. Adams, "A State's Well-Oiled Injustice," *World Press Review* 43, no. 1 (January 1996): 14–15; D. Pypke, "Partners in Crime," *World Press Review* 43, no. 1 (January 1996): 16; H. Harington, "A Continent's New Pariah," *Banker* 145, no. 838 (December 1995): 63–64; D. Knott, "Shell the Target after Nigerian Executions," *Oil and Gas Journal* 93, no. 47 (November 20, 1995): 37; A. Anderson, "A Day in the Death of Ideals," *New Scientist* 148, no. 2005 (November 25, 1995): 3. Guy Arnold, *Third World Handbook* (London: Cassell, 1996), and Yozo Yokota, "International Justice and the Global Environment," *Journal of International Affairs* 54, no. 2 (spring 1999): 583–599. See also D. Kupfer, "Worldwide Shell Boycott," *Progressive* 60, no. 1 (January 1996): 13; Andrew Rowell and Andrea Goodall, *Shell Shocked* (Amsterdam: Greenpeace, 1994); www.greenpeace.org/~commons/ken/hell.html.

Shell's position is outlined in Shell Nigeria, *Human Rights* (Lagos: Shell Petroleum Development Company of Nigeria, 2001); www.shellnigeria.com/frame.asp?Page=hr. and accessed May 10, 2006, in Sir Mark Moody-Stuart (chair of Shell Committee of Managing Directors), *People, Planets, and Profits* (Lagos: Shell Nigeria, 2001); www.shellnigeria.com/frame.asp?Page=Planets; and in Shell Nigeria, *Compensation* (Lagos: Shell Petroleum Development Company of Nigeria, 2001); www.shellnigeria.com/frame.asp?Page=OgergyInformation AdminisoniIssue–all accessed May 10, 2006.

For information on U.S. value-of-life presuppositions in benefit-cost analysis and regulation, see Shrader-Frechette, *Environmental Justice*, 176, 135. For U.S. government information about Shell, see U.S. Energy Information Administration, *Nigeria Environmental Issues* (Washington, D.C.: DOE, April 2000); www.eia.doe.gov/emeu/cabs/nigonv.html. See also U.S. Energy Information Administration, *Nigeria* (Washington, D.C.: DOE, April 2001); www.eia.doe.gov/emeu/cabs/nigeria.html. For additional Shell information see Shrader-Frechette, *Environmental Justice*, 118–120.

40. Re future oil extraction, see "ExxonMobil Nigeria Targets 1mm bpd Output by 2010," *Alexander's Gas and Oil Connections* 10, no. 14 (July 20, 2005); www.gasandoil.com/goc/company/cna52971.htm; accessed May 10, 2006. Re oil-company behavior, see Human Rights Watch, *Letter to Chevron Nigeria* (New York: Human Rights Watch, 2003), www.hrw.org/press/2003/04/nigeria 040703chevron.htm, and R. Devraj, *Nigeria Women in Oil-Rich Delta Region Protest*, report 2401 (Kuala Lumpur, Malaysia: TWN, 2002); www.sjp.ac.lk/careers/dec17/twn/twnf.htm; all accessed May 10, 2006.

41. The Massachusetts Myanmar information is from Kenny Bruno and Jim Valette, "Cheney and Halliburton: Go Where the Oil Is," *Multinational Monitor* 22, no. 5 (May 2001), http://multinationalmonitor.org/mm2001/01may/may01 corp10.html; accessed May 10, 2006. Other information is from Chris Jochnick, "Amazon Oil Offensive: Human Rights Violations in the Oriente, Ecuador," *Multinational Monitor* 16, nos. 1–2 (January 1995): 12–16. Suzana Sawyer, *The Politics of Petroleum* (Minneapolis: University of Minnesota MacArthur Program,

1997). Mike Tidwell, *Amazon Stranger* (New York: Lyons and Burford, 1996). Jason Clay, "Looking Back to Go Forward," in *State of the Peoples: A Global Human Rights Report on Societies,* ed. Mark Miller (Boston: Beacon Press, 1993), 66. Center for Economic and Social Rights, *Rights Violations in the Ecuadorian Amazon* (New York: Center for Economic and Social Rights, 1994), 1. Project Underground, *Independent Annual Report for the Royal Dutch/Shell Group of Companies* (Berkeley: Project Underground, 1997), 6. Project Underground, *Indigenous Communities at the Edge* (Berkeley: Project Underground, 1998); www.moles.org/ProjectUnderground/motherlode/drilling/sacred.html; accessed May 10, 2006. See also *Amazon Oil,* vol. 16; www.advocacynet.org/news_view/news_188.html all accessed May 10, 2006.

42. See Michael Klare, *Blood and Oil* (New York: Henry Holt, 2004), 113ff and Project Underground: Supporting the Human Rights of Communities Resisting Mining and Oil Exploitation, *Kyoto Oilwatch Declaration* (Berkeley: Project Underground, 1997); www.moles.org/ProjectUnderground/alerts/kyoto .html; all accessed May 10, 2006; see also previous 4 notes.

43. Douglas Koplow and Aaron Martin, *Fueling Global Warming* (Cambridge, Mass.: Industrial Economics, 1998). "Big Oil and Its Subsidies," *Economist* 358, no. 8212 (March 10, 2001): 80.

44. David Malin Roodman, *Paying the Piper: Subsidies, Politics, and the Environment* (Washington, D.C.: Worldwatch, 1996), argues that environmentally destructive subsidies are a net loss and cost consumers and taxpayers more than $500 billion annually. B. Fischlowitz-Roberts, *Restructuring Taxes to Protect the Environment* (Washington, D.C.: Earth Policy Institute, 2002) Others (like Thomas Friedman, "A Million Manhattan Projects," *New York Times* CLV, no. 53,589 (Wednesday May 24, 2006): A27) accept the standard economic dictum that, because governments, like that of the United States, subsidize oil, consumers do not pay the full cost.

45. See note 34.

46. Quotation is from Pogge, *World Poverty and Human Rights,* 25.

47. APHA, "The Health Effects of Militarism," policy 8531; www.apha.org/legislative/policy/policysearch/index.cfm?fuseaction=view&id=1113; accessed March 15, 2006. See R. L. Sivard, *World Military and Social Expenditures* (Washington, D.C.: World Priorities, 1996), 1–10; 30–38, and H. W. Cohen et al, "Bioterrorism Initiatives," *American Journal of Public Health* 89, no. 11 (1999): 1629–31.

48. These different responsibility scenarios mirror Pogge, *World Poverty and Human Rights,* 41–42.

49. Respective quotations are from APHA, "Protecting Health-Care Accessibility and Quality in a Profit-Oriented Market," policy number 9702; www.apha .org/legislative/policy/policysearch/index.cfm?fuseaction=view&id=136; accessed March 15, 2006, and APHA, "Endorsement of Public Interest Law Groups," policy 7431; www.apha.org/legislative/policy/policysearch/index.cfm?fuseaction=view &id=773; accessed same date. The philosophical arguments are in Rawls, *A Theory of Justice,* ch. 5; Aristotle, *Nicomachean Ethics,* trans. A. K. Thomson (Harmondsworth, England: Penguin, 1976), bk. 5, ch. 4; Thomas Campbell, *Justice* (Basingstoke, England: Macmillan, 1988), ch. 8; Judith Jarvis Thomson, *Rights, Restitution and Risk* (Cambridge, Mass.: Harvard University Press, 1986).

50. Examples of APHA statements on health threats from racism, chemical threats, and nuclear technology, respectively, are policies 7425, 8223, 8324,

8325, 8523, 9926, and 20017; 2005-5, 2005-6, 2005-7, 2004-5, 2002-5, 2002-13, 20008, 20009, 9910, 9912, 9909, 9806, 9712, 9607, 9494, 9206, 9205, 8912, 8726, 8714, 8511, 8416; and 2004-06, 2003-24, 2001-19, 200032, 9931, 9932, 9911, 9804, 9605, 8917, 8918, 8715, 8531, 8407, 8307; www.apha.org/legislative/policy/policysearch/; accessed March 15, 2006.

51. See the next 15 notes and Kevin Phillips, *Wealth and Democracy* (New York: Broadway, 2002), 79. APHA recomendations are 20005, 200020, 9811, 9710, 9717, 9611, 9508, and 2005-3, LB-9, 2004-09, 2003-22, 2003-19, 2002-6; www.apha.org/legislative/policy/policysearch; accessed March 15, 2006.

52. Phillips, *Wealth and Democracy*, 151–155; see 47–107. Kevin Phillips, "The Progressive Interview," *Progressive* 66, no. 9 (September 2002): 37 of 33–37. Lawrence Mishel, Jared Bernstein, and John Schmitt, *The State of Working America, 2000/2001* (Ithaca, N.Y.: Economic Policy Institute, Cornell University Press, 2001). Thomas Piketty and Emmanuel Saez, "Income Inequality in the United States, 1913–1998," National Bureau of Economic Research, working paper no. W8467 (Washington, D.C.: National Bureau of Economic Research, 2001).

53. Phillips, *Wealth and Democracy*, 134.

54. Federal Receipts and Outlays, *Economic Report of the President* (Washington, D.C.: U.S. Government Printing Office, 2001); Lewis and Allison, *The Cheating of America* (New York: Harper-Collins, 2002), 135–137. Phillips, *Wealth and Democracy*, 149, 156. I. Shapiro and R. Greenstein, "The Widening Income Gulf," The Center on Budget and Policy Priorities, 9-4-99; www.cbpp.org/9-4-99tax-rep.htm; accessed November 4, 2005; "Taxes: Hidden Treasure," *Economist* 314, no. 7638 (January 20, 1990): 24–25. Phillips, *Wealth and Democracy*, 114, 132, 96, 221–222.

55. For these statistics on U.S. quality of life, manufacturing pay, and human development, see The Economist, *Pocket World in Figures 2007* (London: Profile, 2006), 30, 56–65. David Cay Johnston, "$12 Billion in Profit, No Corporate Taxes," *International Herald Tribune,* October 21, 2000, 16. Iris Marion Young, *Inclusion and Democracy* (New York: Oxford, 2000), 34, 48. See also James Gobert, Maurice Punch, "Whistleblowers, the Public Interest, and the Public Interest Disclosure Act of 1998," *Modern Law Review* 63, no. 1 (January 1, 2000): 25–54. H. Inhaber and S. Carroll, *How Rich Is Too Rich?* (New York: Praeger, 1992), ix. See also Institute on Taxation and Economic Policy, *Tax Expenditures: The Hidden Entitlements* (Washington, D.C., Institute on Taxation and Economic Policy, 1996); Institute on Taxation and Economic Policy, *Corporate Income Taxes in the 1990s* (Washington, D.C., Institute on Taxation and Economic Policy, 2000); and "The Unlikeliest Scourge," *Economist* 364, no. 8281 (13 July 2002): 16–19. See also, for example, R. Marcus, "Judges Take Free Trips in Conflict of Interest," *Seattle Times,* April 9, 1998, A3.

56. House Democratic Policy Committee, *Who Is Downsizing the American Dream?* (Washington, D.C.: US Government Printing Office, 1996), and Phillips, *Wealth and Democracy*, 162–163. Jeff Gates, *Democracy at Risk* (New York: Perseus Books, 2000); Michael Klepper and Robert Gunther, *The Wealthy 100* (Secaucus, N.J.: Citadel Press, 1996).

57. Institute for Research on Poverty, *Who Was Poor in 2004?* (Madison, WI: IRP, 2004). Marc and Marque-Luisa Miringhoff, *The Social Health of the Nation* (New York: Oxford University Press, 1999); Phillips, *Wealth and Democracy*, 344–346, 123, 113; see Lewis Lapham, *Money and Class in America* (New York: Ballantine Books, 1989). See *The Economist* Intelligence Unit's Quality-of-Life

Index, 2005; http://www.economist.com/media/pdf/QUALITY_OF_LIFE.pdf search-%22us%20quality%20of%20life%22; accessed 22 September 2006.

58. Phillips, *Wealth and Democracy*, 79, 111, 361–362, 396, and Andrew Hacker, *Money* (New York; Touchstone, 1997). See chapter 1 statistics.

59. David Cay Johnston, "At the Very Top, a Surge in Income in '03," *New York Times*, CLV, no. 53,358 (October 5, 2005), C4.

60. For infant-mortality data, see U.S. Central Intelligence Agency, *The World Factbook* (Washington, D.C.: U.S. Central Intelligence Agency, 2004); www .cia.gov/cia/publications/factbook/rankorder2091rank.htm; accessed January 21, 2005. U.S. CDC, *Infant Morality Fact Sheet* (Washington, D.C.: CDC, 2005); www.cdc.gov/omh/AMH/factsheets/infant.htm; accessed January 21, 2005. Nicholas D. Kristof, "Health Care? Ask Cuba," *New York Times* CLIV, No. 53,092 (January 12, 2005), A23; nytimes.com/2005/01/12/opinion/12kris.htm?hp.

61. Michael Wolff, Peter Rutten, Albert Bayers, and the World Bank Research Team, *Where We Stand* (New York: Bantam, 1992), 23, Phillips, 124; chapters 1–3 here, and previous sections of this chapter.

62. Wolff et al., *Where We Stand*, 113.

63. CDC, *Vital Statistics* (Washington, D.C.: Government Printing Office, 1992), mortality data for 1950–1991. For black pregnancy statistics, see CDC, *Monthly Vital Statistics Report*, vol. 43, no. 12 (1991).

64. George A. Kaplan et al., "Inequality and Income and Mortality in the United States," *British Medical Journal* 312 (1996): 999–1003.

65. Phillips, *Wealth and Democracy*, 151–155. Kevin Phillips, The Progressive Interview, *Progressive*, 37 of 33–37; Lawrence Mishel et al., *The State of Working America*, and Piketty and Saez, "Income Inequality in the United States, 1913–1998."

66. Phillips, *Wealth and Democracy*, 320, 309. Jon Winokur, *The Rich Are Different* (New York: Random House, 1996).

67. Michael Janofsky, "Big Tobacco, in Court Again. But the Stock Is Still Up," *New York Times* CLIV, no. 53,306 (August 14, 2005), 15A.

68. E.g., Henry Payne, "Environmental Injustice," *Reason* 29, no. 4 (August/September 1997): 53–56. David Friedman, "The Environmental Racism Hoax," *American Enterprise* 9, no. 6 (November/December 1998): 75.

69. For arguments and data showing that the poor do not prefer pollution because of its compensatory benefits, see Shrader-Frechette, *Environmental Justice*, 15–18, chs. 4–5.

70. For discussion of these arguments, see previous note. The compensation objection is discussed partly in Christopher Boerner and Thomas Lambert, "Environmental Injustice," in *Taking Sides*, ed. Theodore Goldfarb (Guilford, Conn.: McGraw-Hill, 1997), 73–75. Regarding medical ethics, see Bruce Jennings, Jeffrey Kahn, Anna Mastroianni, and Lisa Parker, eds. *Ethics and Public Health* (Washington, D.C.: Association of Schools of Public Health, 2003); also National Research Council, *Intentional Human Dosing Studies* (Washington, D.C.: National Academy Press, 2004). Science Advisory Board of the EPA, *Testing Human Subjects*, EPA-SAB-EC-00–017 (Washington, D.C.: EPA, 2000). See also Christopher Oleskey, Alan Fleischman, Lynn Goldman, Kurt Hirschhorn, Philip J. Landrigan, Marc Lappe, Mary Faith Marshall, Herbert Needleman, Rosamond Rhodes, and Michael McCally, "Pesticide Testing in Humans," *Environmental Health Perspectives* 112, no. 8 (June 2004): 914–919.

71. See, for example, D. Harmest and J. Wolfe, "Compensating Wage Differentials," *Journal of Labor Economics* 8, no. 1 (1990): S175–S197.

72. C. Daniel and C. Sofer, "Bargaining, Compensating Wage Differentials, and Dualism of the Labor Market," *Journal of Labor Economics* 16, no. 3 (1998): 546–576. P. Dorman and P. Hagstrom, "Wage Compensation for Dangerous Work Revisited," *Industrial and Labor Relations Review* 52, no. 1 (1998): 116–136. M. Moore, "Unions, Employment Risks, and Market Provision of Employment Risk Differentials," *Journal of Risk and Uncertainty* 10, no. 1 (1995): 57–70; see also Shrader-Frechette, Environmental Justice, 135–162.

73. Shrader-Frechette, *Environmental Justice,* 135–162.

74. Ibid., 17–19; see also David Pimental, "Assessment of Environmental and Economic Impacts of Pesticide Use," in *Technology and Values,* ed. Kristin Shrader-Frechette and Laura Westra (Savage, Md.: Rowman and Littlefield, 1997), 371–414. B. Gerhardson, "Biological Substitutes for Pesticides," *Trends in Biotechnology* 20, no. 8 (August 2007): 338–44.

75. For defense of the argument that economic expansion does not promote equality, see Shrader-Frechette, *Risk and Rationality,* 116–121; for defense of the argument that economic expansion typically does not justify human-rights violations, see 140–142. The point about allowing inequality is in William Frankena, "The Concept of Social Justice," in *Social Justice,* ed. Richard Brandt (Englewood Cliffs, N.J.: Prentice-Hall, 1962), 9–15.

76. Peter Singer, *How Are We to Live,* 106–128.

77. Davis, *When Smoke Ran Like Water,* xix. For APHA statements on pesticide dangers and how they can be reduced, see, for instance, policies 20008, 20009, 9909, 9907, 9511, 8726; www.apha.org/legislative/policy/policysearch/index.cfm?fuseaction=search_results—and insert the search term "pesticide"; accessed May 10, 2006. For defenses of the no-viable-alternatives argument, see Boerner and Lambert, "Environmental Injustice," 76–77 of 67–79. D. Payne and C. Raiborn, "Sustainable Development," *Journal of Business Ethics* 32, no. 2 (July 2001): 157–168.

78. See Pogge, *World Poverty and Human Rights,* 211–213. Shrader-Frechette, *Environmental Justice,* last chapter.

79. Viktor Frankl, *Man's Search for Meaning,* trans. Ilse Lasch (London: Hodder and Stoughton, 1964). Singer, *How Are We to Live,* 211–212, 9, 146–193. Shrader-Frechette, *Environmental Justice,* last chapter.

80. Robert Bellah, Richard Madsen, William Sullivan, Ann Swidler, and Steve Tipton, *Habits of the Heart* (Berkeley: University of California Press, 1985). Robert Coles, *The Call of Service* (Boston: Houghton Mifflin, 1993). Singer, *How Are We to Live,* 235; see also 219ff.

81. Singer, *How Are We to Live,* 154–157.

82. M. Gromyko and A. Hellman (eds.), *Breakthrough* (New York: Walker, 1988).

Chapter 5

1. Jim Schwab, *Deeper Shades of Green* (San Francisco: Sierra Club Books, 1994), 1–3. Bonnie Miller Rubin, "Robbins Has Many Uses for Windfall," *Chicago Tribune* 148, no. 336 (December 2, 1994), sec. 2SW, 1.

2. Schwab, *Deeper Shades of Green*, 4. For the EPA claim, see Jeff Long, "Chicago, Environmental Agency Work on Clean Air Tradeoffs," *Chicago Tribune* 154, no. 252 (Sept. 14, 2000).

3. "Corrections and Clarifications," *Chicago Tribune* 149, no. 153 (June 2, 1995), sec. 1, 3.

4. Mark Care, "Incinerator Vote Stokes Fire for Foes," *Chicago Tribune* 148, no. 244 (September 1, 1994), sec. 2SW, 6; Rubin, "Robbins Has Many Uses for Windfall," 1. See also Mark Care, "Robbins Incinerator Clears Finance Hurdle," *Chicago Tribune* 148, no. 328 (November 24, 1994), sec. 1, 1.

5. Ken O'Brien, "Robbins Burner Gets Boost," *Chicago Tribune* 148, no. 243 (August 31, 1994), sec. 2W, 1.

6. Schwab, *Deeper Shades of Green*, 3–8. See Care, "Robbins Incinerator Clears Finance Hurdle," 1, and "Cleaning the Air Slowly," *Chicago Tribune* 156, no. 176 (July 15, 2002); www.chicago.tribune.com and accessed December 12, 2005. Re U.S. air-pollution standards, see chapter 1.

7. "Robbins Incinerator Foes Are Rejected by High Court," *Chicago Tribune* 148, no. 343 (December 9, 1994), sec. 2, 8. See "Illinois Waste-Burner Put Back on Schedule," *Engineering News Record* 230, no. 9 (1993): 17.

8. Schwab, *Deeper Shades of Green*, 2–43. O'Brien, "Robbins Burner Gets Boost," 1; "Robbins Incinerator Foes Are Rejected by High Court," 8. Rubin, "Robbins Has Many Uses for Windfall," 1.

9. Mark Care, "South Suburban Incinerator Projects Are Lukewarm to Red Hot," *Chicago Tribune* 148, no. 347 (December 13, 1994), sec. 2C, 3. See Laura Westra and Peter Wenz (eds.), *Faces of Environmental Racism* (Lanham, Md.: Rowman and Littlefield, 1995), and Robert Bullard, *Dumping in Dixie* (Boulder, Colo.: Westview, 1990). See Frank Ackerman, *The Political Economy of Inequality* (Washington, D.C.: Island Press, 2000).

10. R. Ladenson, "The Social Responsibilities of Engineers and Scientists," in *Ethical Problems in Engineering*, ed. A. Flores (Troy, N.Y.: Center for Studies in Human Dimensions of Technology, 1980), 241–242. Stephanie Bird, "Responsibilities of Scientists and Engineers," *Science and Engineering Ethics* 8, no. 2 (April 2002): 130.

11. W. Frankena, *Ethics* (Englewood Cliffs, N.J.: Prentice-Hall, 1963), 37. W. D. Ross, *The Right and the Good* (London: Oxford University Press, 1973), 18ff. See also Singer, "Famine, Affluence, and Morality," in *Social Ethics*, ed. T. A. Mappes and J. S. Zembaty (New York: McGraw-Hill, 1977), 396–403. H. Jonas, *The Imperative of Responsibility* (Chicago: University of Chicago, 1985), 101ff., 128; Henry Shue, *Basic Rights* (Princeton: Princeton University Press, 1980), 139. Gerald Dworkin (ed.), *Mill's "On Liberty"* (Lanham, Md.: Rowman and Littlefield, 1997).

12. Thomas Pogge, *World Poverty and Human Rights* (Cambridge: Polity, 2002), 13, 22–24, makes similar arguments, for duties to prevent famine.

13. M. Bayles, *Professional Ethics* (Belmont, CA: Wodsworth, 1989), ch. 6, especially 142, 7. P. Camenisch, "On Being a Professional, Morally Speaking," in B. Baumrin and B. Freedman, *Moral Responsibility and the Professions* (New York: Haven, 1983), 44–45, 54–55.

14. See, for example, James Childress, "Fairness in the Allocation and Delivery of Health Care," in *A Time to Be Born and a Time to Die*, ed. Barry Kogan (New York: de Gruyter, 1991), 179–204, and Robert Veatch, "Equality, Justice, and Rightness in Allocating Health Care," in Kogan, *A Time to Be Born and a*

Time to Die, 205–218. Much of this discussion is based on Kristin Shrader-Frechette, *Ethics of Scientific Research* (Lanham, Md.: Rowman and Littlefield, 1994), 68–69.

15. Jonas, *The Imperative of Responsibility*, 128, 93ff. See also Singer, "Famine, Affluence, and Morality." Shue, "Exporting Hazards," in Brown and Shue, *Boundaries*, 135ff.; Elmer Hankiss, "The Loss of Responsibility," in *Political Responsibility of Intellectuals*, ed. I. Maclean, A. Montefiore, and P. Winch (Cambridge: Cambridge University Press, 1991), 29–52. Shrader-Frechette, *Ethics of Scientific Research*, 67–68, on which this discussion is based. Peter Singer, "Living High and Letting Die," *Philosophy and Phenomenological Research* 59, no. 1 (1999): 183–187. Peter Singer, *How Are We to Live?* (New York: Oxford University Press, 1997). For evaluations, see Dale Jamieson (ed.), *Singer and His Critics* (Oxford: Blackwell, 1999).

16. R. K. Colwell, "Natural and Unnatural History," in W. R. Shea and B. Sitter (eds.), *Scientists and Their Responsibility* (Canton, Mass.: Watson, 1989), 17. F. Von Hippel and J. Primack, "Public Interest Science," *Science* 177 (1972): 1169.

17. APHA, "Nestle Boycott," policy 8126; www.apha.org/legislative/policy/policysearch/index.cfm?fuseaction=view&id=998; all accessed March 14, 2006. Ian Brown quoted in Gavin Yamek, "Pop Musicians Boycott Promotion," *British Medical Journal* 322, no. 7280 (2001): 191. See also B. Exeter, "Campaigners for Breast Feeding Claim Partial Victory," *British Medical Journal* 322, no. 7280 (2001): 191.

18. Many of these arguments are in Kristin Shrader-Frechette, *Risk and Rationality* (Berkeley: University of California Press, 1991), 159–166, and Shrader-Frechette, *Ethics of Scientific Research*, 63–100. See J. Lichtenberg, "National Boundaries and Moral Boundaries," in Brown and Shue, *Boundaries*, 80ff. See J. Rawls, *The Law of Peoples* (Cambridge, Mass.: Harvard University Press, 1999), and J. Rawls, *A Theory of Justice*, rev. ed. (Cambridge, Mass.: Harvard University Press, 1999). See David B. Brushwood, "Riff v. Morgan Pharmacy," *Law, Medicine, and Health Care* 14, nos. 3–4 (September 1986): 202–205, and W. Feinberg (ed.), *Pharmacy Law Update 2003* 25, no. 1 (January 2003); www.wfprofessional.com/documents/January%202003.pdf search=%22Riff%20%20%22Morgan%20Pharmacy%22%22, accessed September 17, 2006.

19. American Association for the Advancement of Science, *Principles of Scientific Freedom and Responsibility* (Washington, D.C.: American Association for the Advancement of Science, 1980), 2. See also Institute of Electrical and Electronics Engineers, Committee on the Social Implications of Technology, *Ethical Problems in Engineering*, ed. R. Baum (Troy, N.Y.: Center for the Study of the Human Dimensions of Science and Technology, 1980), 88–90.

20. American Society of Biological Chemists, "Bylaws," 1977. National Society of Professional Engineers, "Criticism of Engineering in Products, Board of Ethical Review, Case No. 76.10," in Flores, *Ethical Problems in Engineering*, 206. Office of Government Ethics, *Standards of Ethical Conduct for Employees of the Executive Branch: Executive Order 12674—Principles of Ethical Conduct for Government Officers and Employees* (Washington, D.C.: Internal Revenue Service, 1993), 35042. See Bayles, *Professional Ethics*, 94, 109.

21. C. I. Jackson, *Honor in Science* (New Haven: Sigma Xi, 1986), 33. See also Steve Clark, "Informed Consent in Medicine," *Southern Journal of Philosophy* 39, no. 2 (2001): 169–187. Regarding professionals' responsibilities,

see Bayles, *Professional Ethics*, 4; Edsall et al., *Scientific Freedom and Responsibility*, 45.

22. American Association for the Advancement of Science, *Principles of Scientific Freedom and Responsibility*, rev. draft (Washington, D.C.: American Association for the Advancement of Science, 1980), 1, 6. Some of this discussion is from Shrader-Frechette, *Ethics of Scientific Research*, 64–67. S. Bok, "Whistleblowing and Professional Responsibilities," in *Engineering Professionalism and Ethics*, ed. J. Schaub, K. Pavlovic, and M. Morris (New York: Wiley, 1983), 413.

23. This point also is in J. Fishkin, *The Limits of Obligation* (New Haven: Yale University Press, 1982). See T. Nagel, *Mortal Questions* (New York: Cambridge University Press, 1979), 84. See also D. Lyons, "Review of *The Limits of Obligation* by J. Fishkin," *Ethics* 94, no. 2 (January 1984): 328–329, and Peter French, *The Spectrum of Responsibility* (New York: St. Martin's Press, 1991), 20; F. Feldman, "Comments on *Living High and Letting Die*," *Philosophy and Phenomenological Research* LIX, no. 1 (1999): 201, and Brad Hooker, "Sacrificing for the Good of Strangers—Repeatedly," *Philosophy and Phenomenological Research* LIX, no. 1 (1999): 180–181.

24. Joel Feinberg, *Doing and Deserving* (Princeton: Princeton University Press, 1970). See Shrader-Frechette, *Ethics of Scientific Research*. See note 23.

25. Joanna Armstrong Schellenberg, Cesar G. Victoria, Adiel Mushi, Don de Savigny, David Schellenberg, Hassan Mshinda, and Jennifer Bryce, "Inequities among the Very Poor," *Lancet* 361 (2003): 561–566. See notes 15, 23–24, 38, and later notes.

26. TV statistics are from U.S. Department of Education, National Center for Education Statistics, *The Condition of Education 2001* (Washington, D.C.: Government Printing Office, 2001), Donald F. Roberts, Ulla G. Foehr, Victoria J. Rideout, and Mollyann Brodie, *Kids and Media at the New Millennium* (Menlo Park, Calif.: Kaiser Family Foundation, November 1999), and U.S. Department of Education, National Center for Education Statistics, *Education in States and Nations* (Washington, D.C.: Government Printing Office, July 1996). See also Jerry Mander, "Who Benefits Most?" *Resurgence* 208 (September/October 2001): 12–15, and Jo Anne Grunbaum, Laura Kann, Steven A. Kinchen, Barbara Williams, James G. Ross, Richard Lowry, and Lloyd Kolbe, Centers for Disease Control and Prevention, U.S. CDC, Division of Adolescent and School Health, Youth Risk Behavior Surveillance System, *Youth Risk Behavior Surveillance 2001* (Washington, D.C.: CDC, 2002). Coffee statistics are from www.coffeeresearch.org/market/usa.htm and E Imports, "Specialty Coffee Statistics"; www.e-importz.com/Support/specialty_coffee.htm; both accessed December 3, 2005.

27. Henry Shue, "The Burdens of Justice," *Journal of Philosophy* 80, no. 30 (October 1983): 600–608, see 602ff., and H. Shue, "Exporting Hazards," in *Boundaries*, ed. P. Brown and H. Shue, *Boundaries* (Totowa, N.J.: Rowman and Littlefield, 1981), 135. See J. Sterba, *The Demands of Justice* (Notre Dame, Ind.: University of Notre Dame Press, 1980), chs. 2 and 6, for arguments for the rights of distant persons. See G. Brock and H. Brighouse (eds.) *The Political Philosophy of Cosmopolitanism* (Cambridge: Cambridge University Press, 2005).

28. In the very *general* sense understood here, methodological values include both tacit and conscious judgments, especially because they can be tied to *actions* as well as rules; indeed, value judgments made unintentionally are perhaps the most dangerous. See Helen Longino, *Science as Social Knowledge* (Princeton:

Princeton University Press, 1990), for Korenbrot information. For examples from the history of science, see Harold I. Brown, *Perception, Theory and Commitment* (Chicago: University of Chicago Press, 1977), 97–100, 147; Kristin Shrader-Frechette, "Recent Changes in the Concept of Matter," in *Philosophy of Science Association 1980*, ed. D. Asquith and R. N. Giere (East Lansing, Mich.: Philosophy of Science Association, 1980), 1:302ff.; and Kristin Shrader-Frechette, "Radiobiological Hormesis, Methodological Value Judgments, and Metascience," *Perspectives on Science* 8, no. 4 (2000): 367–379.

29. See Shrader-Frechette, *Science Policy, Ethics, and Economic Methodology* (Boston: Reidel, 1985), 73–74. Kristin Shrader-Frechette, "Scientific Method and the Objectivity of Epistemic Value Judgments," in *Logic, Methodology, and the Philosophy of Science*, ed. J. Fenstad, R. Hilpinen, and I. Frolov (New York: Elsevier Science, 1989), 373–389.

30. M. Midgley, *Wisdom, Information, and Wonder* (London: Routledge, 1991), 176.

31. M. Scriven, "The Exact Role of Value Judgments in Science," in *Introductory Readings in the Philosophy of Science*, ed. E. Klemke, R. Hollinger, and A. Kline (Buffalo: Prometheus, 1982), 277, and T. Nagel, *The View from Nowhere* (New York: Oxford University Press, 1986), 143–153. For more on those who seek infallibility, see K. Popper, *The Open Society and Its Enemies* (Princeton: Princeton University Press, 1950), 403–406. K. Popper, *The Logic of Scientific Discovery* (New York: Harper, 1965), 56. P. Feyerabend, "Changing Patterns of Reconstruction," *British Journal for the Philosophy of Science* 28, no. 4 (1977): 368.

32. See Shrader-Frechette, *Science Policy, Ethics, and Economic Methodology*, 183; Robert Audi, *The Structure of Justification* (New York: Cambridge University Press, 1993); Joseph Margolis, "On the Ethical Defense of Violence and Destruction," in *Philosophy and Political Action*, ed. Virginia Held, Kai Nielsen, and Charles Parsons (New York: Oxford University Press, 1972), 52–71. On Graham, see Sheldon Krimsky, *Science in the Private Interest* (New York: Rowman and Littlefield, 2003), 39–41.

33. See H. Siegel, "What Is the Question Concerning the Rationality of Science?" *Philosophy of Science* 52, no. 4 (1985): 524–526; R. Rudner, *Philosophy of Social Science* (Englewood Cliffs, N.J.: Prentice Hall, 1966), 4–5. See also W. H. Newton-Smith, "Popper, Science, and Rationality," *Philosophy*, supp. 39 (1995): 13.

34. See R. M. Hare, *Moral Thinking: Its Levels, Methods and Point* (Oxford: Oxford University Press, 1981).

35. On case studies and objectivity, see Shrader-Frechette, *Risk and Rationality*, 39–65, and Kristin Shrader-Frechette and Earl D. McCoy, *Method in Ecology* (Cambridge: Cambridge University Press, 1993), esp. 80–239. See also R. Newell, *Objectivity, Empiricism, and Truth* (New York: Routledge and Kegan Paul, 1986), and Frederick Stortland, "Wittgenstein," *Philosophical Investigations* 21, no. 3 (1998): 203–331.

36. Philip Kitcher, "The Division of Cognitive Labor," *Journal of Philosophy* 87, no. 1 (January 1990): 5–22. Because it is focused on answering the neutrality objection, this discussion avoids details of the complex debate over value judgments in science. See Philip Kitcher, *The Advancement of Science* (Oxford: Oxford University Press, 1995). Kitcher, *Science, Truth, and Democracy* (Oxford: Oxford University Press, 2001). Helen Longino, "Multiplying Subjects and the

Diffusion of Power," *Journal of Philosophy* 88, no. 11 (November 1991): 666–674; Helen E. Longino, *The Fate of Knowledge* (Princeton: Princeton University Press, 2001). Helen E. Longino, *Science as Social Knowledge* (Princeton: Princeton University Press, 1990). Kristin Shrader-Frechette, "Feminist Epistemology and Its Consequences for Policy," *Public Affairs Quarterly* 9, no. 2 (April 1995): 155–174. John Stuart Mill, *On Liberty* (Buffalo: Prometheus, 1986), 60–61. See Popper, *Conjectures and Refutations* (London: Routledge and K. Paul, 1969), especially ch. 11, and Popper, *The Logic of Scientific Discovery*, 106.

37. Israel Scheffler, "Discussion," *Philosophy of Science* 39, no. 3 (1972): 369. See Popper, *The Open Society and Its Enemies*, 403–406; Popper, *Conjectures and Refutations*, 63; I. Maso (ed.), *Openness in Research* (Assen: Gorcum, 1995). Some of this discussion relies on Shrader-Frechette, *Ethics of Scientific Research*, 55–61; National Research Council, *Science and Judgment in Risk Assessment* (Washington, D.C.: National Academy Press, 1996). Daniel Kahneman, Paul Slovic, and Amos Tversky (eds.), *Judgment under Uncertainty* (Cambridge: Cambridge University Press, 1982); Kahneman and Tversky (eds.), *Choices, Values and Frames* (Cambridge: Cambridge University Press, 2000). Anthony Kenny, *The Ivory Tower* (London: Blackwell, 1985), 41.

38. Re the uncertainty objection, see Singer, *One World* (New Haven: Yale University Press, March 2004); Singer, *Practical Ethics* (Cambridge: Cambridge University Press, 1993); Singer, *How Are We to Live*, and Singer, *Writings on an Ethical Life* (New York: Ecco, 2001). See also Peter Unger, *Living High and Letting Die* (Oxford: Oxford University Press, 1996), 6, for his discussion of the factual particulars of Third World child vaccination, mentioned here.

39. Aristotle, *Nicomachean Ethics*, bk. III, trans. W. D. Ross (Oxford: Oxford University Press, 1980). See also Joseph DeMarco, "Competence and Paternalism," *Bioethics* 16, no. 3 (2002): 231–245.

40. See Thomas Kerns, *Environmentally Induced Illnesses* (London: McFarland, 2001), 127, 136–144, 150–170; Devra Davis, *When Smoke Ran Like Water* (New York: Basic Books, 2002), 277; APHA, "Policy Statement 9606: The Precautionary Principle and Chemical Exposure Standards for the Workplace," *American Journal of Public Health* 87, no. 3 (March 1997): 500–501. For these arguments, see Shrader-Frechette, *Risk and Rationality*, 102, 131–145. See also Shrader-Frechette and McCoy, *Method in Ecology*, chs. 7–10. See, for example, National Research Council, *Science and Judgment in Risk Assessment*, 85–105. This discussion relies on Shrader-Frechette, *Ethics of Scientific Research*, 82–96. See also Ted Lockhart, *Moral Uncertainty and Its Consequences* (New York: Oxford University Press, 2000). Carl F. Cranor, "Learning from the Law to Address Uncertainty in the Precautionary Principle," *Science and Engineering Ethics* 7, no. 3 (2001): 313–326. See also Krimsky, *Science in the Private Interest*, 13–132. Bayles, *Professional Ethics*, 99ff. and Carl Cranor, *Regulating Toxic Substances* (New York: Oxford University Press, 1991), and Carl Cranor, *Toxic Torts* (Cambridge: Cambridge University Press, 2006).

41. Unger, "Replies," *Philosophy and Phenomenological Research* LIX, no. 1 (March 1999): 215 of 203–216.

42. Karl Jaspers, *The Question of German Guilt*, trans. E. B. Ashton (New York: Capricorn Books, 1961), 36.

43. Jean-Paul Sartre, *What Is Literature*, trans. Bernard Frechtman (London: Methuen, 1950), 45. Simone de Beauvoir, *The Ethics of Ambiguity*, trans. Bernard Frechtman (New York: Citadel Press, 1949).

44. Jean-Paul Sartre, *Anti-Semite and Jew*, trans. George J. Becker (New York: Schocken Books, 1965), 90; L. May, *Sharing Responsibility* (Chicago: University of Chicago Press, 1992), 146–151.

45. Aristotle, *Nicomachean Ethics*, 63. See Christopher Kutz, *Complicity* (Cambridge: Cambridge University Press, 2000). See L. May, "Ethics and Law for a Collective Age," *Philosophical Review* 111, no. 3 (July 2002): 483–486. M. Gilbert, "Ethics and Law for a Collective Age," *Philosophical and Phenomenological Research* 67, no. 1 (July 2003): 236–239. J. Gardner, "Ethics and Law for a Collective Age," *Ethics* 114, no. 4 (July 2004): 827–830.

46. May, *Sharing Responsibility*, and Hannah Arendt, *Eichmann in Jerusalem* (New York: Viking Press, 1963). See also Dianna Taylor, "Hannah Arendt on Judgment," *International Journal of Philosophical Studies* 10, no. 2 (2002): 151–169. Arne Johan Vetlesen, "Hannah Arendt on Conscience and Evil," *Philosophy and Social Criticism* 27, no. 5 (2001): 1–33.

47. Arguments are from Kristin Shrader-Frechette, "Flawed Attacks on Contemporary Human Rights," *Human Rights Review* 7, no. 2 (2005): 92–110, and in K. Shrader-Frechette, *Science Policy, Ethics, and Economic Methodology*, 121–151, 210–312. For a Kantian perspective see John Martin Gillroy, *Justice and Nature* (Washington, D.C.: Georgetown University Press, 2000).

48. For this objection, see next note and Cass Sunstein, *Risk and Reason* (New York: Cambridge University Press, 2000), 136. Heather Beal, "Ecotourism as a Model for Sustainable Development," *National Forum* 75, no. 4 (Fall 1995): 8–9. Anita Pleumarom, "The Political Economy of Tourism," *Ecologist* 24, no. 4 (July 1994): 142. Joan Giannecchini, "Ecotourism," *Conservation Biology* 7, no. 2 (June 1993): 429–432. P. Nijkamp (ed.), *Sustainable Tourist Development* (Brookfield, VT: Ashgate, 1995). Erlet Cater and G. Lowman (eds.), *Ecotourism* (New York: Wiley, 1994). Elizabeth Boo, *Ecotourism* (Washington, D.C.: World Wildlife Fund, 1990). Stephen Foehr, *Eco-Journeys* (Chicago: Nobel Press, 1992). J. Gordon Nelson, "The Spread of Ecotourism," *Environmental Conservation* 21, no. 3 (Autumn 1994): 248–255. K. Lindberg and D. E. Hawkins (eds.), *Ecotourism* (North Bennington, Vt.: Ecotourism Society, 1993). T. Whelan, *Nature Tourism* (Washington, D.C.: Island Press, 1991). E. L. Shafer, R. Carline, W. R. Guldin, and H. K. Cordell, "Economic Amenity Values of Wildlife," *Environmental Management* 17, no. 5 (1993): 669–682. W. Whitlock, K. Van Romer, and R. H. Becker, *Nature Based Tourism* (Clemson, S.C.: Strom Thurmond Institute, 1991). Peter Frank and Jon Bowermaster, "Can Ecotourism Save the Planet?" *Conde Nast Traveler* 29, no. 12 (December 1994): 134–139. See also Shrader-Frechette and McCoy, *Method in Ecology*, chs. 7–10; J. Park and M. Honey, "The Paradox of Paradise," *Environment* 41, no. 8 (1999): 4–5; M. S. Honey, "Treading Lightly?" *Environment* 41, no. 5 (1999): 45ff. For reasons that maximizing economic welfare might not maximize human and environmental welfare, see next note and E. J. Mishan, *The Costs of Economic Growth* (New York: Praeger, 1967), 109–137. See also J. A. Hobson, *Confessions of an Economic Heretic* (Sussex, England: Harvester Press, 1976), 171, 208–209; A. V. Kneese and C. L. Schultze, *Pollution, Prices, and Public Policy* (Washington, D.C.: Brookings Institution, 1975), 109. Frank Ackerman et al. (eds.), *Human Well-Being and Economic Goals* (Washington, D.C.: Island Press, 1997); John Broome, *Ethics out of Economics* (Cambridge: Cambridge University Press, 1999), and Frank Ackerman, *The Political Economy of Inequality* (Washington, D.C.: Island Press, 2000).

49. US National Research Council, *Valuing Ecosystem Services* (Washington, D.C.: National Academies Press, 2004); www.nap.edu/books/03090938X/html/ and accessed August 28, 2006.

50. See, for example, R. O. Zerbe and L. J. Graham, "The Role of Rights in Benefit-Cost Methodology," *Washington Law Review* 74, no. 3 (1999): 763–797.

51. H. D. Lewis, "The Non-moral Notion of Collective Responsibility," in *Individual and Collective Responsibility*, ed. Peter A. French (Rochester, N.Y.: Schenkman Books, 1995), 122, 171. See R. Baum, *Ethical Problems in Engineering* (Troy, N.Y.: Rensselaer Polytechnic, 1980), 4. See also J. Ladd, "Philosophical Remarks on Professional Responsibility in Organizations," in Flores, *Ethical Problems in Engineering*, 193–194. See also Seumas Miller, "Collective Responsibility," *Public Affairs Quarterly* 15, no. 1 (2001): 65–82.

52. Larry May, *The Morality of Groups* (Notre Dame: University of Notre Dame Press, 1987), 3–111. Peter French, *Collective and Corporate Responsibility* (New York: Columbia University Press, 1984). Michael Zimmerman, "Sharing Responsibility," *American Philosophical Quarterly* 22 (1985): 115–122. On questioning collective responsibility, see J. Raikka, "On Disassociating Oneself from Collective Responsibillity," *Social Theory and Practice* 23, no. 1 (1997): 93–108, and E. F. Paul, F. D. Mikller, and J. Paul, *The Welfare State* (New York: Cambridge University Press, 1997). See also N. Rescher, "Collective Responsibility," *Journal of Social Philosophy* 29, no. 3 (1998): 46–58 and earlier notes, esp. 15.

53. May, *Sharing Responsibility*, 152. Joel Feinberg, *Doing and Deserving* (Princeton: Princeton University Press, 1970), 248.

54. Quoted in Terry O'Neill, "It's Dark, It's Cold, and Outside the Window a Woman Is Screaming. What Would You do?" *Report/News Magazine,* national ed., 30, no. 2 (2003): 33. See May, *Sharing Responsibility*. H. Danner, "Existential Responsibility," *Studies in Philosophy and Education* 17, no. 4 (1998): 261–270.

55. Arendt is quoted in May, *Sharing Responsibility*, xi. See also James G. Hart, "Hannah Arendt," in *Phenomenological Approaches to Moral Philosophy*, ed. John Drummond (Dordrecht: Kluwer Academic, 2002). Gandhi quote is from Dennis Goulet, *The Cruel Choice* (New York: Atheneum, 1971), 133.

56. Similar insights are echoed by Roger Crisp, "Review of *How Are We to Live?*" by Peter Singer, *Ethics* 107, no. 2 (1997): 344–345.

57. May, *Sharing Responsibility*, 3. For an exception, see G. Melleman, *Collective Responsibility* (Amsterdam: Rodopi, 1997).

58. See, for example, Michael Stocker, "The Schizophrenia of Modern Moral Theories," *Journal of Philosophy* 73, no. 14 (August 1976): 453–466. See May, *Sharing Responsibility*, 4, 10. See also Peter Singer (ed.), *Applied Ethics* (Oxford: Oxford University Press, 1986). David Copp, "Can a Random Collection Be Responsible?" *Journal of Philosophy* 67, no. 14 (1970): 471–481. See Larry May and Stacey Hoffman (eds.), *Collective Responsibility* (Savage, Md.: Rowman and Littlefield, 1991). David Copp, "Responsibility for Collective Inaction," *Journal of Social Philosophy* 22, no. 2 (fall 1991): 71–80. See D. Cooper, "Collective Responsibility," *Philosophy* 43, no. 165 (1968): 258–268; D. Cooper, "Collective Responsibility," *Philosophy* 44, no. 168 (1969): 153–155; R. Downie, "Collective Responsibility," *Philosophy* 44, no. 167 (1969): 67–69. R. Hardin, *Collective Action* (Baltimore: Johns Hopkins Press, 1982); M. Olson, *The Logic of Collective Actions*

(Cambridge, Mass.: Harvard University Press, 1971). Larry May, "Collective Inaction and Shared Responsibility," *Nous* 24, no. 2 (April 1990): 269–277. Kenneth Kipnis, "Collective Responsibility," *Ethics* 103, no. 4 (July 1993): 845. See also S. Miller, "Individualism, Collective Responsibility, and Corporate Crime," *Business and Professional Ethics Journal* 16, no. 4 (1997): 19–46.

59. Robert Goodin, *Protecting the Vulnerable* (Chicago: University of Chicago Press, 1985), 137. APHA, "Endorsement of Public-Interest Law Groups," policy 7431; www.apha.org/legislative/policy/policysearch/index.cfm?fuseaction=view&id=773; accessed March 16, 2006. APHA quotations are from its policy 9702, "Protecting Health Care Accessability"; www.apha.org/legislative/policy/policysearch/index.cfm?fuseaction=view&id=136 and accessed March 16, 2006.

60. May, *Sharing Responsibility*, 105ff. See Larry May, "Groups and Democratic Theory," in *Groups and Group Rights,* ed. Christine Sistare (Lawrence: University Press of Kansas, 2001), 117–123.

61. K. Jaspers, *The Question of German Guilt* (Ashton, N.Y.: Dial, 1947), 32. See Copp, "Responsibility for Collective Inaction," 77. See James R. Otteson, "Limits on Our Obligation to Give," *Public Affairs Quarterly* 14, no. 3 (2000): 183–203. For other discussions of the "Failure Objection," see Pogge, *World Poverty and Human Rights*, 7–8.

62. Charles McCarrey, *Citizen Nader* (New York: Saturday Review Press, 1972), 29, 115, 138; Jennifer Scarlott, "Ralph Nader," in *Leaders from the 1960s,* ed. David De Leon (London: Greenwood Press, 1994), 330; Thomas Stewart, "The Resurrection of Ralph Nader," *Fortune* 119, no. 11 (May 22, 1989), 106. For defenses of Nader, see T. Gitlin, "Ralph Nader and the Will to Marginality," *Dissent* 51, no. 2 (spring 2004): 5–7. For criticisms, see J. B. Judis, "Seeing Green: Ralph Nader Betrays Himself," *New Republic* 222, no. 22 (May 2000): 25–27.

63. Karl E. Weick, "Small Wins," *American Psychologist* 39, no. 1 (January 1984): 40–49, esp. 40. See also Karl Weick, "Sensemaking as an Organizational Dimension of Global Change," in *Sensemaking in Organizations*, ed. Gillian Dickens (London: Sage, 1995), 39–56. See also Weick, "Sensemaking as an Organizational Dimension of Global Change," in *Organizational Dimensions of Global Change,* ed. David Cooperrider and Jane Dutton (London: Sage, 1999), 39–56. See Karl Weick (ed.), *Making Sense of the Organization* (Oxford: Blackwell, 2001).

64. Weick, "Small Wins," 40–41, 4; quotation is from 40. Saul Alinsky, *Rules for Radicals* (New York: Vintage, 1972), 114–115.

65. Weick, "Small Wins," 42.

66. For Toxics Release Inventory underreporting, Joe Truini, "Toxic Release Report Paints Murky Picture," *Waste News* 10, no. 5 (2004): 1–27. P. Starke, "The Loopholes," *Environmental Action* 23, no. 3 (1991): 20.

67. Weick, "Small Wins," 43–46; Alinsky, *Rules for Radicals*.

68. Weick, "Small Wins," 46–48. S. C. Kobasa, "Stressful Life Events, Personality, and Health," *Journal of Personality and Social Psychology* 37, no. 1 (1979): 1–11, and S. C. Kobasa, S. R. Maddi, and S. Kahn, "Hardiness and Health," *Journal of Personality and Social Psychology* 42, no. 1 (1982): 168–177.

69. Thucydides, *The History of the Peloponnesian War*, bk. I, sec. 141.

Chapter 6

1. Quoted by Lois Gibbs, foreword to Jim Schwab, *Deeper Shades of Green* (San Francisco: Sierra Club Books, 1994), xii. See Joanna Grant, *Ella Baker* (New York: Wiley, 1998).

2. Schwab, *Deeper Shades of Green*, 44–45.

3. Marilyn Martinez, "Legacy of a Mother's Dedication," *Los Angeles Times*, CIX, no. 2, section B (September 7, 1995), B3; see also B1.

4. Schwab, *Deeper Shades of Green*, 44–45, 55–58. "Mothers' Group Fights Back in Los Angeles," *New York Times*, CXXXIX, no. 48,075 (December 5, 1989), A32. Martinez, "Legacy of a Mother's Dedication," B1; "Mothers of Prevention," *Time*, 137, no. 23 (June 10, 1991), 25; Michael Quintanilla, "The Earth Mother," *Los Angeles Times*, CXIV, no. 142, Section E (April 24, 1995), E1, E5.

5. Martinez, "Legacy of a Mother's Dedication," B3. See Hugh Dellies, "Group Preaches Gospel of Water Conservation," *Chicago Tribune*, 149, no. 79 (March 20, 1995), sec. 1, 3. See also Michel Gelobter, "Have Minorities Benefitted? A Forum," *EPA Journal* 18, no. 1 (March/April 1992): 32–36.

6. Iris Marion Young, *Inclusion and Democracy* (New York: Oxford University Press, 2000), 52–63, 69, makes many of the same points. On 61–70, she points out that narrative and rhetoric have political and strategic roles in developing deliberative democracy.

7. See Plato, *The Republic*, 2nd ed., trans. Desmond Lee (Middlesey, England: Harmondsworth, 1984), book ii, 360. Much of this discussion relies on Peter Singer, *How Are We to Live?* (Amherst, Mass.: Prometheus, 1995), 206–218. For the game-theory material, see Singer, *How Are We to Live*, 129–138, 147, 153. Robert Ayelrod, *The Evolution of Cooperation* (New York: Basic Books, 1984), 27–54, 99. Richard Dawkins, *The Selfish Gene* (Oxford: Oxford University Press, 1976). See also M. Midgley, *The Myths We Live By* (London: Routledge, 2003).

8. Singer, *How Are We to Live*, 212.

9. Robert Bellah, Richard Madsen, William Sullivan, Ann Swidler, and Steven Tipton, *Habits of the Heart* (Berkeley: University of California Press, 1985).

10. See, for example, Bread for the World at www.bread.org/. or Physicians for Social Responsibility at www.psr.org.

11. Young, *Inclusion and Democracy*, 41–46.

12. Young, *Inclusion and Democracy*, 73, 77ff.

13. See Paul Harris (ed.), *Civil Disobedience* (Lanham, Md.: University Press of America, 1989). John Rawls, *A Theory of Justice* (Cambridge, Mass.: Harvard University Press, 1971), 307, 363–368, 389. Martin Luther King, "Letter from Birmingham Jail," in Harris, *Civil Disobedience*, 57–71. A. Sabl, "Looking Forward to Justice," *Journal of Political Philosophy* 9, no. 3 (2001): 307–30.

14. See Myron Glazer and Penina Glazer, *The Whistleblowers* (New York: Basic Books, 1991). M. Davis, "Whistleblowing," in H. LaFollette (ed.) *Oxford Handbook of Practical Ethics* (New York: Oxford University Press, 2003), 539–66.

15. See Young, *Inclusion and Democracy*, 112–114. For the American Public Health Association (APHA) self-description of its activities, see www.apha.org/about/. Quoted examples of its promoting organized action and advocacy are from APHA, "Protecting Health Care Accessibility," policy 9702; www.apha.org/legislative/policy/policysearch/index.cfm?fuseaction=view&id=136; and from

policy 7324, quoted in note 54. Calls for citizen advocacy occur in many APHA documents, such as 9910. For APHA, "Endorsement of Public-Interest Law Groups," see policy 7431; www.apha.org/legislative/policy/policysearch/index.cfm ?fuseaction=view&id=773. All accessed March 10, 2006.

16. Kai Nielsen, "On the Choice between Reform and Revolution," in *Philosophy and Political Action*, ed. Virginia Held, Kai Nielsen, and Charles Parsons (New York: Oxford University Press, 1972), 24; see also 17–51. See Young, *Inclusion and Democracy*, 165, 188–189, and Robert Putnam, *Making Democracy Work* (Princeton: Princeton University Press, 1993).

17. Karl Popper, *Conjectures and Refutations* (London: Routledge and Kegan Paul, 1969), 361.

18. See Young, *Inclusion and Democracy*. See D. Williams and C. Collins, "Racial Residential Segregation," *Public Health Reports* 116, no. 5 (Sept–Oct 2001): 404–16.

19. Nielsen, "On the Choice between Reform and Revolution," 49.

20. Popper, *Conjectures and Refutations*, 355–363.

21. Respective recommendations are APHA, "Affirming the Necessity of a Secure, Sustainable, and Health-Protective Energy Policy," 2004, policy 2004–06; www.apha.org/legislative/policy/policysearch/index.cfm?fuseaction=view&id=1289, "Preventing Human Methymercury Exposure," 1999, policy 9912; www .apha.org/legislative/policy/policysearch/index.cfm?fuseaction=view&id=181; "Preventing Environmental and Ocupational Health Effects of Diesel Exhaust," policy 9912; www.apha.org/legislative/policy/policysearch/index.cfm?fuseaction=view&id=183; "Reducing Occupational Exposure to Benzene," 2005, policy 2005–6; www.apha.org/legislative/policy/policysearch/index.cfm?fuseaction=view&id=1322. "Protecting Human Milk from Persistent Toxic Chemical Contaminants," policy 2005–6; www.apha.org/legislative/policy/policysearch/index.cfm? fuseaction=view&id=1321; "Toxics Reduction as a Means of Pollution Prevention," 1992, policy 9206; www.apha.org/legislative/policy/policysearch/index.cfm? fuseaction=view&id=57; "Protecting Children from Overexposure to Lead," 2005, policy 2005–7; www.apha.org/legislative/policy/policysearch/index.cfm? fuseaction=view&id=181; "Declare Proposed National Permanent Nuclear Waste Repository Site Unsafe," 2000, policy 0011; www.apha.org/legislative/policy/policysearch/index.cfm?fuseaction=view&id=182; all accessed March 18, 2006.

22. See C. Stracke, "Mexico," *World Policy Journal* 20, no. 2 (Summer 2003): 29–36. Robert Hetzel, "Free Trade Debate," *Economic Quarterly* 80, no. 2 (Spring 1994): 39–59; Barry Bosworth, "Debate over NAFTA," *Brookings Review* 11, no. 4 (Fall 1993): 48; Diane Davis, "New-Age Politics Drives NAFTA," *Forum for Applied Research and Public Policy* 10, no. 2 (summer 1995): 43–49. Lori Wallach and Michelle Sforza, *Whose Trade Organization?* (Washington, D.C.: Public Citizen, 1999), 54–55. Regarding NAFTA "Fast Track," see David Firestone, "Senate Approves Bill to Give Bush Trade Authority," *New York Times*, August 2, 2002, A1; Brink Lindsey, "Mixed Signals on Trade Barriers," *Wall Street Journal*, July 30, 2002, A14. Ruth Papazian, "Forbidden Fruit?" *Harvard Health Letter* 19 (1994): 6–8. See also H. Michael Wehr, "Pesticide Residue Regulations and the Pacific Rim," *Food Technology* 46, no. 3 (March 1992): 77–79, and Judith Foulke, "Three Thousand Tons of Peanuts Detained," *FDA Consumer* 26, no. 9 (November 1992): 44. See also Dolores J. Katz, et al., "An Outbreak of Typhoid Fever in Florida Associated with an Imported Frozen Fruit," *Journal of Infectious Diseases* 186, no. 2 (2002): 234–239. Robert Scott, "Will CAFTA Be a Boon to

Farmers and the Farm Industry?" *Economic Policy Institute Issue Brief* 210 (June 2005). Jill Hodges and Ann Marie Kimball, "The Global Diet," *Globalization and Health* 1, no. 4 (2005); available only online at www.globalizationandhealth.com/content/1/1/4. Kelley Lee and Meri Koivusalo, "Trade and Health," *Public Library of Science* 2, no. 1 (2005); http://medicine.plosjournals.org/perlserv/?request=get-document&doi=10%2E1371%2Fjournal%2Epmed%2E0020008 and accessed October 15, 2006. APHA recommendations on such trade agreemeents include "Threats to Global Health and Equity: The General Agreement on Trade in Services (GATS) and the Free Trade Area of the Americas (FTAA)," policy 200121; www.apha.org/legislative/policy/policysearch/index.cfm?fuseaction=view&id=260; all accessed March 18, 2006.

23. J. T. Mathews et al., *World Resources 1986* (New York: Basic Books, 1986), 48–49. See also C. Smith, "Pesticide Exports from U.S. Ports, 1997–2000," *International Journal of Occupational and Environmental Health* 1, no. 4 (2001): 266–74. R. Repetto, *Paying the Price: Pesticides in Developing Countries*, research report no. 2 (Washington, D.C.: World Resources Institute, 1985), 3. See also "Eco-Update," *Acres (USA)* 27, no. 3 (March 1997): 4. W. A. Alarcon et al., "Acute Illnesses Associated with Pesticide Exposure at Schools," *Journal of the American Medical Association* 294, no. 4 (2005): 455–465. Paul Thacker, "Pesticide Risks Remain Uncalculated," *Environmental Science and Technology* 39, no. 7 (2005): 145–146. See notes 24 and 36.

24. U.S. General Accounting Office (GAO), *Pesticides*, report no. GAO/RCED-94-1 (Washington, D.C.: U.S. GAO, 1993); U.S. GAO, *Food Safety: USDA's Role under the National Residue Program Should be Reevaluated* (Washington, D.C.: U.S. GAO, 1994). See also U.S. FDA, "Pesticide Program," *Journal Association of Official Analytical Chemists International* 77, no. 5 (September/October 1994): 161A–185A; Andrew Davis, "Can Congress Close Off the Circle of Poison?" *Business and Society Review* 82 (Summer 1992): 36–40; and Hilary F. French, "The GATT Blunder," *World Watch* 7, no. 2 (March/April 1994): 2. See also March Hellman, "News from Around: Hazardous Pesticide Exports High and on the Rise," *Journal of Pesticide Reform* 16, no. 2 (1996): 13; Wallach and Sforza, *Whose Trade Organization*, 181–186 and 59–61. Michele Late, "Risks of Pesticides Weighed as Chemicals Linger in Human Blood," *Nations Health* 35, no. 7 (2005): 1–17.

25. APHA, "Reducing and Monitoring the Use of Toxic Materials," policy 9205; www.apha.org/legislative/policy/policysearch/index.cfm?fuseaction=view&id=56; accessed March 18, 2006. Re white-collar crime, see ch. 2, sec. 5, notes 53–54.

26. K. Shrader-Frechette, *Environmental Justice: Creating Equality, Reclaiming Democracy* (New York: Oxford University Press, 2002) 131–132. APHA, "Nuclear Accident Liability," policy 8124; www.apha.org/legislative/policy/policysearch/index.cfm?fuseaction=view&id=996; accessed March 22, 2006.

27. For reform see Carl Cranor, *Toxic Torts* (Cambridge: Cambridge University Press, 2006), and Carl Cranor, *Regulating Toxic Substances* (New York: Oxford University Press, 1993); Thomas Kerns, *Environmentally Induced Illnesses* (London: McFarland, 2001), 183–190. Kristin Shrader-Frechette, *Risk and Rationality* (Berkeley: University of California Press, 1991), 198–206. Carl Cranor and David Eastmond, "Scientific Ignorance and Reliable Patterns of Evidence in Toxic Tort Causation," *Law and Contemporary Problems* 64, no. 4

(2001): 5. "Make It Hurt," *Economist* 319, no. 7705 (1991): 71. Allen Kanner, "Equity in Toxic Tort Litigation," *Law and Policy* 26, no. 2 (2004): 209–230. Gary Edmond and David Mercer, "Daubert and the Exclusionary Ethos," *Law and Policy* 26, no. 2 (2004): 231. Re toxic-tort reform see APHA, "Strengthening Worker/Comunity Right to Know," 1987, policy 8714; www.apha.org/legislative/policy/policysearch/index.cfm?fuseaction=view&id=1143.

28. Kerns, *Environmentally Induced Illnesses*, 183. See next four notes.

29. APHA, "Policy Statement 9606: The Precautionary Principle and Chemical Exposure Standards for the Workplace," *American Journal of Public Health* 87, no. 3 (March 1997): 500–501. APHA, "Recognizing and Addressing the Environmental and Occupational Health Problems Posed by Chlorinated Organic Chemicals," 1993, policy 9304; www.apha.org/legislative/policy/policysearch/index.cfm?fuseaction=view&id=88; APHA, "The Precautionary Principle and Children's Health," 2000, policy 200011; www.apha.org/legislative/policy/policysearch/index.cfm?fuseaction=view&id=216; APHA, "The Precautionary Principle and Chemical Exposure Standards for the Workplace," 1996, policy 9606; www.apha.org/legislative/policy/policysearch/index.cfm?fuseaction=view&id=124; all accessed March 19, 2006.

30. Nicholas Ashford and C. S. Miller, *Chemical Exposures* (New York: Van Nostrand and Wiley, 1998), 232–234. See Nicholas Ashford, *Monitoring the Worker for Exposure and Disease* (Baltimore: Johns Hopkins University Press, 1990).

31. See Kerns, 129, 191–192; Christopher Oleskey, Alan Fleischman, Lynn Goldman, Kurt Hirschhorn, Philip J. Landrigan, Marc Lappe, Mary Faith Marshall, Herbert Needleman, Rosamond Rhodes, and Michael McCally, "Pesticide Testing in Humans," *Environmental Health Perspectives* 112, no. 8 (June 2004): 914–919. NRC, Intentional Human Dosing; Science Advisory Board of the U.S. EPA, *Testing Human Subjects*, EPA-SAB-EC-00–017 (Washington, D.C.: EPA, 2000). APHA, "Protection of Child and Adolescent Workers," 2001, policy 20019; www.apha.org/legislative/policy/policysearch/index.cfm?fuseaction=view&id=248; accessed March 14, 2006.

32. Shrader-Frechette, *Environmental Justice*, ch. 3, and Kristin Shrader-Frechette, "Property Rights and Genetic Engineering," *Science and Engineering Ethics* 11, no. 1 (2005): 137–149; see Kerns, *Environmentally Induced Illnesses*, 141–143. APHA, "Precautionary Moratorium on New Concentrated Animal Feed Operations," 2003, policy 20037; www.apha.org/legislative/policy/policysearch/index.cfm?fuseaction=view&id=1243; and APHA, "Creating Policies on Land Use," 2004, policy 2004–04; www.apha.org/legislative/policy/policysearch/index.cfm?fuseaction=view&id=1282; accessed March 14, 2006.

33. See Devra Davis, *When Smoke Ran Like Water* (New York: Basic Books, 2002), 276–277; Kerns, *Environmentally Induced Illnesses*, 92–94, 230–243; APHA, "Policy Statement 9606: The Precautionary Principle and Chemical Exposure Standards for the Workplace," 1996, 501. Regarding prevention see, for example, APHA, "Preventing Human Methyl Mercury Exposure," 1999, policy 9910; www.apha.org/legislative/policy/policysearch/index.cfm?fuseaction=view&id=18; and APHA, "Policy Statement on Prevention," 1976, policy 7633; www.apha.org/legislative/policy/policysearch/index.cfm?fuseaction=view&id=835; all accessed March 14, 2006. Regarding racism and environmental justice, see APHA, "Research and Intervention on Racism as a Fundamental Cause of

Ethnic Disparities in Health," 2001, policy 20017; www.apha.org/legislative/policy/policysearch/index.cfm?fuseaction=view&id=246; all accessed March 10, 2006.

34. See notes 28–33 regarding the APHA recommendation for using the precautionary principle. For an attack on it, see Cass Sunstein, *Laws of Fear* (Cambridge: Cambridge University Press, 2005). For an attack on this attack, see Kristin Shrader-Frechette, "Review of *Laws of Fear* by Cass Sunstein," *Ethics and International Affairs* 20, no. 1 (2006): 123–125. Regarding white-collar crime, see earlier chapters. See also Kerns, *Environmentally Induced Illnesses*, 205. French, "The GATT Blunder." Wallach and Sforza, *Whose Trade Organization*. Joseph DiMento, "Criminal Enforcement of Environmental Law," *Annals of the American Academy of Political and Social Science* 525, no. 1 (1993): 134–147. Mary Clifford, *Environmental Crime* (Gaithersburg, Md.: Aspen, 1998).

35. See Kerns, *Environmentally Induced Illnesses*, 127, 136–144, 150–170. Davis, *When Smoke Ran Like Water*, 277; APHA, "Policy Statement 9606: The Precautionary Principle and Chemical Exposure Standards for the Workplace." See also John Herrick, "Federal Project Financing Incentives for Green Industries," *Natural Resources Journal* 43, no. 1 (2003): 77–111. Robert Anex, "Stimulating Innovation in Green Technology," *American Behavorial Scientist* 44, no. 2 (2000): 188–213.

36. See note 23 and K. Goldberg, "Efforts to Prevent Misuse of Pesticides Exported to Developing Countries," *Ecology Law Quarterly* 12, no. 4 (1985): 1025–51. See U.N. Organization for Economic Cooperation and Development (OECD), *Guidance Document for 111 Pesticides* (Paris: OECD, 1997). See also prior notes for APHA statements on international trade pacts such as NAFTA, and see APHA, "Policy Statement on International Health," 1976, policy 7632; www.apha.org/legislative/policy/policysearch/index.cfm?fuseaction=view&id=834; see also APHA, "Nestle Boycott," 1981, policy 8126; www.apha.org/legislative/policy/policysearch/index.cfm?fuseaction=view&id=998; all accessed March 14, 2006.

37. For sweatshop information, see Anna Yesilevsky, "The Case against Sweatshops," *Humanist* 64, no. 3 (2004): 20–46. Also see Ellen Rosen, *Making Sweatshops* (Berkeley: University of California Press, 2002), and the Worker Rights Consortium website; www.workersrights.org/.

38. See H. Shue, *Basic Rights* (Princeton: Princeton University Press), pt. 3; see also H. Kuflick, "Review of *Basic Rights* by Henry Shue," *Ethics* 94, no. 2 (January 1984): 319–324.

39. Rebecca M. Summary, "The Overseas Private Investment Corporation and Developing Countries," *Economic Development and Cultural Change* 42, no. 4 (July 1994): 817–828. See also Ann L. Brownson (ed.), *1995 Federal Staff Directory* (Mount Vernon, Va.: Staff Directories, 1995), 909. D. R. Obey, "Export of the Hazardous Industries," *Congressional Record*, 124, part 15, 95th Congress, 2nd sess., June 29, 1978, vol. 124, pt. 15, 19763, 19765. See also H. Shue, "Exporting Hazards," in P. Brown and H. Shue, *Boundaries* (Lanham, MD: Rowman & Littlefield, 1981), 137–138, 144. U.S. Congress, House of Representatives, Committee on Education and Labor, *Hearing on H.R. 4376, The OPIC Abolition*, 102nd Congress, 2nd Session, May 27, 1992 (Washington, D.C.: Government Printing Office, 1992). OPIC, *OPIC Highlights* (Washington, D.C.: OPIC, 1997). U.S. Congress, House of Representatives, Committee on International Relations, *The Future of the Overseas Private Investment Corporation*,

105th Congress, 1st Session, February 12, 1997 (Washington, D.C.: U.S. Government Printing Office, 1998).

40. See Peter Van Ness (ed.), *The Human Rights Debate* (New York: Routledge, 1999).

41. Ibid.

42. Regarding OPIC, see note 39. Patrick M. Regan, "U.S. Economic Aid and Political Repression," *Political Research Quarterly* 48, no. 3 (September 1995): 613–628. Carroll J. Doherty, "This Year, Aid Is a Weapon," *Congressional Quarterly Weekly Report* 53, no. 24 (June 17, 1995), 1763. "Cleaning Up," *Economist* 366, no. 8318 (April 5, 2003): 55–56. Michael E. O'Hanlon, *Enhancing U.S. Security through Foreign Aid* (Darby, PA: Diane, 1994). John McCain, "A World Safe for the U.S.," *Freedom Review* 26, no. 3 (May 1995): 12. Ian Vasquez, "U.S. Aid," *Human Events* 51, no. 16 (April 28, 1995): 18–20. N. M. Khilji and E. M. Zampelli, "The Fungibility of U.S. Military and Non-military Assistance and the Impacts on Expenditures of Major Aid Recipients," *Journal of Development Economics* 43, no. 2 (April 1994): 345–362. Sheila Kaplan, "Porkbarrel Politics at U.S. Aid," *Multinational Monitor* 14, no. 9 (September 1993): 10–15. "Two Well-to-Do Countries Get Most of U.S. Aid," *National Catholic Reporter* 29, no. 42 (October 1, 1993): 5, 20. Edward D. Breslin, "U.S. Aid, the State, and Food Insecurity in Rural Zimbabwe," *Journal of Modern African Studies* 32, no. 1 (March 1994): 81–110. "The Politics of Aid," *Scientist* 6, no. 7 (March 1992): 1. J. Seiberling and C. Schneider, "How Congress Can Help Developing Countries Help Themselves," *Journal '86: Annual Report of the World Resources Institute* (Washington, D.C.: World Resources Institute, 1986), 57, 59. See also Peter H. Koehn and Olatunde J. B. Ojo (eds.), *Making Aid Work* (Lanham, Md.: University Press of America, 1999). Roger Bate, "USAID and Fighting Malaria," U.S. Senate Committee on Homeland Security and Government affairs, Congressional Testimony, May 12, 2005; www.aei.org/publications/pubID.22508,filter.all/pub_detail.asp; accessed September 24, 2006.

43. See note 42. See also Robert Watson, "U.S. Aid to the Third World," *Journal of Third World Studies* 11, no. 2 (Fall 1994): 202–239. M. Bhattacharya, "USAID," *Economic and Political Weekly* 29, no. 37 (1994): 2401. Andrew Cohen, "The Help That Hurts," *Progressive* 58, no. 1 (January 1994): 27. Joseph R. Biden Jr., "U.S. Senator Discusses the Need for an Environmental Aid and Trade Act That Would Help Americans Use the Job Opportunities Created by the Demand for Environmental Protection," *Environmental Law* 23, no. 2 (1993): 687–696.

44. See note 42. J. Brian Atwood, "U.S. Foreign Assistance Program Reform," *U.S. Department of State Dispatch* 6, no. 1 (January 2, 1995): 9–12. Gary Posz, "Redesigning U.S. Foreign Aid," *SAIS Review* 14, no. 2 (Summer/Fall 1994): 159–170. Dick Kirschten, "Rethinking Foreign Aid," *National Journal* 25, no. 9 (February 27, 1993): 541. S. Poe, S. Pilatovsky, B. Miller, and A. Ogundele, "Human Rights and U.S. Foreign Aid Revisited," *Human Rights Quarterly* 16, no. 3 (1994): 539–558. B. A. Abrams and K. A. Lewis, "Human Rights and the Distribution of U.S. Foreign Aid," *Public Choice* 77, no. 4 (December 1993): 815. Jan Narveson, "The Ethics of Aid and Trade," *Canadian Journal of Agricultural Economics* 41, no. 2 (July 1993): 233. Steven C. Poe, "Human Rights and U.S. Foreign Aid," *Human Rights Quarterly* 12, no. 4 (November 1990): 499–512. See also L. Brown and E. Wolf, "Reversing Africa's Decline," in L. Brown (ed.), *State of the World 1986* (New York: Norton, 1986), 182. For criticisms of the

World Bank and suggestions for reform, see Devesh Kapur, *The State in a Changing World: A Critique* (Cambridge, Mass.: Weatherhead Center of Harvard University, 1998); Jonathan A. Fox and L. David Brown (eds.), *The Struggle for Accountability* (Cambridge, Mass.: MIT Press, 1998); Joan M. Nelson, *Reforming Health and Education* (Washington, D.C.: Overseas Development Council, 1999); and Shahrukh Rafi Khan, *Do World Bank and IMF Policies Work?* (New York: St. Martin's Press, 1999). "Dithering on Debt," *Economist* 375, no. 8423 (2005): 13–14. James Henry and Laurence Kotlikoff, "Why Can't the World Bank Be More Like a Bank?" *Wall Street Journal*, 245, no. 106 (2005), A20. For reform of U.S. foreign-aid policies, see APHA, "Foreign Assistance Act," policy 8926; www.apha.org/legislative/policy/policysearch/index .cfm?fuseaction=view&id=1205; accessed March 10, 2006.

45. APHA, "Increasing Worker and Community Awareness of Toxic Hazards," policy 8416; www.apha.org/legislative/policy/policysearch/index.cfm? fuseaction=view&id=1078. Other APHA policies protecting right to know include 2005-6, 2002-5, 9503, 9494, 9302, 9206, 9205, 8714, 8607, 8696; all accessed March 11, 2006.

46. John Robbins, *The Food Revolution* (York Beach, Me.: Conari, 2001), 339; see Kerns, *Environmentally Induced Illnesses*, 170–180. See APHA, "Supporting a Nationwide Environmental Health Tracking Network," policy 20038; www.apha.org/legislative/policy/policysearch/index.cfm?fuseaction=view&id= 1244; and APHA, "Support of the Labeling of Genetically Modified Foods," policy 200111; www.apha.org/legislative/policy/policysearch/index.cfm?fuseaction= view&id=250; all accessed March 10, 2006.

47. APHA, "Food Marketing and Advertising Directed at Children," policy 200317; www.apha.org/legislative/policy/policysearch/index.cfm?fuseaction= view&id=1255; "Alcohol and Tobacco Outdoor Advertising," policy 8921; www .apha.org/legislative/policy/policysearch/index.cfm?fuseaction=view&id=1200; "Alcohol and Tobacco Industry Product Placement in Feature Films," policy 8920; www.apha.org/legislative/policy/policysearch/index.cfm?fuseaction=view&id= 1199; "Advertising and America's Drug Dilema," policy 7108; www.apha.org/ legislative/policy/policysearch/index.cfm?fuseaction=view&id=673; all accessed March 12, 2006.

48. Donald Collins, "Dictating Content," in *We the Media*, ed. Don Hazen and Julie Winokur (New York: Norton, 1997), 57. FAIR is Fairness and Accuracy in Reporting.

49. APHA, "Threats to Public Health Science," policy 2004-1; www.apha .org/legislative/policy/policysearch/index.cfm?fuseaction=view&id=1297. APHA, "Increasing Research Funds for Environmental and Occupational Health," policy LB-7; www.apha.org/legislative/policy/policysearch/index.cfm?fuseaction=view &id=1317; "OMB Abuse of the Paperwork Reduction Act," policy 8716; www.apha.org/legislative/policy/policysearch/index.cfm?fuseaction=view&id= 1145; "Support for Community-Based Participatory Research in Public Health," policy 2004-12; www.apha.org/legislative/policy/policysearch/index.cfm?fuseac tion=view&id=1298; "Strengthening the Public Health Work Force," policy 2005-12; www.apha.org/legislative/policy/policysearch/index.cfm?fuseaction=view &id=1306--all accessed March 12, 2006.

50. The educational statistics are from Sam Dillon, "At Public Universities, Warnings of Privatization," *New York Times* CLV, no., 53,369 (October 16, 2005), A12.

51. APHA, "Supporting Legislation for Independent Post-marketing (Phase IV) Comparative Evaluation of Pharmaceuticals," policy 20031; www.apha .org/legislative/policy/policysearch/index.cfm?fuseaction=view&id=1265; "Concern about the Food and Drug Administration's Drug Approval Process," policy 9915; www.apha.org/legislative/policy/policysearch/index.cfm?fuseaction=view &id=186; "Establishment of an Independent Laboratory to Test the Efficacy of Chemical Germicides," policy 9113; http://www.apha.org/legislative/policy/ policysearch/index.cfm?fuseaction=view&id=40; all accessed March 10, 2006. Quotation is from APHA, "Threats to Public Health Science," cited in note 49. For adversary assessment and other improvements in benefit-cost analysis and quantitative risk assessment, see Kristin Shrader-Frechette, *Risk and Rationality* (Berkeley: University of California Press, 1991), 169–218. For conflicts of interest that require adversary assessment see S. Krimsky, *Science in the Private Interest* (New York: Rowman and Littlefield, 2003); M. Wadman, "Study Discloses Financial Interests behind Papers," *Nature* 385, no. 6615 (January 30, 1997): 376, and H. T. Stelfox et al., "Conflicts of Interest in the Debate over Calcium-Channel Antagonists," *New England Journal of Medicine* 338, no. 2 (January 1998): 101–107.

52. Krimsky, *Science in the Private Interest.* See Kerns, *Environmentally Induced Illnesses,* 110–111, 197–201. APHA, "Ensuring the Scientifc Credibility of Government Public Health Advisory Committees," policy 20036; www.apha .org/legislative/policy/policysearch/index.cfm?fuseaction=view&id=1242--accessed March 12, 2006.

53. U.S. National Research Council, *Understanding Risk in a Democracy* (Washington, D.C.: National Academy Press, 1996). The APHA promotes attention to stakeholder deliberation in many documents, as in APHA, "Action Needed on Multiple Chemical Sensitivity Report," policy 9909; www.apha.org/ legislative/policy/policysearch/index.cfm?fuseaction=view&id=180, and in its policy statements on trade (9494), on land use (2004–04), on consumer choice in health care (20003), and on consent (7839). Quotations are from APHA, "The Precautionary Principle and Chemical Exposure Standards," policy 9606; www .apha.org/legislative/policy/policysearch/index.cfm?fuseaction=view&id=124. All documents were accessed March 13, 2006.

54. See Kerns, *Environmentally Induced Illnesses,* 172–178; similar points are made in Shrader-Frechette, *Risk and Rationality,* 86–87. APHA, "Support for Community-Based Participatory Research," policy 2004–12; www.apha.org/ legislative/policy/policysearch/index.cfm?fuseaction=view&id=1298; "Prevent, Response and Training for Emerging and Re-Emerging Infectious Diseases," policy 200016; www.apha.org/legislative/policy/policysearch/index.cfm?fuseaction =view&id=222; "Environmental Quality, Environmental Health," policy 7325; www.apha.org/legislative/policy/policysearch/index.cfm?fuseaction=view&id= 742. Quotation is from APHA, "Principles of Comprehensive Health Planning," policy 7324; www.apha.org/legislative/policy/policysearch/index.cfm?fuseaction= view&id=741. All accessed March 14, 2006. APHA, "Support for Culturally and Linguistically Appropriate Services," policy 200120; www.apha.org/legislative/ policy/policysearch/index.cfm?fuseaction=view&id=259; "Worker Notification and Institutional Review," policy 9503; www.apha.org/legislative/policy/ policysearch/index.cfm?fuseaction=view&id=98; "The Right to Informed Consent," policy 7839; www.apha.org/legislative/policy/policysearch/index.cfm?fuse action=view&id=916; "Funding for the Consumer Product Safety Commission,"

policy 8914; www.apha.org/legislative/policy/policysearch/index.cfm?fuseaction=view&id=1193; all accessed March 17, 2006.

55. See APHA sources in note 15.

56. Sue Shaw, "Celebrities Who Care: Actors, Singers, Musicians Step Forward to Save the Planet and Animals," *Saving Our Resources Today*, July 1, 2002; www.sort.org. "Star Power Lights the Way," *TIME Europe* 155, no. 16A (April/May 2000): 80. For information about retirees and their volunteering, see Anne Field, "Work Still Does a Body Good," *Business Week*, no. 3761 (December 10, 2001), 98. See also Daniel Kadlec, "The Right Way to Volunteer," *TIME* 168, no. 10 (September 4, 2006): 76.

57. Robert Coles, *The Call of Service* (Boston: Houghton Mifflin, 1993), 57–64.

58. For Bono, see James Traub, "The Statesman," *New York Times Magazine* CLV, no. 53,341 (September 18, 2005), 8–89, 96. For Sheen and La Duke, see Brooks Biggs and Anita Roddick, *Brave Hearts and Rebel Spirits* (Chichester, England: Roddick Books, 2003), 50–51, 76–79.

59. David Barsamian, "Danny Glover," *Progressive* 66, no. 12 (December 2002): 35–38.

60. David Kupfer, "Martin Sheen," *Progressive* 67, no. 7 (July 2003): 35–39.

61. See note 57.

62. The examples of Taylor and Bauer come from Bellah et al., *Habits of the Heart*, 190–195, 214. The example of Dennis Grover is from Kristin Shrader-Frechette, personal communication.

63. See David Korten, "Compassionate Capitalism," in *A Revolution in Kindness*, ed. Anita Roddick (Chichester, England: Roddick Books, 2003), 78–79. See also Biggs and Roddick, *Brave Hearts and Rebel Spirits*, and www.Anita Roddick.com.

64. For the Neuhaus quotation, see Richard Neuhaus, "Indefensible Ethics, Debating Peter Singer," *Dignity*, 8, no. 2 (Summer 2002): 1; www.cbhd.org/resources/bioethics/neuhaus_2002-summer.htm; accessed September 29, 2006. For the Vonnegut quotation, see Kurt Vonnegut, "Cold Turkey," *In These Times* 28, no. 12 (May 10, 2004): 32.

65. For information on on Maguire and Sheen, respectively, see Biggs and Roddick, *Brave Hearts and Rebel Spirits*, 220–227, 50–51.

66. The examples in this and the next paragraph come from the author.

67. Bellah et al., *Habits of the Heart*, 214–216, 249, 258–271, 277–296; Michael Harrington, *Decade of Decision* (New York: Simon and Schuster, 1980).

68. Singer, *How Are We to Live*, 163.

69. Singer, *How Are We to Live*, 164–166. "Giving Your All?" *Economist* 351, no. 8121 (May 29, 1999): 29.

70. For information on national service programs, see Sara Hebel, "National-Service Program Turns Critics into Fans," *Chronicle of Higher Education*, April 26, 2002, A24–26. John McCain and Evan Bayh, "A New Start for National Service," *New York Times*, November 6, 2001, A21. Michael M. Johns, "Mandatory National Health Service," *Journal of the American Medical Association* 269 (1993): 3156–57. Doug Bandow, "National Service: Utopias Revisited," in *Cato Institute Policy Analysis*, no. 190 (Washington, D.C.: Cato Institute 1993). Gary L. Yates, "Mandatory National Service" (Woodland Hills, Calif.: California Wellness Foundation, 2003); www.tcwf.org. David Brooks, "As Parties

Grow Weary, Time for an Insurgency," *New York Times*, October 9, 2005, sec. 4, 12.

71. Coles, *The Call of Service*, 256.
72. Coles, *The Call of Service*, 277–278, 284.
73. Sam Keen, *Fire in the Belly* (New York: Bantam, 1991), 121.